Women's Health

Guest Editors

JOEL J. HEIDELBAUGH, MD
WENDY S. BIGGS, MD

PRIMARY CARE: CLINICS IN OFFICE PRACTICE

www.primarycare.theclinics.com

Consulting Editor
JOEL J. HEIDELBAUGH, MD

March 2009 • Volume 36 • Number 1

SAUNDERS an imprint of ELSEVIER, Inc.

W.B. SAUNDERS COMPANY
A Division of Elsevier Inc.

1600 John F. Kennedy Boulevard, Suite 1800 ● Philadelphia, PA 19103-2899

http://www.theclinics.com

PRIMARY CARE: CLINICS IN OFFICE PRACTICE Volume 36, Number 1
March 2009 ISSN 0095-4543, ISBN-13: 978-1-4377-0532-4, ISBN-10: 1-4377-0532-4

Editor: Barbara Cohen-Kligerman
Developmental Editor: Donald Mumford

Primary Care: Clinics in Office Practice (ISSN: 0095–4543) is published quarterly by Elsevier Inc., 360 Park Avenue South, New York, NY 10010-1710. Months of issue are March, June, September, and December. Business and Editorial Offices: 1600 John F. Kennedy Blvd., Suite 1800, Philadelphia, PA 19103-2899. Customer Service Office: 6277 Sea Harbor Drive, Orlando, FL 32887–4800. Periodicals postage paid at New York, NY and additional mailing offices. Subscription prices are $176.00 per year (US individuals), $296.00 (US institutions), $89.00 (US students), $215.00 (Canadian individuals), $348.00 (Canadian institutions), $140.00 (Canadian students), $268.00 (foreign individuals), $348.00 (foreign institutions), and $140.00 (foreign students). Foreign air speed delivery is included in all *Clinics* subscription prices. All prices are subject to change without notice. POSTMASTER: Send address changes to *Primary Care: Clinics in Office Practice*, Elsevier Periodicals Customer Service, 11830 Westline Industrial Drive, St. Louis, MO 63146. Customer Service (orders, claims, online, change of address): Elsevier Periodicals Customer Service, 11830 Westline Industrial Drive, St. Louis, MO 63146. Tel: 1-800-654-2452 (U.S. and Canada); 314-453-7041 (outside U.S. and Canada). Fax: 314-453-5170. E-mail: journalscustomerservice-usa@elsevier.com (for print support); journalsonlinesupport-usa@elsevier.com (for online support).

Reprints. For copies of 100 or more, of articles in this publication, please contact the Commercial Reprints Department, Elsevier Inc., 360 Park Avenue South, New York, NY 10010-1710. Tel. (212) 633-3812; Fax: (212) 482-1935; E-mail: reprints@elsevier.com.

Primary Care: Clinics in Office Practice is covered in *MEDLINE/PubMed (Index Medicus)* and *EMBASE/ Excerpta Medica, Current Contents/Clinical Medicine,* and *ISI/BIOMED.*

Printed and bound in the United Kingdom
Transferred to Digital Print 2011

Contributors

CONSULTING EDITOR

JOEL J. HEIDELBAUGH, MD
Clinical Assistant Professor, Departments of Family Medicine and Urology; Clerkship Director, Department of Family Medicine, University of Michigan Medical School, Ann Arbor; Ypsilanti Health Center, Ypsilanti, Michigan

GUEST EDITORS

JOEL J. HEIDELBAUGH, MD
Clinical Assistant Professor, Departments of Family Medicine and Urology; Clerkship Director, Department of Family Medicine, University of Michigan Medical School, Ann Arbor; Ypsilanti Health Center, Ypsilanti, Michigan

WENDY S. BIGGS, MD
Assistant Professor, Department of Family Medicine, Michigan State University College of Human Medicine, East Lansing; Associate Director, Midland Family Medicine Residency, Midland, Michigan

AUTHORS

WENDY S. BIGGS, MD
Assistant Professor, Department of Family Medicine, Michigan State University College of Human Medicine, East Lansing; Associate Director, Midland Family Medicine Residency, Midland, Michigan

AMY R. BLAIR, MD
Assistant Professor, Department of Family Medicine, Loyola University, Chicago Stritch School of Medicine, Maywood, Illinois

CHEYANNE M. CASAS, MD
Assistant Professor, Department of Family Medicine, Loyola University, Chicago Stritch School of Medicine, Maywood, Illinois

AMY C. DENHAM, MD, MPH
Assistant Professor, Department of Family Medicine, University of North Carolina School of Medicine, Chapel Hill, North Carolina

LINDA FRENCH, MD
Professor and Chair, Department of Family Medicine, University of Toledo, College of Medicine, Toledo, Ohio

HEIDI GULLETT, MD, MPH
Physician, Dayspring Family Health Center, Jellico, Tennessee

R. VAN HARRISON, PhD
Professor of Medical Education, Department of Medical Education, University of Michigan Medical School, Ann Arbor, Michigan

DIANA L. HEIMAN, MD
Assistant Professor, Department of Family Medicine, University of Connecticut School of Medicine, Farmington; Family Medicine Center at Asylum Hill, Hartford, Connecticut

JULIE E. HERINGHAUSEN, BSN
University of Michigan Medical School, Ann Arbor, Michigan

VALERIE J. KING, MD, MPH
Associate Professor, Department of Family Medicine, Oregon Health and Science University, Portland, Oregon

ROBERT W. LASH, MD
Associate Professor of Medicine, Division of Metabolism, Endocrinology and Diabetes, Department of Internal Medicine, University of Michigan Medical School, Ann Arbor, Michigan

SHEILA M. MARCUS, MD
Clinical Associate Professor, Department of Psychiatry, University of Michigan; Director, Child and Adolescent Psychiatry, University of Michigan Health System, University of Michigan, Ann Arbor, Michigan

JANE McCORT, MD
Assistant Professor of Medicine, Division of General Medicine, University of Michigan Medical School, Ann Arbor, Michigan

CATHLEEN MORROW, MD
Associate Professor; Predoctoral Director, Department of Community and Family Medicine, Dartmouth Medical School, Lebanon, New Hampshire

SAUDIA MUSHKBAR, MD
Neighborhood Health Clinic, Fort Wayne, Indiana

ELIZABETH H. NAUMBURG, MD
Associate Dean of Advising; Professor, Department of Family Medicine, University of Rochester School of Medicine and Dentistry, Highland Family Medicine Center, Rochester, New York

JANE M. NICHOLSON, MD
Assistant Professor of Obstetrics and Gynecology, Department of Obstetrics and Gynecology, University of Michigan Medical School, Ann Arbor, Michigan

KEVIN PHELPS, DO
Assistant Professor, Department of Family Medicine, University of Toledo, College of Medicine, Toledo, Ohio

NAGESWAR RAO POTHULA, MD, MHA
Department of Family Medicine, University of Toledo, College of Medicine, Toledo, Ohio

ANN M. RODDEN, DO, MS
Assistant Professor, Department of Family Medicine, Medical University of South Carolina, Charleston, South Carolina

LOURDES VELEZ, MD
Assistant Professor of Family Medicine, Department of Family Medicine, University of Michigan Medical School, Ann Arbor, Michigan

JOHANNA B. WARREN, MD
Assistant Professor, Department of Family Medicine, Oregon Health and Science University, Portland, Oregon

AMY WEIL, MD
Associate Professor, Department of Medicine, Division of General Medicine and Epidemiology; Co-director, Beacon Child and Family Program, University of North Carolina School of Medicine, Chapel Hill, North Carolina

DAVID G. WEISMILLER, MD, ScM
Associate Professor of Family Medicine, Department of Family Medicine, The Brody School of Medicine; Associate Provost – Institutional Planning, Assessment and Research, East Carolina University, Greenville, North Carolina

ALAN M. WEISS, MD, MBA
Staff Physician, Cleveland Clinic Main Campus, Cleveland, Ohio

RACHEL M. WILLIAMS, MD
Family Physician, Covenant Health Care, Saginaw, Michigan

ADAM J. ZOLOTOR, MD, MPH
Assistant Professor, Department of Family Medicine, University of North Carolina School of Medicine; Injury Prevention Research Center, University of North Carolina, Chapel Hill, North Carolina

Contents

Diana L. Heiman

Amenorrhea is a complicated and common problem encountered by primary care physicians. Performing a thorough history and physical examination can often narrow the differential diagnosis considerably. The addition of basic determinations of serum FSH and LH or other tests as indicated by abnormalities on the history or examination can then make the diagnosis more clear. In all cases of primary amenorrhea, treatment is directed by the diagnosis. The primary goal of treatment is to facilitate the normal sexual development through gentle coaxing into puberty. In secondary amenorrhea, there is a greater focus on fertility and prevention of complications from the associated abnormal hormone levels. Probability of conception is dictated by the reversibility of the cause of the amenorrhea.

Cathleen Morrow and Elizabeth H. Naumburg

Primary dysmenorrhea is commonly a straightforward diagnosis that can be made accurately with an attentive history. In young women who have classic symptoms and no specific indication, a pelvic examination is often unnecessary in the initial evaluation. The opportunity for primary care practitioners to support women in unearthing the best approach to this chronic recurrent discomfort to minimize adverse life impact is significant and valuable. Identification of patients who are incapacitated by their symptoms or have symptoms that represent underlying pathology is a critical component of a careful history. The wide range of treatments available for primary dysmenorrhea virtually ensures that all females troubled by the symptoms can find relief with safe and inexpensive treatments while limiting negative side effects.

Office visits centering on preventive and gynecologic concerns compose a significant proportion of any primary care practice. The detection and prevention of gynecologic cancers are topics that often predominate such visits. The trend of increasing obesity in the general population and the exploding public awareness of the prevalence of human papillomavirus are examples of topics that affect the primary care physician's approach toward gynecologic cancer screening for women. Changing incidence rates in endometrial cancer and cervical cancer challenge the traditional approach to screening, guiding the primary care physician to consider individual risk factors during the routine health maintenance examination. In this article, the epidemiology, screening guidelines, and a review of management are presented for vulvar, cervical, ovarian, and endometrial cancer.

Cervical cancer and its dysplasia precursors account for significant morbidity and mortality in women worldwide. Human papillomavirus infection is common, preventable, and now widely accepted as the causative agent with oncogenic potential in the development of cervical cancer. Screening via Papanicolaou testing is critical, and interpretation of test results with knowledge of patient risk factors is imperative. Many evidence-based guidelines for screening, interpretation, and management have been developed and are widely available for use.

Prevalence studies show that one in five women experience an episode of major depressive disorder during their lifetime. It is important for health care providers to be aware of (1) the frequency of depression in this population; (2) signs, symptoms, and appropriate screening methods; and (3) health risks for the mother and growing fetus if depression is undetected or untreated. Because management of depressed pregnant women also includes care of a growing fetus, treatment may be complicated and primary care providers should consider a multidisciplinary approach, including an obstetrician, psychiatrist, and pediatrician, to provide optimal care.

> Intimate partner violence (IPV) is a common problem, affecting large numbers of women, men, and children who present to primary care practices. It takes on many forms, including psychologic/emotional, physical, and sexual abuse, and its effects on the health of victims and their children are varied. Although many primary care physicians may be uncomfortable inquiring about IPV, a knowledge of patients' IPV victimization may help physicians develop a better understanding of patients' presenting symptoms and health risks, form more effective therapeutic relationships, and work toward reducing the myriad health risks associated with IPV.

> Osteoporosis is a common disorder with significant morbidity and mortality. Clinical risk factors can identify patients most likely to have osteoporosis. Patients who have decreased bone mass are candidates for calcium and vitamin D supplementation; those who have more severe bone loss should be screened for secondary causes and started on medical therapy. First-line therapy most often is a bisphosphonate. Estrogen reduces hip fractures in women. Recombinant parathyroid hormone is reserved for patients who have failed or are not candidates for bisphosphonate therapy. Follow-up dual-emission x-ray absorptiometry is reserved for when a change in bone mineral density will make a difference in therapy.

> Public awareness of the benefits of a healthy transition through menopausal and postmenopausal stages offers women a new perspective on aging and empowers them to take greater responsibility for their own health and well-being. Primary care physicians are a chief influence on information regarding health behaviors, risk assessment, and medical interventions that preserve health and that prevent premature death and disability. Clinicians can help identify therapy goals for short-term relief of menopausal symptoms and long-term relief and prevention of osteoporosis and fractures. Physicians must consider individual needs and concerns and be cognizant that because a woman's needs can change, re-evaluation is needed.

THE CLINICS ARE NOW AVAILABLE ONLINE!

Access your subscription at:
www.theclinics.com

Foreword

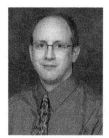

Joel J. Heidelbaugh, MD
Consulting Editor

Welcome! This volume marks the 36th year of existence for *Primary Care: Clinics in Office Practice*, one of the longest running and most successful publications in the *Clinics of North America* program. This volume also serves as my debut as consulting editor, a challenging position that I am honored to undertake.

Primary care providers face an enormous challenge in everyday practice: how can we balance increasingly busy office practices *and* keep our medical knowledge current through reading? More medical journals exist today than a decade ago, and somehow the time we reserve to read and gather new knowledge seems to be increasingly encroached upon. The *Clinics* have enjoyed resounding success across all of their specialty volumes, focusing on the creation and delivery of concise, practical books that are considered to be leading references.

The principal goal of this series is to select common topics that are timely and frequently encountered in the ambulatory care setting. The creation of each issue will be driven by a guest editor of suitable expertise and academic credentials who has selected authors to provide detailed, systematic reviews of the current literature on each subtopic, diagnostic and therapeutic algorithms where applicable, and current summaries of the latest patient-oriented practice recommendations highlighted in tables and figures. We are dedicated to keeping the *Clinics* format accessible and portable, while always striving to match advances in technology and meet the needs of our readers.

It is a great honor to serve as consulting editor for the *Primary Care: Clinics in Office Practice* series. I offer my sincere thanks to Ms. Barbara Cohen-Kligerman, senior clinics editor, and the editorial staff at Elsevier for their support and guidance. Together, we greatly appreciate the loyalty of our dedicated subscribers and look

Prim Care Clin Office Pract 36 (2009) xiii–xiv
doi:10.1016/j.pop.2008.10.014
0095-4543/08/$ – see front matter © 2009 Elsevier Inc. All rights reserved.

primarycare.theclinics.com

forward to bringing readers, old and new, the very best in evidence-based reviews on primary care topics.

Joel J. Heidelbaugh, MD
Departments of Family Medicine and Urology
Department of Family Medicine
University of Michigan Medical School
Ann Arbor, MI

Ypsilanti Health Center
200 Arnet, Suite 200
Ypsilanti, MI 48198

E-mail address:
jheidel@umich.edu (J.J. Heidelbaugh)

Preface

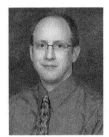 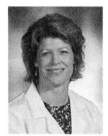

Joel J. Heidelbaugh, MD   Wendy S. Biggs, MD
Guest Editors

The term "women's health" encompasses a wide spectrum of normal events, diseases, disorders, and concerns throughout the female lifespan. Recent decades have fostered a need to provide a greater awareness of these unique issues. In fact, in 1991, the US Department of Health and Human Services created a vision to ensure that "all women and girls are healthier and have a better sense of well being" with its mission to "provide leadership to promote health equity for women and girls through sex/gender-specific approaches."[1] Throughout primary care, more nurse practitioners, physician assistants, family physicians, internists, and pediatricians are turning their desire for clinical practice toward creating a niche in caring for female patients of all ages and engaging in research centered on healthcare disparities.

Over the age of 18, more women seek preventive healthcare services than men in the US.[2] Still, an astonishing one in five US women will die from cardiovascular disease, and nearly one in six women will get breast cancer in their lifetime. Osteoporosis accounts for significant morbidity in elderly women, yet there is often poor attention toward prevention and screening in clinical practice. Routine health maintenance examinations provide solid opportunities to discuss primary and secondary prevention of these and many other important health risks. While the Papanicolau test has provided a landmark screening tool for cervical cancer, we now have the promise of significantly decreasing the incidence of the human papillomavirus through vaccination of young women between the ages of 9 and 26. Certainly, cancer is a great concern for every woman, yet many common and, fortunately, non–life-threatening issues may never enter into discussion during preventive or routine office visits due to embarrassment: menopausal symptoms, urinary complaints, fear of vaginal infection, dysmenorrhea and depression. The rate of violence against women continues to grow at an alarming pace, pressing primary care providers to consider screening women and offer appropriate interventions.

In reviewing numerous primary care and specialty-oriented journals and texts with a focus on women's health, we saw a growing need for the primary care provider to have a current, easy-to-access, and evidence-based reference suitable for approaching many of the common dilemmas encountered in caring for women in our practices.

Prim Care Clin Office Pract 36 (2009) xv–xvi
doi:10.1016/j.pop.2008.10.013
0095-4543/08/$ – see front matter © 2009 Elsevier Inc. All rights reserved.
primarycare.theclinics.com

Diagnostic and therapeutic algorithms are presented throughout many of the articles in this issue of *Primary Care: Clinics in Office Practice* to provide a quick reference for the busy clinician and to serve as excellent teaching tools for our varied learners. The collection of authors assembled herein represents a cohort of nationally recognized academic clinicians and scholars with years of practical expertise and a solid knowledge of the current literature, as evidence by their reviews. We would like to offer sincere gratitude to all of the authors who gave their valuable time and energy to participate in this project. Dr. Grant Greenberg, clinical assistant professor of Family Medicine at the University of Michigan Medical School, merits special consideration for his assistance in author recruitment. Lastly, we thank Ms. Barbara Cohen-Kligerman, senior clinics editor, and her wonderful staff at Elsevier for their support and assistance in the publication of this issue.

Joel J. Heidelbaugh, MD
Departments of Family Medicine and Urology
Department of Family Medicine
University of Michigan Medical School
Ann Arbor, MI

Ypsilanti Health Center
200 Arnet, Suite 200
Ypsilanti, MI 48198

Wendy S. Biggs, MD
Office of Medical Education
4005 Orchard Drive
Midland, MI 48640

E-mail addresses:
jheidel@umich.edu (J.J. Heidelbaugh)
wendy.biggs@midmichigan.org (W.S. Biggs)

REFERENCES

1. The National Women's Health Information Center. US Department of Health and Human Services. Available at: http://www.4woman.gov/. Accessed August 31, 2008.
2. Heron M. Deaths: leading causes for 2004. Natl Vital Stat Rep 2007;56(5):1–95.

Amenorrhea

Diana L. Heiman, MD[a,b,*]

KEYWORDS

- Amenorrhea • Polycystic ovary syndrome
- Ovarian failure—premature • Gonadal dysgenesis
- Anovulation

Key Points	Evidence Level
The most common cause of primary amenorrhea is constitutional delay of growth and puberty.	C
The primary goal of primary amenorrhea treatment is the gradual initiation of pubertal development.	C
All patients who have secondary amenorrhea should be evaluated for pregnancy.	C
All patients who have polycystic ovary syndrome should be evaluated for the metabolic syndrome, specifically focusing on glucose intolerance.	C
Athletes who have the female athlete triad should be treated for bone loss with calcium and vitamin D in addition to correcting the amenorrhea with an increase in calories and/or decrease in physical activity.	C

Amenorrhea is a common problem evaluated in primary care. Primary amenorrhea, by definition, is either the absence of menses by age 16 if normal development and sexual characteristics are present or the absence of menses by age 14 if no secondary sexual characteristics have developed. Secondary amenorrhea is by far more common and is defined as the absence of menses for 3 months in a woman who had previously regular menses or for 9 months in a woman who had previous oligomenorrhea.[1–3] The prevalence of secondary amenorrhea in the general population has been cited to be as high as 5%, with the prevalence in some groups, including competitive athletes, as high as almost 80%.[4] The most common cause of secondary amenorrhea is

[a] Department of Family Medicine, University of Connecticut School of Medicine, Farmington, CT, USA
[b] Family Medicine Center at Asylum Hill, 99 Woodland Street, Hartford, CT 06105, USA
* Family Medicine Center at Asylum Hill, 99 Woodland Street, Hartford, CT 06105.
E-mail address: dheiman@stfranciscare.org

Prim Care Clin Office Pract 36 (2009) 1–17
doi:10.1016/j.pop.2008.10.005
0095-4543/08/$ – see front matter © 2009 Elsevier Inc. All rights reserved.

pregnancy. The evaluation for the nonpregnant patient involves a thorough look at a complex system. In either case, a thorough history and physical examination can assist in narrowing the differential diagnosis before obtaining laboratory tests or investigational studies.

NORMAL MENSTRUAL CYCLE AND SEXUAL DEVELOPMENT

The normal progression of puberty has traditionally been measured with Tanner staging (**Table 1**).[5] Puberty begins with the initiation of a growth spurt between ages 6 and 8 years. After the growth spurt has begun, breast bud formation (thelarche) occurs. Adrenarche, the activation of the adrenal glands producing androgens, then occurs resulting in the growth of axillary and pubic hair within a 2-year period. At the time of gonadarche, or initiation of sex hormone production, longitudinal growth is at its maximum and the uterus and vagina grow to their normal adult size. Finally, menarche begins at an average age of 12.8 years.[5] The typical time course from thelarche to menarche is 3 years. The total time of pubertal changes, including the accelerated growth phase, typically is 4.5 years.[5] Delayed puberty occurs, by definition, in children who fall two standard deviations below the mean age of pubertal development for their peers. In the United States, this correlates to absence of breast development by the age of 13.5 years, pubic hair by age 14 years, and menses by age 16 years.[6,7] These age recommendations may change with a younger age now being seen with normal pubertal development.[8] Primary amenorrhea also exists if there is no menarche within 5 years after thelarche. When children fall outside the range that is considered normal, investigation is warranted.

The normal menstrual cycle involves a complex interaction between the hypothalamic-pituitary axis and the ovaries and outflow tract. The hypothalamus secretes pulsatile gonadotropin releasing hormone (GnRH), which in turn stimulates the anterior pituitary to produce follicle stimulating hormone (FSH) and luteinizing hormone (LH). FSH acts on the ovaries to induce the formation of follicles, whereas LH maintains the growth of the follicles, which in turn secrete estrogen. A peak in estrogen secretion occurring midcycle stimulates an LH surge that triggers ovulation. With ovulation, there is formation of a corpus luteum cyst that produces progesterone and leads to endometrial growth. If the oocyte is not fertilized, the corpus luteum dissipates after which menses occurs. Any disruption in the hypothalamic-pituitary axis can result in abnormal menses.[3]

Table 1						
Normal female pubertal development by Tanner staging						
Age Range (y)	8–10 Initial Growth Acceleration	9–11 Thelarche	9–11 Adrenarche	11–13 Peak Growth	12–14 Menarche	13–16 Adult Characteristics
Tanner staging						
Breast development	1	2	2	3	4	5
Pubic hair development	1	1	2	3	4	5

Data from Speroff L, Glass RH, Kase NG. Normal and abnormal sexual development. In: Clinical gynecologic endocrinology and infertility. 6th edition. Baltimore (MD): Lippincott Williams & Wilkins, 1999:339–79.

PRIMARY AMENORRHEA
Cause

There are numerous causes of primary amenorrhea (**Box 1**).[2,6,9,10] It is easiest to evaluate a woman for the cause in the context of presence or absence of pubertal changes. In all cases, a thorough history and physical examination (**Box 2**) should be performed focusing on secondary sexual characteristic development, family history, and symptoms of cyclic abdominal pain or breast tenderness.[2,6,9,10] **Fig. 1** highlights an approach to the evaluation of primary amenorrhea.[1,6,11,12] If secondary sexual characteristics are present, pregnancy should be ruled out. Laboratory and radiographic evaluation of suspected systemic diseases should be performed as indicated. Routine radiographic studies are not recommended because they are generally not useful or required to make an accurate diagnosis.[6]

Presence of Secondary Sexual Characteristics

If the woman has the presence of breast development with only minimal or no pubic hair, she is classified with the diagnosis of androgen insensitivity syndrome.[1] The patient is a genetic male with undescended testes and is phenotypically female. A karyotype must be performed to guide proper treatment, and the testes must be surgically removed as soon as possible because of the high chance of developing a malignancy after puberty.[1]

In the presence of normal secondary sexual characteristics, including pubic hair, the first step in the evaluation is to perform an ultrasound evaluation to determine if the patient has a uterus. Müllerian agenesis, congenital absence of the vagina and abnormal uterine development, is the most common anatomic cause of primary amenorrhea and second most common cause of primary amenorrhea accounting for approximately 15% of cases.[1,9,13] Activation of anti-müllerian hormone is believed to be the cause of the abnormality, leading to malformation of the female genital tract.[6,13] Patients may complain of cyclic abdominal pain if there is endometrial tissue in the rudimentary uterus and mittelschmerz or breast tenderness because of the presence of functioning ovaries and cyclic hormonal changes. An absent or truncated vagina and absence of normal adult uterus confirm the diagnosis. Karyotyping should be performed to confirm that the patient is genetically female.[13]

In the presence of a normal uterus, outflow tract obstruction must be considered in cases of primary amenorrhea. When the outflow tract is patent, an evaluation for secondary amenorrhea should proceed and pregnancy should be ruled out. Congenital outflow tract obstruction has several causes, including imperforate hymen and transverse vaginal septum. Both causes are typically associated with cyclic abdominal pain attributable to the accumulation of blood within the uterus and vagina.[1]

Absence of Secondary Sexual Characteristics

When evaluating patients who lack secondary sexual characteristics, the diagnosis is primarily based on laboratory values. Serum FSH and LH levels and a karyotype can aid in the diagnosis. With low FSH and LH levels resulting in hypogonadotropic hypogonadism, constitutional delay of growth and puberty (CDGP) is the most common cause.[9,14] The delayed growth is often familial and may be discovered by obtaining a detailed family history. The hypogonadotropic hypogonadism of CDGP is indistinguishable from that of hypothalamic/pituitary failure.[11] In CDGP, bone age is greater than one standard deviation below chronologic age, and history and physical examination are normal.[6] Height in these patients may be normal or less than normal and the patients generally tend to be lean. A recent case series found that 22% of the boys and

Box 1
Causes of primary amenorrhea

Absent secondary sexual characteristics
Constitutional delay of growth and puberty
Hypogonadotropic hypogonadism
    Gonadal dysgenesis
        Turner syndrome
        Others
    Chronic illness
        Diabetes
        Thyroid disease
        Inflammatory bowel disease
        Chronic renal insufficiency
        Depression/severe psychosocial stressors
        Chronic liver disease
        Immunodeficiency
        Anorexia nervosa
        Many others
    Kallmann syndrome
    Cranial radiation
    Idiopathic
Hypergonadotropic hypogonadism
    Ovarian failure
    Chemotherapy
    Pelvic radiation
Present secondary sexual characteristics
Pregnancy
Hypogonadotropic hypogonadism
    Chronic illness
    Central nervous system tumor
    Hypothalamic/pituitary destruction
    Cranial radiation
Hypergonadotropic hypogonadism
    Ovarian failure
    Chemotherapy
    Pelvic radiation
Eugonadotropic
    Androgen insensitivity syndrome
    Müllerian agenesis
    Polycystic ovary syndrome

Data from Refs.[2,6,9,10]

girls who had CDGP had a body mass index greater than or equal to the 85th percentile for age. These patients tended to be taller and have bone ages that were less delayed than the lean patients.[14] CDGP is a normal variant and watchful waiting is appropriate. Another congenital cause of hypogonadotropic hypogonadism is Kallmann syndrome, which is associated with anosmia.[15]

The causes of hypergonadotropic hypogonadism (elevated serum FSH and LH) in primary amenorrhea are gonadal dysgenesis and premature ovarian failure (POF). Turner syndrome (45,XO) is the most common form of female gonadal dysgenesis. Physical findings in Turner syndrome include webbing of the neck, widely spaced nipples, and short stature. Mosaic inheritance occurs in approximately 25% of these patients and is associated with a more normal phenotype and spontaneous onset of puberty and menarche.[16] Rarely, pure gonadal dysgenesis can occur with a 46,XX or 46,XY genotype.[6] POF is discussed in more detail in the setting of secondary amenorrhea.

Treatment

Treatment of primary amenorrhea depends on the cause. The primary goal is to ensure normal puberty is occurring. Secondary goals include addressing fertility issues and avoiding complications of the hypoestrogenic state. If CDGP is present, watchful waiting with follow-up is indicated. When chronic diseases are uncovered, treatment of the underlying problem typically results in progression of puberty along its normal course. With Müllerian agenesis, psychologic support of the patient and her family are warranted. Also, surgical or nonsurgical creation of a vagina should be undertaken at the time of desired sexual intercourse.[13] In girls who have gonadal failure, initiation of pubertal development and menses with very low doses of estrogen, followed by estrogen and progesterone or combination oral contraceptive pills, results in normal growth and development and osteoporosis prevention. Fertility does not return except in rare cases. These women can conceive with the assistance of donated ova and in vitro fertilization.

In girls who have a permanent deficiency of estrogen, restriction of growth and decreased bone density occur. It therefore becomes important to coax these patients gently into puberty with the initiation of low-dose estrogen and then combined estrogen and progesterone, or oral contraceptive pills, when menarche occurs. It is believed that peak bone density can be achieved in these girls with proper hormonal therapy.[6]

SECONDARY AMENORRHEA

After evaluating for pregnancy, thyroid disease, and hyperprolactinemia, the remaining causes of secondary amenorrhea can be divided into normogonadotropic amenorrhea, hypergonadotropic hypogonadism, or hypogonadotropic hypogonadism. Common specific causes of each of these classes are discussed later. Evaluation should begin with determination of serum thyroid stimulating hormone (TSH) and prolactin levels (**Fig. 2**). Abnormalities in either the TSH or prolactin are discussed. If they are both normal, a progestogen challenge should be performed (**Table 2**).[3,17]

DIFFERENTIAL DIAGNOSIS
Hypothyroidism

Few patients have amenorrhea attributable to hypothyroidism. Often before the onset of amenorrhea, hypothyroidism is already clinically apparent because of other

Box 2
History and physical examination in primary amenorrhea

History

Sexual activity

Prescription drug use

Illicit drug use

Previous chemotherapy or radiation

Current or previous chronic illness

Psychosocial stressors

Nutritional history

Exercise history

Family history

Menarche and menstrual history of mother/sisters

Pubertal/growth delay

Genetic defects

Chronic illness

Infertility

Review of systems

Vasomotor symptoms

Galactorrhea

Hirsutism

Acne

Hair pattern/balding

Cyclic abdominal pain or breast changes

Symptoms of hypo/hyperthyroidism

Anosmia

Physical examination

Vital signs

Anthropomorphic measurements

    Body mass index

    Growth chart

    Tanner staging

Dysmorphic features

    Webbed neck

    Barrel chest

    Widely spaced nipples

Skin examination

    Hirsutism/virilization

    Acne

    Striae

    Buffalo hump

Abdominal/pelvic examination

    External genital appearance

    Pubic hair

    Vaginal septum

    Imperforate hymen

    Presence of uterus

    Clitoral hypertrophy

    Inguinal mass (undescended testes)

Neurologic examination

Breast examination

Thyroid examination

Data from Refs.[2,6,9,10]

symptoms. In many cases, however, the treatment of hypothyroidism restores normal menses and often in a few months resolves associated galactorrhea.[18]

Hyperprolactinemic Amenorrhea

For patients who have elevated prolactin levels or evidence of galactorrhea, headaches, or visual disturbances on history or physical examination, an MRI study of the pituitary gland is important to rule out a pituitary tumor. Adenomas are the most common source of anterior pituitary dysfunction; other causes are listed in **Box 3**.[19] If the prolactin levels are greater than 100 ng/mL or symptoms of an intracranial mass are present, an MRI should be considered.

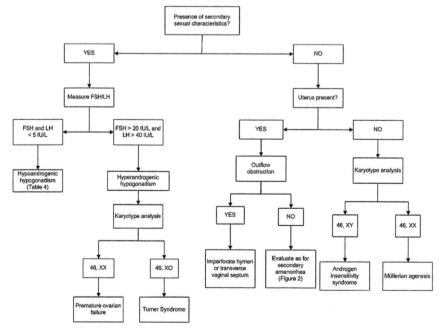

Fig. 1. Evaluation of primary amenorrhea. (*Data from* Refs.[1,6,11,12].)

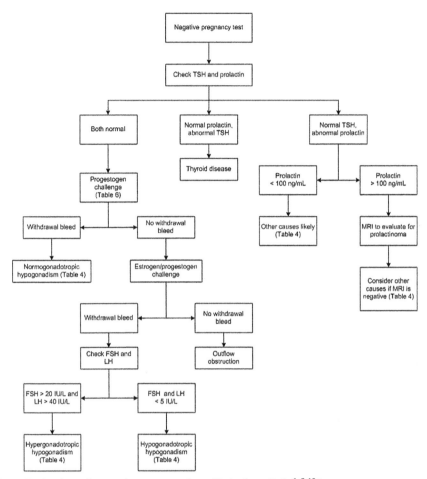

Fig. 2. Evaluation of secondary amenorrhea. (*Data from* Refs.[1–3,10].)

Medications, such as tricyclic antidepressants, opiates, cimetidine, calcium channel blockers, and estrogens can also cause an elevation of prolactin levels, although not typically greater than 100 ng/mL.[19] Prolonged hypothyroidism may also result in elevated prolactin levels and galactorrhea. In rare cases, ectopic production of prolactin can occur from tissue in the hypopharynx, from bronchogenic carcinoma, renal cell carcinoma, gonadoblastoma, or a prolactinoma in an ovarian dermoid cyst or teratoma.[19]

Adenomas are the most likely cause of anterior pituitary dysfunction, although empty sella syndrome, other tumors such as meningiomas, craniopharyngiomas or metastases, tuberculosis, sarcoidosis, cysts, and fatty deposits can cause dysfunction also.[19] Sheehan syndrome, known as hypopituitarism due to postpartum hemorrhage and resultant lack of blood flow to the pituitary, can also occur in the presence of obstetric hemorrhage and presents with problems in the postpartum period.

Microadenomas (those <10 mm in diameter) found on MRI in the absence of any intracranial symptoms can be followed with repeat prolactin levels and imaging every few years. Microadenomas are slow growing and are rarely malignant. About one third of patients who have secondary amenorrhea have a pituitary adenoma.[19] Treatment of

Table 2
Progestogen and estrogen/progestogen challenge test procedures

Progestogen Challenge		Estrogen/Progestogen Challenge
Medication	Duration	
Medroxyprogesterone acetate (Provera) 10 mg once daily, orally	7–10 d	Conjugated equine estrogen 1.25 mg OR estradiol 2 mg on days 1 to 21, followed by a progestational agent for 10–14 days (doses at left)
Norethindrone acetate (Aygestin), 5 mg once daily, orally	7–10 d	
Progesterone 200 mg (intramuscular oil), parenterally	Single dose	
Micronized progesterone (Prometrium) 400 mg daily, orally	7–10 d	
Micronized progesterone vaginal gel 4% or 8% (Crinone), intravaginally	Every other day for six applications	

Data from Speroff L, Fritz MA. Amenorrhea. In: Clinical gynecologic endocrinology and infertility. 7th edition. Philadelphia, PA: Lippincott Williams & Wilkins, 2005;401–64; and Warren MP, Biller BM, Shangold MM. A new clinical option for hormone replacement therapy in women with secondary amenorrhea: effects of cyclic administration of progesterone from the sustained-release vaginal gel Crinone (4% or 8%) on endometrial morphologic features and withdrawal bleeding. Am J Obstet Gyn 1999;180:42–8.

microadenomas should be directed at treatment of infertility or galactorrhea and breast discomfort. Dopamine agonists, including bromocriptine and cabergoline, are used to decrease symptomatology and improve infertility and are the current treatments of choice. Macroadenomas often need to be treated more aggressively with shrinkage with dopamine agonists or consideration of transsphenoidal neurosurgery.[19]

Normogonadotropic Anovulation

Hyperandrogenic chronic anovulation

Polycystic ovarian syndrome (PCOS) is the most common cause of hyperandrogenic chronic anovulation. PCOS affects a minimum of 6% of women of reproductive age.[20,21] Although there is no universally accepted definition, there are three sets of diagnostic criteria. The National Institutes of Health 1990 criteria define it as a diagnosis of chronic anovulation with hyperandrogenism in which other secondary causes have been excluded.[22] The Rotterdam 2003 criteria refined the NIH criteria to be diagnostic if two of the following are present: clinical or biochemical signs of hyperandrogenism, oligo- or anovulation, and polycystic ovaries, and the exclusion of other causes (congenital adrenal hyperplasia [CAH], androgen-secreting tumors, Cushing syndrome).[23] In 2006, the Androgen Excess Society proposed their diagnostic criteria, which include presence of all of the following: hirsutism or hyperandrogenemia, oligo-ovulation or polycystic ovaries, and exclusion of other androgen excess or related disorders (possibly excluding 21-hydroxylase deficient nonclassical adrenal hyperplasia, androgen-secreting neoplasms, androgenic/anabolic drug use or abuse, Cushing

Box 3
Causes of amenorrhea

Hyperprolactinemic

Prolactin >100 ng/mL

    Pituitary adenoma

    Empty sella syndrome

Prolactin 20–100 ng/mL

    Pregnancy

    Breast stimulation

    Breastfeeding

    Hypothyroidism

    Medications

        Oral contraceptive pills

        Antipsychotics

        Antidepressants

        Antihypertensives

        H2 receptor blockers

        Opiates, cocaine

    Ectopic production

        Renal cell carcinoma

        Ovarian dermoid cyst

        Teratoma

        Hypopharynx

        Gonadoblastoma

        Bronchogenic carcinoma

    Altered metabolism

        Renal failure

        Liver failure

Normogonadotropic

Hyperandrogenic anovulation

    Polycystic ovary syndrome

    Thyroid disease

    Cushing obesity

    Exogenous androgens

    Androgen secreting ovarian or adrenal tumor

    Acromegaly

    Nonclassic congenital adrenal hyperplasia

Outflow tract obstruction

    Asherman syndrome

    Cervical stenosis

    Imperforate hymen[a]

Vaginal septum[a]

Congenital

Androgen insensitivity syndrome[a]

Müllerian agenesis[a]

Hypogonadotropic hypogonadism

Hypothalamic amenorrhea[a]

Chronic illness

Diabetes

Thyroid disease

Inflammatory bowel disease

Chronic renal insufficiency

Depression/severe psychosocial stressors

Chronic liver disease

Immunodeficiency

Anorexia nervosa

Bulimia

Excessive exercise

Excessive weight loss/malnutrition

Cranial radiation

Central nervous system tumor

Hypothalamic/pituitary destruction

Sheehan syndrome

Constitutional delay of growth and puberty[a]

Kallmann syndrome[a]

Hypergonadotropic hypogonadism

Premature ovarian failure

Autoimmune

Genetic

Galactosemia

17-Hydroxylase deficiency

Chemotherapy

Pelvic radiation

Mumps

Idiopathic

Postmenopausal ovarian failure

Gonadal dysgenesis[a]

Turner syndrome[a]

Others[a]

[a] Cause of primary amenorrhea only.
Data from Refs.[2,3,12,13]

syndrome, the syndromes of severe insulin resistance, thyroid dysfunction, and hyperprolactinemia).[23]

The primary cause of PCOS is unknown, but insulin resistance is believed to be a fundamental component to the disease process. The differential diagnosis for the patient who has hyperandrogenism and chronic anovulation is listed in **Box 3**.[3,4,10] The diagnosis of PCOS is primarily clinical; however, additional laboratory work may be necessary to rule out secondary causes of hyperandrogenism. Patients who have PCOS often have signs of androgenism, such as acne, hirsutism, and obesity; however, rapid virilization or evidence of clitoromegaly, temporal balding, or deepening of the voice should prompt the search for an alternate diagnosis.

PCOS is associated with abnormal gonadotropin secretion (**Box 4**).[2,10] There is preliminary suggestion that measurement of the prostate-specific antigen (PSA) may also help identify patients who have PCOS. The level of PSA increases with exposure to excess androgens and progestins and has been found to be elevated in patients who have hyperandrogenism due to PCOS.[24,25] Patients who have PCOS may also have slightly elevated levels of testosterone and dehydroepiandrosterone sulfate (DHEA-S). Although there are no levels that definitively indicate or rule out tumors or pathology, significantly elevated levels of serum total testosterone (greater than 200 ng/dL) indicate a possible androgen-secreting tumor, and elevated levels of DHEA-S (greater than 700 ng/dL) are suggestive of an adrenal tumors. Serum 17-hydroxyprogesterone levels can also be assayed to evaluate for adult-onset CAH, most often due

---

Box 4
Laboratory evaluation of hyperandrogenism

Serum testosterone (normal 20–80 ng/dL)

<200 ng/dL: evaluate for hyperandrogenic chronic anovulation[a]

>200 ng/dL: evaluate for androgen-secreting tumor

Serum dehydroepiandrosterone sulfate (normal 250–300 ng/dL)

<700 ng/dL: consider hyperandrogenic chronic anovulation[a]

>700 ng/dL: evaluate for adrenal or ovarian tumor

Serum 17-hydroxyprogesterone (normal <2 ng/mL)

Draw morning level during follicular phase of menstrual cycle

>4 ng/mL consider adrenocorticotropic stimulation test to diagnose congenital adrenal hyperplasia

Consider a dexamethasone suppression test if clinically indicated[b]

Morning cortisol level >5 μg/dL consider Cushing disease

[a] These values are not specific for diagnosis of hyperandrogenic chronic anovulation.
[b] An overnight dexamethasone suppression screening test can be administered by giving 1 mg of dexamethasone between 11 PM and midnight and drawing a single blood sample for serum cortisol at 8 AM the following day. In healthy individuals who have an intact hypothalamic pituitary axis, the serum cortisol level should be suppressed to <5 μg/dL. If the morning cortisol level is >5 μg/dL, then Cushing disease should be suspected and further testing done to confirm it. There is some variability in the cut off values that can affect sensitivity and specificity of the test.
Data from American College of Obstetricians and Gynecologists. ACOG practice bulletin. Clinical management guidelines for practicing obstetrician-gynecologists: number 41. December 2002;100(6):1389–402; and Kiningham RB, Apgar BS, Schwenk TL. Evaluation of amenorrhea. Am Fam Physician 1996:53:1185–94.

to a 21-hydoxylase deficiency. 17-Hypdroxyprogesterone levels greater than 4 ng/mL suggest CAH. An abnormal test for CAH should be followed by an adrenocorticotropic stimulation test.[22]

Cushing disease is also common in the differential diagnosis of hyperandrogenism but is relatively uncommon at an estimated prevalence of 1:1,000,000. Routine testing for Cushing disease may not be necessary and should be considered in those patients who have stigmata of the disease, including striae, cervicodorsal fat, significant central obesity, easy bruising, hypertension, and proximal muscle weakness. Cushing disease is most commonly evaluated by a dexamethasone suppression test. A morning cortisol level less than 5 µg/dL with the dexamethasone suppression test rules out Cushing disease.[20,22]

Patients who have untreated PCOS have large amounts of unopposed circulating estrogens associated with a theoretic increased risk for development of endometrial cancer. A true increased incidence has not been seen epidemiologically.[23] Associated with the insulin resistance that is seen with PCOS is also a threefold to sevenfold increased risk for developing diabetes mellitus and subsequent inherent health risks. There have been no prospective studies to document a definitive increased risk in patients who have PCOS for coronary artery disease, yet abnormal serum lipid profiles and diabetes are prevalent in patients who have PCOS and studies looking at surrogate endpoints for coronary artery disease suggest that patients who have PCOS may be at increased risk for heart disease. There is, however, a slightly elevated incidence of stroke seen in women who have PCOS.[23,26] A more recently identified association seen in women who have PCOS is nonalcoholic fatty liver disease (NAFLD). These two conditions share insulin resistance as a primary feature and although no definitive cause and effect relationship has been proved, an increased frequency of NAFLD in women who have PCOS versus controls has been observed.[27]

The primary treatment strategy of PCOS involves weight loss, diet, and exercise. A weight loss as small as 5% can make a significant difference in lowering androgen levels and improving hirsutism, resumption of normal menses, and decreasing insulin resistance, although it may take months to see these results. In all patients, routine screening for serum lipid profiles and screening for insulin resistance and diabetes mellitus with a 2-hour glucose tolerance test should be considered.[22]

Maintenance of a normal endometrium may be accomplished with the use of oral contraceptive pills or cyclic progesterone. The best regimen of cyclic progesterone to prevent endometrial cancer is not known, but typically a 10- to 14-day course each month has been advocated. Hirsutism may be treated with antiandrogens, such as spironolactone, flutamide, or finasteride. All of these medications have potential for teratogenicity, and should be used cautiously or concomitantly with the oral contraceptive pill.[22] In addition to the previously mentioned lifestyle changes, insulin-sensitizing agents, such as metformin and the thiazolidinediones, can be considered for reducing insulin resistance, hirsutism, and ovulation.[28] Treatment for patients who have PCOS desiring conception is beyond the scope of this article, but potential regimens including the use of clomiphene citrate and metformin have been successful.[22,29,30]

Outflow tract obstruction

The most common outflow tract obstruction to cause secondary amenorrhea is Asherman syndrome. This syndrome is most often a result of excessive endometrial curettage resulting in intrauterine synechiae and scarring. Diagnosis can be made with a hysterogram or hysteroscopy; the latter is more accurate at detecting small adhesions.[3]

Hypergonadotropic Hypogonadism

Ovarian failure

Ovarian failure can occur because of natural menopause or premature ovarian failure (POF). Normal menopause occurs on average at age 50 years and is due to ovarian follicle depletion. POF is a condition involving amenorrhea, hypoestrogenism, and elevated gonadotropins before the age of 40 years.[31] It affects approximately 0.1% of women by age 30 and 1% of women by age 40.[32] POF is not always an irreversible condition like natural menopause. In approximately 50% of women, POF is characterized by intermittent ovarian functioning. Women who have POF have an approximated 5% to 10% chance of natural conception.[32] Premature ovarian failure does carry an increased risk for osteoporosis and heart disease, however.[32–34] One survey of 19,000 women indicated that ovarian failure occurring before age 40 was associated with an increased mortality from heart disease, stroke, cancer, and all other causes of death.[32] Treatment should be aimed at reducing these risks. Estrogen supplementation has not been proved to be beneficial in either inducing ovulation or in preventing cardiovascular mortality, but does seem to improve bone mineral density.[35,36]

POF may occur because of ovarian follicle dysfunction or depletion and has several causes (**Box 3**). It has also been associated with autoimmune endocrine disorders, such as Addison disease, diabetes mellitus, and most commonly hypothyroidism.[31,32] Patients younger than age 30 years who have premature ovarian failure should have a karyotype performed to rule out the presence of a Y chromosome and the need for removal of gonadal tissue.[32] Because of the association with other disorders, fasting serum glucose, TSH, free thyroxine, and morning cortisol levels should be drawn in women who have premature ovarian failure. Further laboratory evaluation should be considered on an individual basis and should include a complete blood count, erythrocyte sedimentation rate, total serum protein, anti-nuclear antibody, and rheumatoid factor assays, and a corticotropin stimulation test.[36,37] Approximately 20% to 40% of women who have premature ovarian failure develop another autoimmune disorder; therefore, if initial laboratory evaluation is within normal limits, periodic screening should be considered. Ovarian biopsy and anti-ovarian antibody testing have not been shown to be of clinical benefit in premature ovarian failure.[32]

Hypogonadotropic Hypogonadism

Hypothalamic amenorrhea

Hypothalamic amenorrhea is characterized by abnormalities in GnRH pulsatile secretion with resultant disruption of the hypothalamic-pituitary-ovarian axis. This disruption is often due to weight loss with disordered eating, such as anorexia nervosa and bulimia nervosa, excessive exercise, and psychologic stress (see **Box 3**). The exact mechanism of how stress or weight loss affects the secretion of GnRH is unknown. Leptin, a protein produced by the obesity gene, seems to have some association with weight loss and amenorrhea and osteoporosis. Leptin levels seem to be regulated by energy intake and correlate well with body mass index in humans, serving as a regulator of basal metabolic rate. Low leptin levels or the loss of the usual diurnal secretion of leptin has been noted in patients who have amenorrhea. Leptin receptors are present in bone also, suggesting that leptin may be instrumental in bone mass regulation.[38–40]

Treatment of patients who have hypothalamic amenorrhea depends on the cause. Patients who have excessive weight loss need to be screened for disordered eating and those who have a diagnosis of anorexia nervosa or bulimia nervosa should be treated for these disorders. Return of normal menses may occur with the successful treatment of the underlying disorder and return of a reasonable body weight.[40]

Athletes who have the triad of disordered eating, amenorrhea, and osteoporosis fit into the category of the female athlete triad. Many athletes experience amenorrhea at some time in their athletic careers but the exact prevalence of the female athlete triad is unknown.[41] In patients who have the female athlete triad, a modest increase in caloric intake and 10% decrease in training is often adequate for the resumption of menses. Athletes who have continued amenorrhea are at risk for bone loss and osteoporosis. This bone loss may not be reversible and is occurring at a time when peak bone mass should be developing.[41,42] Weight-bearing exercise in athletes may be partially protective against bone loss, but treatment is still needed.[43] This early bone loss places them at greater risk for osteoporosis as they age.

In women who are unable to alter their eating or training habits to resume normal menses, treating the amenorrhea and hypoestrogenism with the oral contraceptive pill may be considered. Only small, nonrandomized studies have examined the benefits of the oral contraceptive pill on bone mass. In general, it seems that the use of the oral contraceptive pill may prevent further loss, but it does not appreciably reverse the loss of bone in these patients.[42] Other agents, such as used for the treatment of postmenopausal osteoporosis, have not been studied in women of reproductive age because they have a potential for teratogenicity (eg, bisphosphonates, selective estrogen receptor modulators). Adequate calcium and vitamin D intake should be recommended also.

SUMMARY

Amenorrhea is a complicated and common problem encountered by primary care physicians. Performing a thorough history and physical examination can often narrow the differential diagnosis considerably. The addition of basic determinations of serum FSH and LH or other tests as indicated by abnormalities on the history or examination can then make the diagnosis more clear. In all cases of primary amenorrhea, treatment is directed by the diagnosis. The primary goal of treatment is to facilitate the normal sexual development through gentle coaxing into puberty. In secondary amenorrhea, there is a greater focus on fertility and prevention of complications from the associated abnormal hormone levels. Probability of conception is dictated by the reversibility of the cause of the amenorrhea.

REFERENCES

1. The practice committee of the American Society for Reproductive Medicine. Current evaluation of amenorrhea. Fertil Steril 2006;86(Suppl 4):S148–55.
2. American College of Obstetricians and Gynecologists. Amenorrhea. (ACOG technical bulletin 128). Washington, DC: ACOG; 1989.
3. Speroff L, Fritz MA. Amenorrhea. In: Speroff L, Fritz MA, editors. Clinical gynecologic endocrinology and infertility. 7th edition. Philadelphia: Lippincott Williams & Wilkins; 2005. p. 401–64.
4. Warren MP, Ramos RH, Bronson EM. Exercise associated amenorrhea: are altered leptin levels an early warning sign? Phys Sportsmed 2002;30(10): 41–6.
5. Speroff L, Glass RH, Kase NG. Normal and abnormal sexual development. In: Seifer DB, Speroff L, editors. Clinical gynecologic endocrinology and infertility. 6th edition. Baltimore (MD): Lippincott Williams & Wilkins; 1999. p. 339–79.

6. Pletcher JR, Slap GB. Menstrual disorders. Pediatr Clin North Am 1999;46(3): 505–18.

7. Marshall WA, Tanner JM. Variations in patterns of pubertal changes in girls. Arch Dis Child 1969;44(235):291–303.

8. Herman-Giddens ME, Slora EJ, Wasserman RC, et al. Secondary sexual characteristics and menses in young girls seen in office practice: a study from the pediatric research in office settings network. Pediatrics 1997;99:505–12.

9. Reindollar RM, Byrd JR, McDonough PG. Delayed sexual development: a study of 252 patients. Am J Obstet Gynecol 1981;140:371–80.

10. Kiningham RB, Apgar BS, Schwenk TL. Evaluation of amenorrhea. Am Fam Physician 1996;53:1185–94.

11. Albanese A, Stanhope R. Investigation of delayed puberty. Clin Endocrinol (Oxf) 1995;43:105–10.

12. McIver B, Romanksi SA, Nippoldt TB. Evaluation and management of amenorrhea. Mayo Clin Proc 1997;72:1161–9.

13. Folch M, Pigem I, Konje JC. Müllerian agenesis: etiology, diagnosis, and management. Obstet Gynecol Surv 2000;55(10):644–9.

14. Sedlmeyer IL, Palmert MR. Delayed puberty: analysis of a large case series from an academic center. J Clin Endocrinol Metab 2002;87(4):1613–20.

15. Traggiai C, Stanhope R. Delayed puberty. Best Pract Res Clin Endocrinol Metab 2002;16(1):139–51.

16. Simpson J, Rajkovic A. Ovarian differentiation and gonadal failure. Am J Med Genet 1999;89:186–200.

17. Warren MP, Biller BM, Shangold MM. A new clinical option for hormone replacement therapy in women with secondary amenorrhea: effects of cyclic administration of progesterone from the sustained-release vaginal gel Crinone (4% or 8%) on endometrial morphologic features and withdrawal bleeding. Am J Obstet Gynecol 1999;180(pt 1):42–8.

18. Kalro B. Impaired fertility caused by endocrine dysfunction in women. Endocrinol Metab Clin North Am 2003;32:573–92.

19. Pickett CA. Diagnosis and management of pituitary tumors: recent advances. Prim Care 2003;30(4):765–89.

20. Solomon C. The epidemiology of polycystic ovary syndrome; prevalence and associated disease risks. Endocrinol Metab Clin North Am 1999;28(2):247–63.

21. Trivax B, Azziz R. Diagnosis of polycystic ovary syndrome. Clin Obstet Gynecol 2007;50(1):168–77.

22. American College of Obstetricians and Gynecologists. Clinical management guidelines for practicing obstetrician-gynecologists: number 41. ACOG practice bulletin 2002;100(6):1389–402.

23. The Rotterdam ESHRE/ASRM-Sponsored PCOS consensus working group. Revised 2003 consensus on diagnostic criteria and long-term health risks related to polycystic ovary syndrome. Fertil Steril 2004;81(1):19–25.

24. Vural B, Özkan S, Bodur H. Is prostate-specific antigen a potential new marker of androgen excess in polycystic ovary syndrome? J Obstet Gynaecol Res 2007; 33(2):166–73.

25. Burelli A, Cionini R, Rinaldi E, et al. Serum PSA levels are not affected by the menstrual cycle or the menopause, but are increased in subjects with polycystic ovary syndrome. J Endocrinol Invest 2006;29(4):308–12.

26. Mather KJ, Kwan F, Corenblum B. Hyperinsulinemia in polycystic ovary syndrome correlates with increased cardiovascular risk independent of obesity. Fertil Steril 2000;73(1):150–6.

27. Cerda C, Pérez-Ayuso RM, Riquelme A, et al. Nonalcoholic fatty liver disease in women with polycystic ovary syndrome. J Hepatol 2007;47:412–7.
28. Setji TL, Brown AJ. Polycystic ovary syndrome: diagnosis and treatment. Am J Med 2007;120:128–32.
29. Velazquez E, Acosta A, Mendoza SG. Menstrual cyclicity after metformin therapy in polycystic ovary syndrome. Obstet Gynecol 1997;90(3):392–5.
30. Kolodziejczyk B, Duleba AJ, Spacsynski RZ, et al. Metformin therapy decreases hyperandrogenism and hyperinsulinemia in women with polycystic ovary syndrome. Fertil Steril 2000;73(6):1149–54.
31. Anasti JN. Premature ovarian failure: an update. Fertil Steril 1998;70(1):1–15.
32. Kalantaridou S, Davis SR, Nelson LM. Premature ovarian failure. Endocrinol Metab Clin North Am 1998;27(4):989–1006.
33. van der Schow Y, van der Graaf Y, Steyerberg EW, et al. Age at menopause as a risk factor for cardiovascular mortality. Lancet 1996;347:714–8.
34. Jacobsen BK, Nilssen S, Heuch I, et al. Does age at natural menopause, affect mortality from ischemic heart disease? J Clin Epidemiol 1997;50:475–9.
35. Taylor A, Adams J, Mulder J, et al. A randomized, control trial of estradiol replacement therapy in women with hypergonadotropic amenorrhea. J Clin Endocrinol Metab 1996;81:3615–21.
36. Kalantaridou S, Naka KK, Papanikolaou E, et al. Impaired endothelial function in young women with premature ovarian failure: normalization with hormone therapy. J Clin Endocrinol Metab 2004;89:3907–13.
37. Kim TJ, Anasti JN, Flack MR, et al. Routine endocrine screening for patients with karyotypically normal spontaneous premature ovarian failure. Obstet Gynecol 1997;89(5 pt 1):777–9.
38. Miller KK, Parulekar MS, Schoenfeld E, et al. Decreased leptin levels in normal weight women with hypothalamic amenorrhea: the effects of body composition and nutritional intake. J Clin Endocrinol Metab 1998;83:2309–12.
39. Welt CK, Chan JL, Bullen J, et al. Recombinant human leptin in women with hypothalamic amenorrhea. N Engl J Med 2004;351:987–97.
40. Mitan LA. Menstrual dysfunction in anorexia nervosa. J Pediatr Adolesc Gynecol 2004;17:81–5.
41. Drinkwater BL, Nilson K, Chesnut CH III, et al. Bone mineral contents of amenorrheic and eumenorrheic athletes. N Engl J Med 1984;311(5):278–81.
42. Robinson TL, Snow-Harter C, Taaffe DR, et al. Gymnasts exhibit higher bone mass than runners despite similar prevalence of amenorrhea and oligomenorrhea. J Bone Miner Res 1995;10(1):26–35.
43. Hergenroeder AC, Smith EO, Shypailo R, et al. Bone mineral changes in young women with hypothalamic amenorrhea treated with oral contraceptives, medroxyprogesterone or placebo over 12 months. Am J Obstet Gynecol 1997;176:1017–25.

Dysmenorrhea

Cathleen Morrow, MD[a,*], Elizabeth H. Naumburg, MD[b]

KEYWORDS

- Cramping • Menstrual pain • Menstrual flow
- Pelvic pain • Treatment of dysmenorrhea

Dysmenorrhea is the most common gynecologic condition experienced by menstruating women. The term dysmenorrhea is derived from the Greek words *dys* (difficult, painful, or abnormal), *meno* (month), and *rrhea* (flow). It is characterized by crampy lower abdominal pain that can range widely in severity and associated symptoms, yet its overall impact often has significant medical and psychosocial implications. Dysmenorrhea is potentially the most underdiagnosed gynecologic condition because of common societal beliefs regarding a lack of effective treatments and expectations about the burden of menstruation. The hallmark of primary (spasmodic) dysmenorrhea is painful menses in the absence of any associated macroscopic pathologic process, whereas secondary (congestive) dysmenorrhea implies painful menses with associated organic pelvic pathology.[1] The focus of this article is on primary dysmenorrhea.

EPIDEMIOLOGY

The prevalence of primary dysmenorrhea peaks in the second and third decades of life and decreases in frequency with advancing age as the prevalence of secondary dysmenorrhea increases. A recent systematic review of worldwide literature on chronic pelvic pain reports a prevalence of dysmenorrhea at 17% to 80%.[2] The most recent studies conducted on adolescent women report a prevalence range from 20% to 90%.[3,4] The precise prevalence of dysmenorrhea is difficult to discern because of variations in definitions and survey methodology. A population-based survey conducted in Sweden nearly 2 decades ago found that 10% to 24% of women who had dysmenorrhea admitted that symptoms interfered with their daily function, 51% missed work or school because of their symptoms, and only 31% had reported their symptoms to their physician.[5] Women often do not seek medical evaluation for their symptoms of dysmenorrhea, despite a common negative impact on their quality of life.

---

[a] Department of Community and Family Medicine, Dartmouth Medical School, DHMC HB #7015, 1 Medical Center Drive, Lebanon, NH 03756, USA
[b] Department of Family Medicine, University of Rochester School of Medicine and Dentistry, Highland Family Medicine Center, 777 South Clinton Avenue, Rochester, New York 14620, USA
* Corresponding author.
E-mail address: cathleen.morrow@dartmouth.edu (C. Morrow).

Prim Care Clin Office Pract 36 (2009) 19–32
doi:10.1016/j.pop.2008.10.004
0095-4543/08/$ – see front matter © 2009 Elsevier Inc. All rights reserved.

primarycare.theclinics.com

NATURAL HISTORY

Most sources agree that primary dysmenorrhea is associated with ovulatory cycles, so symptoms typically do not begin with the first menstrual cycles. As menses due to ovulation ensues, associated with the maturation of the hypothalamic-pituitary-gonadal axis, the symptoms of dysmenorrhea are more likely to present. Generally, it is believed that ovulation becomes associated with menstrual cycles 2 to 4 years after menarche in most women, but there is some evidence to suggest that ovulatory cycles may start within months or even with the onset of menses.[6] The diagnosis of primary dysmenorrhea is thus suggested by the onset of symptoms coinciding with the natural history of ovulation.

For any given menstrual cycle, there may be a wide variation in the degree of symptomatology from woman to woman. Adverse symptoms generally begin within hours after the onset of menstrual flow and can last for up to 72 hours, typically peaking in the first 24 to 48 hours of the menstrual cycle. The experienced pain is commonly in the lower abdominal or suprapubic region, is described as crampy or waxing and waning in intensity, and may radiate to the lower back or inner thighs. Associated symptoms are common and may include nausea, vomiting, diarrhea, headache, malaise, or fatigue. The specific pattern of symptoms and relationship to menstrual onset may become consistent for an individual patient.

The intensity of symptoms of primary dysmenorrhea tends to diminish with advancing age and following childbirth. A cohort study of the natural history of dysmenorrhea in nulliparous women in China found that diminished symptoms occurred in women who had more frequent intercourse, less frequent associated symptoms, and increased age. By the time most women in this cohort reached age 40, symptoms of primary dysmenorrhea were virtually absent.[7]

The natural history of secondary dysmenorrhea varies from the typical pattern of primary dysmenorrhea in one or more features. The onset of symptoms may occur later in a woman's menstrual history, presenting many years to decades after menarche. The associated pain may have different characteristics and can occur at times other than concomitant with menstrual flow or it may be associated with other factors. In these cases, the clinician must be astute to consider underlying gynecologic pathology, including uterine fibroids, endometriosis, adenomyosis, and chronic pelvic inflammatory disease. Consideration should also be given to non-gynecologic pathology that is exacerbated with menses, such as irritable bowel syndrome, interstitial cystitis, or migraines.

PATHOPHYSIOLOGY

An excess or imbalance of prostaglandins, vasopressin, and chemical substances derived from phospholipids is a commonly proposed cause for dysmenorrhea that is no longer heavily disputed. Evidence for this theory includes measurements of the prostaglandins PGF2 and PGE2 and vasopressin in menstrual fluid that correlate with adverse symptoms of dysmenorrhea. In addition, these chemicals are known to cause symptoms of increased uterine contractility and cramping, nausea, vomiting, and diarrhea in other clinical situations. Finally, there is solid evidence that blocking the synthesis of prostaglandins with cyclooxygenase inhibitors is associated with lower levels of prostaglandins found in menstrual fluid and a clinically significant decrease in symptoms.[8]

The association of primary dysmenorrhea with ovulation makes sense on a physiologic level because of the normal sequence of cyclical endometrial growth. The increase in serum progesterone following ovulation causes an increase in arachidonic acid, which is a precursor to prostaglandins, prostacyclin, and thromboxane A2, all of which promote uterine contractions and act as potent vasoconstrictors.[9] The biologic effects of these substances vary, yet prostaglandins PGF2 and PGE2 have been proved to be higher in concentration in the endometrium and menstrual fluid of women who have primary dysmenorrhea.

The mechanism by which elevations in prostaglandins and other chemical mediators lead to crampy pelvic pain is further postulated to be due to myometrial contraction strength and ischemia. Older studies have demonstrated that the uterine contraction pattern in women who have dysmenorrhea is different.[10] Newer studies have supported the difference in myometrial contractions in primary dysmenorrhea compared with eumenorrheic women. Specifically, a change in the intensity of uterine contractions as measured by MRI and intrauterine pressure recordings has been postulated as one of the mechanisms by which oral contraceptives relieve dysmenorrhea.[11] There are also studies that implicate the role of ischemic uterine myometrium in the pathophysiology of menstrual cramps. Studies using Doppler flow have demonstrated higher arterial resistance in patients who have dysmenorrhea.[12] It has also been shown that vasopressin plays a role in the pathophysiology of dysmenorrhea.[13] Although the specific contributions of these various mechanisms are not yet perfectly understood, the pathophysiology of dysmenorrhea has solidly moved beyond a psychosomatic cause.

RISK FACTORS

Numerous factors have been associated with an increased risk for primary dysmenorrhea, yet the literature contains a limited consensus (**Box 1**).[14,15] Some of this confusion is secondary to a failure to distinguish primary from secondary dysmenorrhea, which clearly has different risk ranges. A study of gynecologic complaints in women who have dysmenorrhea and menorrhagia discovered a relationship between the number of gynecologic complaints and risk for sexual assault.[16] Childbirth and

---

Box 1
Risk factors for dysmenorrhea

Adolescence

Anxiety or stress

Body mass index <20 or >30 kg/m²

Depression, especially if associated with an eating disorder

Disrupted social networks

Family history, especially in a first-degree relative

Menarche at a young age

Menorrhagia

Metrorrhagia

Nulliparity

Smoking

Data From French, L. Dysmenorrhea. Am Fam Physician 2005;71(2):285–91; with permission; and Andresch B, Milsom I. An epidemiologic study of young women with dysmenorrhea. Am J Obstet Gynecol 1982;144:655–60.

exercise have been linked to improved symptoms or lower risk for dysmenorrhea, but current data are inconsistent and conflicting with regard to outcomes. It stands to reason that primary dysmenorrhea might be particularly bothersome and disruptive to a woman who has multiple social, emotional, psychologic, financial, or family stressors. What is experienced as a relative inconvenience to one woman may be experienced as severely painful and disruptive to another, depending on various multiple social and health circumstances.

EVALUATION AND DIFFERENTIAL DIAGNOSIS

Evaluation of dysmenorrhea begins with a careful and detailed history of symptomatology. In young women, the distinct cyclic pain pattern varies from woman to woman in detail but is essentially pathognomonic for the disorder. Typically, the onset of pain is described as crampy, achy, or dull; located in the midline suprapubic region with or without radiation into the back, legs, and abdomen; may begin hours before the actual appearance of menstrual flow; and often persists for 24 to 72 hours. Many young women require education and counseling regarding the normalcy of their cyclic pain associated with the menstrual cycle, particularly when it is experienced as severe, or when the patient has limited female family or social networks, which serve as the usual source of education for young women with regard to their menses.

Painful menses occurring within the first 6 months to 1 year of menarche is often of the most concern, creating fear and anxiety that there must be "something wrong," given the intensity experienced by some young women. Reassurance by trusted family members and clinicians can serve as powerful treatment. As always, reassurance can only be given and received after careful inquiries have been made into the duration, nature, location, severity, and treatments attempted thus far. Without this, the clinician risks failing to recognize the need for further evaluation and treatment. The abdominal and pelvic examinations should, by definition, be normal in primary dysmenorrhea. Abnormalities in pelvic structures, adnexal pain, pelvic fullness, or evidence of cervical stenosis or irregularity should prompt consideration for the diagnosis of secondary dysmenorrhea and evaluation by a gynecologist. If the clinical picture is consistent and there are no other concerning findings, however, laboratory testing or imaging have no significant role in making an accurate diagnosis of primary dysmenorrhea.

Secondary dysmenorrhea is associated with underlying pelvic pathology and necessitates further evaluation to determine its cause. A key differentiating factor in secondary dysmenorrhea is the presence of symptoms of pain and menstrual bleeding that persist beyond the normal menstrual cycle. The differential diagnosis includes endometriosis, salpingitis, and pelvic inflammatory disease, and with advancing age, leiomyomas and adenomyosis. Less commonly, structural abnormalities of the uterus, including a bicornuate uterus or blind uterine horn, may be determined as the cause of dysmenorrhea, yet these are more likely to be diagnosed in younger women in the peri-reproductive period. Extrauterine pathology must also be considered and associated pelvic, bladder, and abdominal structural problems may present with chronic pelvic pain syndromes that suggest dysmenorrhea.

TREATMENT

The array of potential treatments for primary dysmenorrhea is extensive and diverse (**Table 1**). The most commonly used pharmacologic agents are nonsteroidal anti-inflammatory drugs (NSAIDs), and these medications compose the most extensive supportive data in the literature for their use. An estimated 10% to 25% of women either do not respond to NSAIDs or choose not to use them because of side effect profiles,

Table 1	
Treatments for dysmenorrhea	
Intervention	**Strength of Recommendation**
Effective	
NSAIDs	A
Probably effective	
Extended cycle OCs	B
Danazol, leuprolide	B
Hysterectomy	B
Depo-Provera; Mirena IUS	B
Topical heat	B
Possibly effective	
Acupuncture/acupressure	B
Behavioral interventions, exercise	B
Chinese herbs	B
Fish oil supplements	B
Low-fat vegetarian diets	B
Oral contraceptives	B
Thiamine supplementation	B
TENS (transcutaneous electric nerve stimulation)	B
Uncertain effectiveness	
Nifedipine	C
Surgical interventions (LUNA, PSN)	C
Terbutaline	C
Transdermal	C
Ineffective	
Spinal manipulation	B

A, B, and C refer to SORT evidence recommendations used by the *American Family Physician*. *Data from* French, L. Dysmenorrhea. Am Fam Physician 2005;71(2):285–91.

intolerance, or discomfort with medication usage. Millions of women seek alternative, complementary, or natural remedies for the discomfort of menstrual pain and there are numerous effective treatments that can offer relief.

Many of the modalities reviewed here have little to no supporting data to corroborate their efficacy, yet many women use them successfully. Several therapeutic options are difficult to study in controlled trials and may not have inherent financial incentives that promote study interest and sponsorship, yet the absence of rigorous supporting literature should not dissuade the clinician from considering them as viable options. The task of the primary care provider in this setting is to educate patients regarding the current literature and level of demonstrated effectiveness, and to respect women's values and empower individual choices, particularly in light of the harmless nature of most of alternative modalities and their tendency to promote overall health and well-being.

Education and Support

Often neglected, the discussion of normal menstrual cycling, inquiring into symptoms associated with each woman's cycle, and basic education regarding the physiology of menses and the pathophysiology of cramps should be a part of every young female's primary care. The extent and detail of such education varies from woman to woman depending on interest and degree to which symptoms affect quality of life. The woman who identifies lost days of school, work, or significant depressed mood associated with dysmenorrhea bears more detailed consideration and education. Context relative to symptoms bears consideration; that is, the woman who presents with a chief complaint of menstrual pain is approached differently than one seen for routine well woman care.

Prostaglandin Inhibitors

The mainstay of pharmacologic treatment of primary dysmenorrhea spans across the several classes of prostaglandin synthetase inhibitors, including aspirins, fenamates, and nonsteroidal anti-inflammatory medications (NSAIDs) (**Table 2**).[17,18] Considerable data attest to their effectiveness in diminishing the intensity of symptoms associated with high levels of endometrial prostaglandins. Their effectiveness results from cyclooxygenase inhibition and a subsequent decrease in prostaglandin production, leading to diminished concentration of prostaglandins in endometrial fluid and decreased uterine tone. In general, approximately 70% of women experience moderate to complete relief of painful cramping with the use of prostaglandin inhibitors, although individual trials show wide variations in range.[19] A Cochrane review examining the use of NSAIDs in primary dysmenorrhea concluded that compared with placebo, the number needed to treat was 2.1 for moderate relief over a period of 3 to 5 days.[20]

Many women find one NSAID to be more effective than another, and tend to try various products before settling on a single effective medication and dosage. Data

Table 2 Nonsteroidal anti-inflammatory drugs		
Medication	**Dosing**	**Relative Costs**
Ibuprofen (Motrin)	200–800 mg tid to qid; max: 2400–3200 mg	$
Mefenamic acid (Ponstel)	500 mg initially; 250 mg qid; max: 1500 mg	$$$$$
Naproxen (Naprosyn, Aleve)	250–500 mg bid; max: 1375 mg	$$$
Diclofenac (Voltaren, Cataflam)	50 mg bid to tid or 75 mg bid; max: 225 mg	$
Diflunisal (Dolobid)	500–1000 mg initially; 250–500 bid to tid; max: 2500 mg	$$$
Etodolac (Lodine)	200–400 mg bid to tid; max: 1200 mg	$$
Flurbiprofen (Ansaid)	50–100 mg bid to qid; max: 300 mg	$
Ketoprofen (Orudis)	25–75 mg tid-qid; max: 300 mg	$$
Ketorolac (Toradol)	10 mg q 4–6 h; max: 40 mg	$$
Nabumetone (Relafen)	1000 mg qd to bid; max: 2000 mg	$$$
Oxaprozin (Daypro)	1200 mg qd; max: 1800 mg	$$$$
Piroxicam (Feldene)	20 mg qd; max: 20 mg	$
Sulindac (Clinoril)	150–200 mg bid; max: 400 mg	$$
COX-2 inhibitor, celecoxib (Celebrex)	200 mg bid; max: 400 mg	$$$$

Data from American Society of Health System Pharmacists. AHFS Drug Information 2008. McEvoy GK, Snow EK, editors. Accessed August 4, 2008; and Treatment guidelines from the medical letter: drugs for pain 2007;5(56):23–5.

suggests that there is little difference in effectiveness between products, yet an extensive Cochrane review recommends ibuprofen, mefenamic acid, and naproxen as first-line treatment based on effectiveness and tolerability.[20] Evidence for increased effectiveness of the newer and more expensive products is limited, although dosing and side effects may prompt a greater search for alternatives. Dosing ranges for NSAIDs vary considerably and counseling women to use the lowest effective dose improves tolerability and minimizes common side effects of nausea, gastrointestinal distress or dyspepsia, drowsiness, fluid retention, and diarrhea. At higher doses, NSAIDs can decrease renal flow by reducing the concentration of vasodilating renal and endometrial prostaglandins and can lead to subsequent renal failure, particularly in higher-risk patients. Long-term use of NSAIDs in higher doses can precipitate esophageal reflux and ulcer formation and lead to upper gastrointestinal bleeding. Most women tolerate these medications well, especially when they are taken with food, and relief normally occurs within the first cycle when they are taken. Generally NSAIDs are taken as needed, although some authors argue (particularly in cases of severe dysmenorrhea) for continuous interval use for the 2 to 5 days during which symptoms persist, suggesting that a steady state of prostaglandin inhibition is more effective than an episodic one.[21] There has been literature to suggest that beginning the medication before the onset of symptoms may be more effective than waiting for symptoms to occur, but there are poor outcome data to substantiate this notion.[22] Clinician advice is useful in initiating NSAID therapy, yet most women ultimately manage their NSAID use as their symptoms and circumstances dictate.

The cyclooxygenase-2 (COX-2) inhibitor celecoxib can provide the advantage of diminished gastrointestinal side effects and once-daily dosing, but its cost argues against its regular use except when conventional NSAIDs have proved to be ineffective or poorly tolerated.[23] Aspirin can be effective for severe uterine pain and cramping but tends to be required in higher doses than most providers recommend. Acetaminophen, although an effective analgesic, is not helpful for symptoms of dysmenorrhea given its lack of prostaglandin inhibition.

Oral Contraceptives

Oral contraceptives (OCs), by their suppression of ovulation and creation of a predictable cyclic pattern of increase and decrease of serum estrogen and progesterone, lead to diminished endometrial thickening and decreased production of prostaglandin-rich endometrial fluid. Given this mechanism, one could consider them to be excellent agents for the treatment of dysmenorrhea, yet solid data to support this contention are limited. Nonetheless, nonsystematic reviews claim that OCs are up to 90% effective in the treatment of dysmenorrhea.[24] Longstanding observational data seem to be the basis for this contention, and one randomized controlled trial (RCT) of women taking desogestrel-based OCs concluded that this regimen was effective in treatment of dysmenorrhea symptoms relative to placebo.[25] A Cochrane review, however, concluded that there was insufficient evidence from RCTs to support the contention that OCs were effective in treating primary dysmenorrhea.[26] Observational studies have suggested that differences in formulation between monophasic and multiphasic OCs offer no appreciable difference in effectiveness of treatment, but data are limited. No clear usefulness for transdermal or vaginal contraceptives in the treatment of dysmenorrhea has been established.

Continual dosing of OCs with limited numbers of withdrawal cycles per year (typically every 3 months) is an increasingly popular method of controlling multiple hormone-related symptoms, including pelvic pain, premenstrual symptoms, menorrhagia, and the inconvenience of monthly cycles. Although it stands to reason that decreased frequency of menstrual periods would lead to diminished dysmenorrhea, there are no data to support this method as an effective treatment.[27]

Hormonal Alternatives

Other hormonally based contraceptive therapeutic options have potential efficacy in the treatment of primary dysmenorrhea for the woman who desires both contraception and pain relief. The levonorgestrel-releasing intrauterine device (Mirena) has demonstrated efficacy in reducing menstrual flow and suppressing endometrial thickening, and has been shown to decrease pain associated with menstruation by as much as 50%.[28] Nonhormonal intrauterine devices, such as the copper-embedded systems (ParaGard), have the tendency to increase menstrual flow and pain associated with menses.

Depot formulations of medroxyprogesterone acetate (Depo-Provera) tend to markedly diminish menstrual flow and most women using this method of contraception are amenorrheic after 6 months from commencement of therapy. Studies have established the usefulness of depot formulations of medroxyprogesterone in treating secondary dysmenorrhea, but have not evaluated efficacy in patients who have primary dysmenorrhea.[29]

More potent hormonal agents, such as the gonadotropin releasing hormone (GnRH) analogs goserelin acetate, leuprolide acetate, and nafarelin acetate, effectively suppress menstruation and induce medical menopause. These agents are used only in cases of severe and refractory dysmenorrhea, are expensive, and have substantial side effects, including hot flashes, decreased libido, vaginal dryness, mood changes, and headache.[30] They are generally not used in standard treatment of primary dysmenorrhea; thus the indications for their use suggest specialty referral and evaluation.

Nonhormonal Medications

Nonhormonal medications have been studied in small uncontrolled trials as potential agents for the treatment of primary dysmenorrhea. These include the calcium channel blockers nifedipine and verapamil, and the beta-adrenergic receptor agonist terbutaline, all proved to directly relax the smooth muscle of the myometrium. Given the availability of other proved medication options, additional and more rigorous trials with viable outcome data would be needed to prove efficacy and superiority over NSAID and hormonal options for symptomatic relief.[31,32]

Use of opioid agonists, particularly in combination with NSAIDs, may play a role in severe cases of primary dysmenorrhea but most authors and clinicians view their usefulness in this setting to be limited. The requirement of narcotics for pain control should suggest concern for the accuracy of the diagnosis of primary dysmenorrhea and prompt evaluation of a potential secondary cause of menstrual pain and consideration for specialty referral.

Currently under investigation are agents that attempt to inhibit leukotrienes in the prostaglandin cascade, and the role of vasopressin in increased muscle contractility. A single RCT using a vasopressin antagonist given up to 3 days before the onset of pain demonstrated significant pain reduction compared with placebo.[33] Nitric oxide is another known smooth muscle relaxant and has been investigated for symptomatic relief of dysmenorrhea with positive effects, but has been limited in practicality by the common side effect of headache.[34]

Nutrition

The role of arachidonic acid as a precursor to prostaglandin formation has led to numerous recommendations about the potential role for dietary control of primary dysmenorrhea. In general, a low-fat diet rich in fish (particularly salmon, tuna, and halibut), beans, seeds (eg, pumpkin, sesame, and sunflower), whole grains, and fruits and vegetables is most conducive to decreased arachidonic acid in the diet. A single RCT showed a reduction in symptoms in women who followed a low-fat vegetarian diet, but was limited by its small size.[35] A systematic review that encompassed nearly 1100 women examined the relationship between diet and dysmenorrhea and concluded that consumption of fish oil had a positive effect on diminishing pain symptoms.[36] These recommendations are difficult to directly study for improving symptoms, but all clinicians should recognize the sound principles of such dietary recommendations for improving health.

Numerous nutritional supplements have been studied in small nonrandomized trials for the treatment of menstrual pain, including vitamin B1 (thiamine), vitamin B3 (niacin), vitamin B6 (pyridoxine), zinc, calcium, magnesium, and omega-3 fatty acids. A single study found that 100 mg of vitamin B1 taken once daily improved symptoms in 87% of patients. Vitamin B6 taken 100 mg once daily either alone or in combination with magnesium led to decreased pain symptoms in women but this finding was difficult to evaluate systematically because of varying forms and dosages of magnesium.[37]

Herbal Remedies

Similar to nutritional supplements, numerous herbal remedies and preparations have been promoted to treat symptoms of primary dysmenorrhea, yet many health food and supermarket formulations target dysmenorrhea in combination with treatment of premenstrual symptoms. The most widely studied formulations have been the Chinese herbal preparations, recently systematically reviewed by the Cochrane group. They concluded that Chinese herbal preparations showed significant promise as a treatment of pain associated with menses, but that studies were limited by poor methodology and absence of consistency across preparations.[38] A woman interested in Chinese herbal treatments for dysmenorrhea would benefit from referral to a trained practitioner, because the range of herbs and combinations of herbal preparations used in traditional Chinese medicine are extensive.

Behavioral Interventions

Behavioral interventions, including relaxation training, biofeedback, and mind-body awareness, have been posited to be effective in treating painful menses, but data supporting these treatments are limited. A Cochrane review found five trials involving 213 women using different modalities for behavior training, primarily focused on progressive muscle relaxation and biofeedback. They concluded that behavioral interventions may be effective but that all of the trials were small, had poor methodology, and needed to be "viewed with caution."[39] Experienced clinicians may be aware of the clinical usefulness of relaxation and biofeedback training in promoting health and well-being for some individuals; thus it is reasonable to encourage such training for interested patients.

Chiropractic and Osteopathic Treatments

Chiropractic and osteopathic manipulative techniques purport to improve symptoms of primary dysmenorrhea by improving overall spine and pelvic alignment, increasing pelvic blood flow, reducing pelvic congestion, and improving sympathetic pathways to the pelvis altered by poor alignment or surrounding musculoskeletal dysfunction. Techniques of manipulation vary considerably among the modalities, involving spinal manipulation in chiropractic treatment and soft tissue manipulation in osteopathic manipulation. A Cochrane review of five RCTs involving spinal manipulation as a modality for treating dysmenorrhea found no significant difference compared with sham manipulation.[40] It is important to appreciate that of the five trials found to be worthy of review, four trials studied high-velocity low-amplitude osteopathic manipulation and only one trial studied the Toftness method (an older chiropractic technique involving spinal manipulation not generally used in present day). Many practitioners of these modalities would argue strenuously with comparison of the two techniques and believe strongly that soft tissue or spinal manipulation can be highly effective for a subset of women who have significant pelvic and low back misalignment.

Acupuncture and Transcutaneous Electrical Nerve Stimulation

The mechanism of action of acupuncture is complex and involves receptor and nerve fiber stimulation in complex interaction with endorphins, serotonin, and likely other neurochemical substances. A Cochrane systematic review found a single RCT that showed significant pain reduction in women who had primary dysmenorrhea but concluded that further research was needed to confirm this.[41] A more recent RCT from Germany that examined 649 women found significant improvement in quality of life and decreased intensity of pain in the acupuncture-treated group relative to controls.[42]

Transcutaneous electrical nerve stimulation (TENS) uses skin stimulation of nerve fibers at varying frequencies and intensities to relieve pain. The previously cited Cochrane review found limited evidence from small trials for pain reduction with a range of 42% to 60% of patients experiencing moderate relief and evidence from a single trial, which led to reduced use of oral analgesics.[41]

Culture and Traditional Remedies

Many, if not most, women do not perceive dysmenorrhea as a serious medical condition, but rather a normal component of menstruation, and most would not consider it a complaint worthy of a medical visit. In virtually all cultures, there is shared knowledge and information passed among women regarding remedies for painful periods. In some African tribes, it is recommended that a warm cloth be applied to the lower abdomen. In Colombia, a warm iron is suggested. In China a "re shui dai" (hot water bottle) placed around the belly button area is favored. Warm alcohol drinks during painful menses is a remedy espoused by many young women, frequently taught to them by their mothers. The limited studies available on this treatment have suggested that although frequent alcohol consumption is associated with a lower overall risk for menstrual cramps, it is associated with more severe cramps and longer duration of pain in women who have dysmenorrhea.[43]

Informally, women also recommend intercourse in general, and orgasm in particular, as helpful for painful menses. Although there exist many cultural prohibitions against sexual activity during menstruation, and some women have negative associations related to sex and menstrual fluid, other women do not, and intercourse around the time of menses is widely viewed as a time when the risk for pregnancy is virtually nonexistent. There is no medical literature to support or refute the efficacy of orgasm in treatment of dysmenorrhea. The increased uterine contractility and increased vascular flow resulting from orgasm is believed to promote efficient menstrual flow and reduce pelvic congestion, suggesting potential mechanisms for diminished symptoms of dysmenorrhea.[44]

Heat

The direct application of heat to the lower abdominal wall is a time-honored home remedy for menstrual cramps that is practiced virtually worldwide. Although rarely studied, Akin and colleagues found that continuous topical heat application was as effective or superior to moderate-dose ibuprofen at 400 mg dosed three times daily for pain relief.[45] Although heat therapy has been used for millennia, its lack of portability and practicality in the modern age has tended to diminish its relevance and has tended to confine its applicability to home usage with hot water bottles, hot baths, and heating pads. Newer modalities, including heat patches and wearable heating devices, make its application more realistic for active women and it should not be dismissed as a viable treatment option, particularly for those women intolerant of the common gastrointestinal side effects of NSAIDs.

Exercise

Exercise is another treatment option held to be efficacious in diminishing the symptoms of primary dysmenorrhea, and there is a widely held belief that people who exercise regularly suffer less pain overall. A comprehensive review of the literature surrounding exercise and menstrual pain concluded that empiric data are minimal and results of observational studies have been mixed. At best, results from controlled trials have suggested that exercise reduces symptoms of dysmenorrhea, but most studies have been small and methodologically flawed.[46] A similar review of the literature 10 years earlier drew the same conclusions about inadequate substantiation.[47]

Surgical Treatments

The two primary surgical treatments for severe refractory dysmenorrhea are laparoscopic uterine nerve ablation (LUNA) by cautery or CO_2 laser, and presacral neurectomy (PSN). LUNA involves transection of afferent pain fibers within the uterosacral ligaments, whereas PSN directly transects the nerve fibers in the pelvis.[48,49] These procedures are only indicated for the rare patient who suffers from severe refractory dysmenorrhea, and such persistent and severe symptoms should prompt reevaluation of the diagnosis, investigation for secondary causes, and specialist referral. A review of RCTs evaluating both procedures included nine trials, two of open PSN and the remainder of the laparoscopic approach, and concluded that at 12 months' follow-up, LUNA had better outcomes in that there were fewer complications compared with control or no treatment, but that PSN was more effective in relief from pain. The presacral procedure had a higher rate of adverse events, including ureteral injury, hemorrhage from the middle sacral vein, and sympathetic bladder and bowel dysfunction.[50]

PREVENTION

Proper nutrition, exercise, tobacco cessation, minimal alcohol intake, and other generally good health habits all potentially contribute to a diminished experience of dysmenorrhea and minimize its inconvenience and unpleasantness. Self-management of discomfort serves to empower young women, specifically giving them a sense of control over bodily functions, which might otherwise overwhelm them or seem mysterious. The clinician's sympathetic education to this end is time well spent with the patient. The level of prostaglandins in any given woman's system may not be alterable or even easily assayed and interpreted, although this goal is the basis for theories centering on proper nutrition as a viable treatment option. Emphasis on the natural course of primary dysmenorrhea, with education about the natural diminution of symptoms with age, provides further reinforcement that, although perhaps not preventable, the symptoms of dysmenorrhea are manageable and will improve over time.

SUMMARY

Primary dysmenorrhea is commonly a straightforward diagnosis that can be made accurately with an attentive history and, in young women who have classic symptoms and no specific indication, a pelvic examination is often unnecessary in the initial evaluation. The opportunity for primary care practitioners to support women in unearthing the best approach to this chronic recurrent discomfort such that it minimizes adverse life impact is significant and valuable. Identification of patients who are incapacitated by their symptoms, or have symptoms that represent underlying pathology, is a critical component of a careful history. The wide range of treatments available for primary dysmenorrhea virtually ensures that all females troubled by the symptoms can find relief with relatively safe and inexpensive treatments while limiting negative side effects. The opportunity to counsel and support healthy lifestyle choices that contribute positively to general health and provide symptom relief are myriad in this condition and should not be overlooked. Like so many disorders encountered in primary care medicine, dysmenorrhea affords clinicians the opportunity to teach, counsel, and support patients toward not only the relief of symptoms but also optimal health.

REFERENCES

1. Dawood MY. Dysmenorrhea. J Reprod Med 1985;30(3):154–67.
2. Latthe P, Latthe M, Say L, et al. WHO systematic review of prevalence of chronic pelvic pain: neglected reproductive health morbidity. BMC Public Health 2006;6: 177.
3. Davis AR, Westhoff CL. Primary dysmenorrhea in adolescent girls and treatment with oral contraceptives. J Pediatr Adolesc Gynecol 2001;14:3–8.
4. Banikarim C, Chacko MR, Kelder SH. Prevalence and impact of dysmenorrhea on Hispanic female adolescents. Arch Pediatr Adolesc Med 2000;154:1226–9.
5. Sundell G, Milsom I, Andersch B. Factors influencing the prevalence and severity of dysmenorrhea in young women. Br J Obstet Gynaecol 1990;97:588–94.
6. Zhang K, Pollack S, Ghoads A, et al. Onset of ovulation after menarche in girls: a longitudinal study. J Clin Endocrinol Metab 2008;93(4):1186–94.
7. Juang CM, Yen MS, Horng HC, et al. Natural progression of menstrual pain in nulliparous women at reproductive age: an observational study. J Chin Med Assoc 2006;69(10):484–8.
8. Dawood MY, Khan-Dawood FS. Effects of naproxen sodium on menstrual prostaglandins and primary dysmenorrhea. Obstet Gynecol 1983;61(3):285–91.
9. Jabbour HN, Sales KJ, Smith OP, et al. Prostaglandin receptors are mediators of vascular function in endometrial pathologies. [Review] [227 refs] Source. Mol Cell Endocrinol 2006;252(1–2):191–200.
10. Csapo A, Pinto–Dantas CR. The cyclic activity of the non-pregnant human uterus. A new method for recording intrauterine pressure. Fertil Steril 1966;17(1):34–8.
11. Hauksson A, Ekstrom P, Juchnicka E, et al. The influence of a combined oral contraceptive on uterine activity and reactivity to agonists in primary dysmenorrhea. Acta Obstet Gynecol Scand 1989;68(1):31–4.
12. Altunyurt S, Gol M, Altunyurt S, et al. Primary dysmenorrhea and uterine blood flow: a color Doppler study. J Reprod Med 2005;50:251–5.
13. Liedman R, Skillern L, James I, et al. Validation of a test model of induced dysmenorrhea. Acta Obstet Gynecol Scand 2006;85(4):451–7.
14. French L. Dysmenorrhea. Am Fam Physician 2005;71(2):285–91.
15. Andresch B, Milsom I. An epidemiologic study of young women with dysmenorrhea. Am J Obstet Gynecol 1982;144:655–60.

16. Golding JM, Wilsnack SC, Learman LA. Prevalence of sexual assault history among women with common gynecologic symptoms. Am J Obstet Gynecol 1998;179(4):1013–9.
17. American Society of Health-System Pharmacists. AHFS Drug Information 2008. McEvoy GK, Snow EK, editors. Accessed August 4, 2008. Treatment guidelines from the medical letter: drugs for pain. 2007;5(56):23–5.
18. Treatment guidelines from the medical letter: drugs for pain 2007;5(56):23–5.
19. Owen PR. Prostaglandin synthetase inhibitors in the treatment of primary dysmenorrhea: outcome trials reviewed. Am J Obstet Gynecol 1984;148:96–103.
20. Marjoribanks J, Proctor ML, Farquhar C. Nonsteroidal anti-inflammatory drugs for primary dysmenorrhea. Cochrane Database Syst Rev 2003;(4): CD001751.
21. Dawood MY, Khan-Dawood FS. Clinical efficacy and differential inhibition of menstrual fluid prostaglandin F2alpha in a randomized, double-blind, crossover treatment with placebo, acetaminophen, and ibuprofen in primary dysmenorrhea. Am J Obstet Gynecol 2007;196(1):35e1–5.
22. Chan WY, Fuchs F, Powell AM. Effects of naproxen sodium on menstrual prostaglandins and primary dysmenorrhea. Obstet Gynecol 1983;61:285–91.
23. Hayes EC, Rock JA. Cox-2 inhibitors and their role in gynecology. Obstet Gynecol Surv 2002;57:768–80.
24. Smith RP. Dysmenorrhea in gynecology for the primary care physician. In: Stovall TG, Ling FW, Zite NB, et al, editors. 2nd edition. Springer; 2008. p. 335–9.
25. Hendrix SL, Alexander NJ. Primary dysmenorrheal treatment with a desogestrel-containing low dose oral contraceptive. Contraception 2002;66:393–9.
26. Proctor ML, Roberts H, Farquhar CM. Combined oral contraceptives for primary dysmenorrhea. Cochrane Database Syst Rev 2001;4:CD002120.
27. Edelman AB, Gallo MF, Jensen JT, et al. Continuous or extended cycle vs. cyclic use of combined oral contraceptives for contraception. Cochrane Database Syst Rev 2005;CD004695.
28. Baldaszti E, Wimmer-Puchinger B, Loschke K. Acceptability of the long-term contraceptive levonorgestrel-releasing intrauterine system: a 3-year follow-up study. Contraception 2003;67:87–91.
29. Kaunitz AM. Injectable depot-medroxyprogesterone acetate contraception: an update for US clinicians. Int J Fertil Womens Med 1998;43:73–83.
30. Nafarelin for endometriosis. The Medical Letter 1990;32(825):81–2.
31. Andersson DE, Ulmsten U. Effect of nifedipine on myometrial activity and lower abdominal pain in women with primary dysmenorrhea. Br J Obstet Gynaecol 1978;85:142–8.
32. Akerlund M, Andersson KE, Ingemarsson J. Effects of terbutaline on myometrial activity, uterine blood flow, and lower abdominal pain in women with primary dysmenorrhea. Br J Obstet Gynaecol 1976;19:303–12.
33. Brourd R, Bossmar T, Fournie-Lloret D, et al. Effect of SR49059, an orally active vasopressin receptor antagonist in the prevention of dysmenorrhea. Br J Obstet Gynaecol 2000;107:614–9.
34. Transdermal Nitroglycerin/Dysmenorrhea Study Group. Transdermal nitroglycerine in the management of pain associated with primary dysmenorrhea: a multinational pilot study. J Int Med Res 1997;25(1):41–4.
35. Barnard ND, Scialli AR, Hurlock D, et al. Diet and sex-hormone binding globulin, dysmenorrhea, and premenstrual symptoms. Obstet Gynecol 2000;95:245–50.
36. Fjerbaek A, Knudsen UB. Endometriosis, dysmenorrhea, and diet – what is the evidence? Eur J Obstet Gynecol Reprod Biol 2007;132(2):140–7.

37. Proctor ML, Murphy PA. Herbal and dietary therapies for primary and secondary dysmenorrhea. Cochrane Database Syst Rev 2001;(2):CD002124.
38. Zhu X, Proctor M, Bensoussan A, et al. Chinese herbal medicine for primary dysmenorrhea. Cochrane Database Syst Rev 2008;2:CD005288.
39. Proctor ML, Murphy PA, Pattison HM, et al. Behavioral interventions for primary and secondary dysmenorrhea. Cochrane Database Syst Rev 2007;(3):CD002248.
40. Proctor ML, Hing W, Johnson TC, et al. Spinal manipulation for primary and secondary dysmenorrhea. Cochrane Database Syst Rev 2006;(3):CD002119.
41. Proctor ML, Smith CA, Farquhar CM, et al. Transcutaneous electrical nerve stimulation and acupuncture for primary dysmenorrhea. Cochrane Database Syst Rev 2002;(1):CD002123.
42. Witt CM, Reinhold T, Brinkhaus B, et al. Acupuncture in patients with dysmenorrhea: a randomized study on clinical effectiveness and cost effectiveness in usual care. Am J Obstet Gynecol 2008;198(2):166–8.
43. Harlow SD, Park M. A longitudinal study of risk factors for the occurrence, duration and severity of menstrual cramps in a cohort of college women. Br J Obstet Gynaecol 1996;103(11):1134–42.
44. Hatcher RA. Counseling couples about coitus during menstrual flow. Contracept Technol Update 1981;2(12):167.
45. Akin MD, Weingand KW, Hengehold DA, et al. Use of continuous low level topical heat in the treatment of dysmenorrhea. Obstet Gynecol 2001;97:343–9.
46. Daley AJ. Exercise and primary dysmenorrhea: a comprehensive and critical review of the literature. Sports Med 2008;38(8):859–70.
47. Golomb LM, Solidum AA, Warren MP. Primary dysmenorrhea and physical activity. Med Sci Sports Exerc 1998;30(6):906–9.
48. Gurgan T, Urman B, Aksu T, et al. Laparoscopic CO_2 laser nerve ablation for treatment of drug resistant primary dysmenorrhea. Fertil Steril 1992;58:422–4.
49. Chen FP, Chang SD, Chu KK, et al. Comparison of laparoscopic presacral neurectomy and laparoscopic uterine nerve ablation for primary dysmenorrhea. J Reprod Med 1996;41:463–6.
50. Laththe PM, Proctor ML, Farquhar CM, et al. Surgical interruption of pelvic nerve pathways in dysmenorrhea: a systematic review of effectiveness. Acta Obstet Gynecol Scand 2007;86(1):4–15.

Common Gynecologic Infections

Wendy S. Biggs, MD[a,b,]*, Rachel M. Williams, MD[c]

KEYWORDS

- Vaginitis • Candidiasis • Bacterial vaginosis
- Trichomonas • Sexually transmitted infection
- Chlamydia • Gonorrhea • Herpes simplex virus

Key Points	Evidence Level
Screening for chlamydia should be performed in all sexually active nonpregnant women 24 years old or younger, or older than age 24 if at high risk for acquiring chlamydia. (USPSTF guideline A recommendation).	A
Asymptomatic pregnant women should not have serologic screening for herpes simplex virus. (USPSTF D recommendation).	B
Routine screening for bacterial vaginosis in asymptomatic pregnant women not at high risk for preterm delivery shows no benefit and is not recommended.	A
Treatment of bacterial vaginosis before 20 weeks' gestation may decrease preterm delivery. (Cochrane Database).	A
Pregnant women who have active herpetic lesions or prodromal symptoms of recurrent herpes at time of delivery should have a caesarean section. (ACOG guideline).	B
Oral acyclovir can be given at 36 weeks' pregnancy in women who have primary HSV outbreaks or are at risk for recurrent herpes. (ACOG guideline).	B
Asymptomatic trichomonas in pregnant women should not be treated.	A
Fluoroquinolones should not be used to treat gonorrhea because of increased resistance. (CDC guideline).	B

[a] Department of Family Medicine, Michigan State University College of Human Medicine, East Lansing, MI, USA
[b] Midland Family Medicine Residency, Midland, MI, USA
[c] Covenant Health Care, Saginaw, MI, USA
* Corresponding author. Office of Medical Education, 4005 Orchard Drive, Midland, MI 48640.
E-mail address: wendy.biggs@midmichigan.org (W.S. Biggs).

Prim Care Clin Office Pract 36 (2009) 33–51
doi:10.1016/j.pop.2008.10.002
0095-4543/08/$ – see front matter © 2009 Elsevier Inc. All rights reserved.

More than one half of the patients seen in primary care practices are women. Although women may seek care from a gynecologist for vulvar or vaginal complaints, family physicians are frequently their first source of health care. Gynecologic infections can occur externally on the vulva, or internally in the vagina, cervix, uterus, and fallopian tubes. Presenting symptomatology can provide clues to aid in making an accurate diagnosis of such infections, yet physical examination and laboratory tests may be necessary to make a definitive diagnosis. Many infections in the female reproductive tract are sexually transmitted, whereas other common infections are due to an overgrowth of the normally colonizing bacteria or yeast in the vagina. Gynecologic infections may adversely affect quality of life by causing discomfort and pain and by negatively affecting normal sexual functioning and reproductive capacity. Primary care clinicians should possess a solid understanding of the differential diagnosis and treatment of common gynecologic infections.

VULVAR INFECTIONS

Women may present with vulvar irritation or ulceration, which may or may not be attributable to infection. Noninfectious vulvar irritation may be due to contact dermatitis from sanitary pads, maceration caused by wetness from urinary incontinence, or allergy from latex condoms. Vulvar ulcers that result from infections may be either painless or painful. A single painless ulcer is a hallmark of the syphilis chancre, whereas painful ulcers may be attributable to the herpes simplex virus or lymphogranuloma venereum (LGV). More than one of these diseases can be present simultaneously in the same patient because they are sexually transmitted. In the United States, herpes simplex virus type 2 (HSV-2) is the most frequent cause of genital ulcers.

Herpes Simplex Virus

HSV-2 infects or has infected an estimated one out of four women in the United States. More than 1.5 million new infections of HSV-2 occur annually with the peak incidence in the 20- to 29-year-old age group.[1] Many cases of HSV-2 may be asymptomatic. Among adults who report never having had genital herpes, the seroprevalence of HSV-2 antibodies is 21.6%.[2] According to the National Health and Nutrition Examination Surveys (NHANES), the overall prevalence of HSV-2 antibodies increased from 16% during 1976 to 1980 (NHANES II) to 21% during 1988 to 1994 (NHANES III),[2] but then decreased to 17% between 1999 and 2004 (NHANES IV).[3] African Americans are more likely to be infected with HSV-2 than other ethnic or racial groups. In the NHANES III study, the seroprevalence of HSV-2 was 55.7% in African American women versus 18.7% in Caucasian women.[2] Across all ethnic and racial groups, the risk for acquiring HSV-2 increases with greater lifetime number of sexual partners.[2]

HSV-1, which commonly causes perioral ulcers, can be transferred to the genital region with oral-genital contact. Many people become infected with HSV-1 as children and carry immunity; thus, acquired HSV-1 genital infections are less inflammatory and tend to recur less frequently than HSV-2. A nonimmune adult who acquires HSV-1 by way of genital transmission may have severe symptoms similar to HSV-2. The prevalence of HSV-1 genital herpes was found to be much lower than the HSV-2 form with a seroprevalence of 1.8% versus 17% in the NHANES IV trial (1999–2004).[3]

Primary HSV infection may be symptomatic, atypical, or asymptomatic. The classic genital herpes infection presents as painful vesiculopustular lesions or genital ulcers and may be associated with constitutional symptoms, including fever, headache, or malaise. More than one half of women may have an atypical presentation with genital itching, irritation, or localized erythema, vulvar fissures, or dysuria.[4] Nearly 90% of patients infected with HSV-2 have at least one subsequent recurrence with varying symptoms. Recurrences tend to be less severe than the initial infection. Many patients have prodromal symptoms before the appearance of genital ulcers, such as burning or irritation. Antiviral medications, including acyclovir, valacyclovir, and famciclovir are used in various regimens to treat primary or recurrent HSV infections and are reasonably effective (**Table 1**). For episodic treatment of recurrences, medications should be started at the first sign of prodromal symptoms or ulcers, ideally within the first 24 hours. Viral shedding can occur during an asymptomatic state, promoting its sexual transmission. HSV-2 shedding has been shown to occur 1% to 8% of days overall, with one half to two thirds within 1 week before or after a clinically recognized episode.[4] Genital HSV-1 sheds virus asymptomatically less frequently compared with HSV-2.[4] For a patient who has frequent recurrences or the desire to reduce the risk for transmission to a sexual partner, antivirals are used for suppressive therapy. For example, valacyclovir 500 mg daily significantly reduced the acquisition of symptomatic HSV-2 infection in sexual partners compared with placebo (hazard ratio 0.25 (0.08–0.75), $P<.008$).[5] Famciclovir at 125 mg or 250 mg three times daily decreased the percentage of days of asymptomatic HSV viral shedding sixfold or more compared with placebo (125 mg TID, odds ratio [OR] 6.1 [95% CI 3.5–10.8, $P<.0001$]; 250 mg TID, OR 7.7 [95% CI 4.0–14.5, $P<.0001$]).[6]

Herpes simplex virus infections in pregnancy

HSV can be transmitted to a newborn at delivery. The risk for transmission is greater with a primary outbreak (30% to 50%) than with recurrent episodes of herpes (less than 1%);[7] however, because most herpetic outbreaks in pregnant women are recurrences, most cases of neonatal herpes infections are due to recurrent herpes. All pregnant women should be asked if they have a history of genital herpes. If a noninfected pregnant woman's partner has known genital herpes, she should avoid sexual

Table 1		
Medications for herpes simplex virus infections		
Clinical Presentation	**Medication**	**Dosage**
Primary infection	Acyclovir (Zovirax)	400 mg orally three times daily for 7–10 d or 200 mg orally five times daily for 7–10 d
	Famciclovir (Famvir)	250 mg orally three times daily for 7–10 d
	Valacyclovir (Valtrex)	1 g orally twice daily for 7–10 d
Recurrent episodes	Acyclovir	400 mg orally three times daily for 5 d or 800 mg orally twice daily for 5 d or 800 mg orally three times daily for 2 d
	Famciclovir	125 mg orally twice daily for five d or 1 g orally twice daily for 1 d
	Valacyclovir	500 mg orally twice daily for 3 d or 1 g orally once daily for 5 d
Suppressive therapy	Acyclovir	400 mg orally twice daily
	Famciclovir	250 mg twice daily
	Valacyclovir	500 mg or 1 g orally once daily

Data from Centers for Disease Control and Prevention. Sexually transmitted diseases treatment guidelines, 2006. MMWR Recomm Rep 2006;55(RR-11):1–94 [Published correction appears in MMWR Recomm Rep 2006;55(36):997].

intercourse during the third trimester, and if her partner has orolabial herpes, oral sexual contact should be avoided.[7] Oral acyclovir may be given to women with the first episode of genital herpes or severe recurrent herpes and may be considered in women at 36 weeks of gestation who have a primary infection of HSV or are at risk for recurrent HSV.[7] At the time of delivery, women who have known HSV should be asked about prodromal symptoms and examined carefully for herpetic lesions. The American College of Obstetricians and Gynecologists (ACOG) recommends caesarean section for women who have active herpes lesions or prodromal symptoms at time of delivery,[7] yet caesarean section may not completely eliminate the transmission of neonatal HSV. The United States Preventive Services Task Force (USPSTF) recommends against serologic screening for HSV in asymptomatic pregnant women (D recommendation), because primary HSV infection may take up to 4 weeks to detect antibodies.[8]

Herpes simplex virus and HIV

HSV infections in immunocompromised patients who have HIV infection tend to be a reactivation of dormant virus. Immunocompromised patients may have extensive mucocutaneous involvement or prolonged outbreaks. Recurrences are often more frequent, more extensive, and of longer duration than in immunocompetent patients. HIV-positive patients should be offered HSV type–specific serologic testing and offered continuous suppressive therapy if found to be seropositive for HSV-2, with the goal of diminishing the frequency and severity of outbreaks.[9] HIV-infected individuals may have prolonged virus shedding and be more contagious than immunocompetent patients who have HSV. The extent to which pharmacologic suppression suppresses viral shedding remains unknown.[9]

Syphilis

The incidence of syphilis is increasing; the Centers for Disease Control and Prevention (CDC) report an increase in the United States every year since 2000, from 2.1 per 100,000 people to 3.7 per 100,000 people, with 36,000 cases in 2006.[9] The largest increases have occurred among men; however, in 2007, the syphilis rate among females increased from 1 per 100,000 people to 1.1 per 100,000 people. This 10% increase marked the third consecutive annual increase. During the previous decade, syphilis rates had declined among women, thus a concerning resurgence of syphilis among women may be occurring.[9] The incidence of syphilis peaks in women between 20 and 24 years of age. The United States distribution of syphilis is geographically localized, with one half of all primary and secondary syphilis reported from major metropolitan areas, such as Los Angeles, Houston, Dallas–Fort Worth, Chicago, San Francisco, and their surrounding counties.[10]

The famous physician William Osler stated "the physician who knows syphilis knows medicine," alluding to the many stages and presentations of the disease. The spirochete Treponema pallidum causes syphilis; the primary infection presents as a painless genital ulcer, known as a chancre, at the infection site. Secondary syphilis occurs 4 to 10 weeks after the primary infection and may present as myalgias, fever, malaise, lymphadenopathy, mucocutaneous lesions, or skin rash, including the soles and palms. If untreated, syphilis then enters a latent phase that may last for years. Tertiary syphilis manifestations may involve any organ with complications of periarteritis, endarteritis, and chronic inflammation. This late reaction produces many different lesions, importantly aortic, cardiac, and ophthalmic lesions, or granulomas (gummas). The central nervous system involvement of neurosyphilis can occur at any stage.[9]

Nontreponemal serologic tests, including the Venereal Disease Research Laboratory (VDRL) and rapid plasma reagin (RPR) assays, do not conclusively diagnosis syphilis. False-positive VRDL or RPR assays are common with other medical conditions, including the autoimmune diseases. The antibody titers correlate with disease activity, and a fourfold change in titer indicates a clinically significant change. After appropriate treatment, the antibody titers usually diminish and the nontreponemal test becomes nonreactive; however, in some patients the titer persists at low levels for lifetime. Treponemal tests, such as the fluorescent treponemal antibody absorbed (FTA-ABS) and *T pallidum* particle agglutination (TP-PA), are often used to confirm a positive nontreponemal serologic test. The treponemal tests remain reactive during a patient's lifetime regardless of treatment; thus, a positive FTA-ABS cannot be used to diagnose a current infection. Only darkfield examination for spirochetes and direct fluorescent antibody tests of tissue or exudate are definitively diagnostic for syphilis.[9]

Penicillin is the mainstay of treatment of syphilis. Benzathine penicillin G 2.4 million units intramuscularly for one dose is the recommended treatment of primary or secondary syphilis; however, the dosage and length of treatment depend on the stage of syphilis and organ involvement. CDC guidelines state that in nonpregnant penicillin-allergic patients, ceftriaxone 1 g intramuscularly or intravenously daily for 8 to 10 days may be considered; however, if the patient has an anaphylactic reaction to penicillin, tetracycline 500 mg four times a day or doxycycline 100 mg twice a day for 14 days is recommended.[9]

Syphilis and pregnancy

All women should be screened early in the prenatal period for syphilis to identify and treat infected women and avoid congenital syphilis. Most often, a nontreponemal test is performed and if positive, confirmed with a treponemal test. High-risk women should be screened each trimester and at delivery. Testing for syphilis should be performed in any intrauterine fetal death before 20 weeks. Parenteral penicillin G is the only documented effective treatment of syphilis during pregnancy. Women who report an allergy to penicillin should undergo allergy skin testing. If a penicillin allergy is proved, patients should be referred for penicillin desensitization.[9]

Syphilis and HIV

Syphilis is diagnosed in HIV-positive patients using nontreponemal and treponemal testing in the same manner as for HIV-negative patients. HIV-positive patients may be at an increased risk for neurosyphilis and treatment failure. Close follow-up with a clinician experienced in HIV and syphilis is recommended.[9]

Chancroid

Chancroid, caused by the bacteria *Haemophilus ducreyi*, is rare in the United States, with fewer than 150 cases reported in 1999.[11] When it occurs, it often is in discrete outbreaks. A painful genital ulcer and tender suppurative inguinal lymphadenopathy suggest chancroid. A definitive diagnosis is made by culture on a special media, which is not readily available. Chancroid can thus be diagnosed clinically by excluding HSV and syphilis.[9]

Treatment of chancroid consists of a single dose of azithromycin 1 g orally or ceftriaxone 250 mg intramuscularly. Ciprofloxacin 500 mg twice a day for 3 days or erythromycin 500 mg three times a day for 1 week can also be used for cases of allergy or intolerance; however, the compliance may be reduced. Patients should be re-examined in 3 to 7 days for clinical improvement. Large ulcers may take up to 2 weeks to heal and large fluctuant lymph nodes may require incision and drainage.[9] All sexual partners with whom patients who have chancroid had contact during the 10 days before the onset of symptoms should be treated, even if asymptomatic. Chancroid is a cofactor for HIV transmission. HIV-positive patients who have chancroid heal more slowly and may require longer courses of antibiotics.[9]

Lymphogranuloma Venereum

LGV is caused by *Chlamydia trachomatis* serovars L1, L2, or L3. LGV is endemic in East and West Africa, India, Southeast Asia, South America, and the Caribbean, with sporadic cases occurring in North America, Australia, and most of Asia.[12] Women who practice receptive anal intercourse are at risk.[9] The initial presentation of LGV is a painless ulcer at the site of inoculation. In women, the ulcer may appear on the vulva, but commonly it is unnoticed, occurring internally on the posterior wall of the vaginal or cervix. Ten to 30 days after exposure, enlarged tender lymph nodes (buboes) appear. In women, the lymph node involvement reflects the location of the inoculation site: inguinal if the primary ulcer was vulvar, versus pelvic or perirectal if the primary lesion was cervical, vaginal, or anal. Rectal exposure also causes proctocolitis, with symptoms of mucoid or bloody rectal discharge, anal pain, tenesmus, and fever.[12]

Diagnosis of LGV is primarily made on a clinical basis. In the presence of large inguinal lymph nodes or symptoms of proctocolitis, history should focus on factors that increase a woman's risk for LGV, including travel to an endemic area, a high number of sexual partners, prostitution, or receptive anal intercourse. Laboratory tests are less helpful because culture and genetic probe (DNA) testing for chlamydia are not specific for LGV.[13] Doxycycline 100 mg orally twice daily for 3 weeks is the treatment of choice, with erythromycin 500 mg orally four times daily for 3 weeks the alternative.[9] Pregnant women should be treated with erythromycin, because doxycycline is contraindicated. HIV-infected individuals should be treated with doxycycline or erythromycin for at least 3 weeks and longer regimens may be required because symptom resolution is slower in these patients.[9]

VAGINAL INFECTIONS

Vaginitis is one of the most common medical problems for which women present to family physicians. An estimated 75% of women have at least one episode of vulvovaginal candidiasis within their lifetime, with 40% to 45% having two or more episodes.[13] The most common causes of vaginitis are bacterial vaginosis (22% to 50%), vulvovaginal candidiasis (17% to 39%), and *Trichomonas vaginalis* (4% to 35%).[14] Patients who have vaginitis often present with vaginal or perineal itching, burning, vulvar or vaginal irritation, and abnormal vaginal discharge. Many women who have bacterial vaginosis and trichomonas may be asymptomatic. Co-infections may exist and the exact cause of vaginal symptoms in a significant proportion of women may remain undiagnosed.

Vulvovaginal Candidiasis

The classic symptom constellation associated with vulvovaginal candidiasis caused by *Candida albicans* is thick, white, "curdy" or "cheesy" discharge, vaginal irritation, or erythema and itching, yet the thick white discharge may only be present in 20% to 60% of cases of candidal vulvovaginitis.[15,16] Although the presence of the thick white discharge is only moderately sensitive and specific, when present, it strongly predicts candidiasis (**Table 2**). Although vulvar or vaginal inflammation is associated with candidiasis, it also frequently can occur in trichomonas, and 50% to 87% of patients who have vaginal candidiasis complain of itching.[14] When itching occurs with a curdy

Table 2
Predictive value of symptoms for vulvovaginal candidiasis

Symptom	Sensitivity (%)	Specificity (%)	Positive Likelihood Ratio (95% CI)	Negative Likelihood Ratio (95% CI)	Reference
Thick, cheesy or curdy discharge	65	73	2.4 (1.4–4.2)	0.48 (0.27–0.86)	Abbott[38]
	—	—	18.2 (9.2–36)	—	Eckert et al[15]
Itching	50	64	1.4 (1.2–1.7)	0.18 (0.05–0.70)	Chandeying
	87	50	1.7 (1.3–2.4)	0.26 (0.09–0.78)	et al[16] Abbott[38]
Curdy discharge with itching	77	100	150 (20–1000)	0.23 (0.14–0.37)	Eckert et al[15]

discharge, the sensitivity for candidiasis is 77% with 100% specificity.[15] Lack of itching decreases the likelihood of candidiasis, whereas lack of odor makes candidiasis more likely.[15] Symptoms alone should not be used to diagnoses vaginal candidiasis definitively, yet this is common practice.

Vulvovaginal candidiasis may be uncomplicated (mild, infrequent infection, nonpregnant patient) or complicated (recurrent, severe symptoms, pregnant or diabetic or immunosuppressed patient). Approximately 10% to 20% of women have complicated vulvovaginal candidiasis. Topical azoles are the mainstay of treatment of this condition,[17] with treatment regimens ranging from 1 day to 1 week with similar efficacy (**Table 3**). Some 80% to 90% of patients who complete therapy achieve relief of symptoms and have negative cultures.[18] Oral fluconazole is more acceptable and convenient for many women, but may cause headache or gastrointestinal side effects and is more expensive. In complicated cases, a second dose of oral fluconazole 150 mg given at day three yields an 80% cure rate versus 67% with a single dose.[19] In women who have recurrent infections (more than four per year), a longer course of oral fluconazole (7 to 14 days) may be needed to suppress the *Candida*. Suppression therapy with fluconazole 150 mg weekly for 6 months controls symptomatic episodes in 90% of women, and one half have prolonged symptom relief.[20] A treatment failure may indicate infection with *Candida glabrata*, which does not respond well to azoles. Boric acid 600 mg capsules given intravaginally for 14 days may be effective.[21]

Bacterial Vaginosis

Bacterial vaginosis (BV) is a polymicrobial vaginal infection that occurs when the hydrogen peroxide–producing lactobacillus normally present in the vagina diminish, allowing other bacteria to proliferate, including anaerobes, *Gardnerella vaginalis*, and *Mycoplasma hominis*. Routine cultures are not helpful in diagnosing bacterial vaginosis because up to 50% of women who harbor *G vaginalis* vaginally are asymptomatic. When symptomatic, a woman may complain of a fishy odor, yellow or grayish discharge, and vaginal irritation. A yellow discharge increases the likelihood of BV fourfold,[22] but also can indicate a trichomonas infection. A white discharge makes BV less likely (**Table 4**).[22] A clinical diagnosis of BV requires three out of four Amsel criteria (**Box 1**), which are 92% sensitive but only 77% specific.[23] Treatment reduces symptoms, yet recurrences are common, with 23% at one month and 58% in 12 months.[24]

Table 3
Treatment of vaginal candidiasis

Drug	Common Name	Dose and Route of Administration	Duration of Treatment	Available Over-the-Counter
Butoconazole 2% cream	Femstat, Mycelex-3	5 g intravaginally	3 d	Yes
Butoconazole 2% cream	Gynazole-1	5 g sustained release intravaginally	1 d	No
Clotrimazole 1%	Gyne-Lotrimin 7	5 g intravaginally	7–14 d	Yes
Clotrimazole 2%	Gyne-Lotrimin 3	5 g intravaginally	3 d	Yes
Clotrimazole vaginal tablet	Mycelex	100 mg intravaginally	7 d	No
Clotrimazole vaginal tablet	Mycelex	200 mg intravaginally	3 d	No
Clotrimazole vaginal tablet	Mycelex	500 mg intravaginally	1 d	No
Miconazole 2% cream	Monistat-7	5 g intravaginally	7 d	Yes
Miconazole suppository	Monistat-7 suppositories	100 mg intravaginally	7 d	Yes
Miconazole suppository	Monistat-3	200 mg intravaginally	3 d	Yes
Miconazole suppository	Monistat-1 combination pack	1200 mg intravaginally, with miconazole 2% cream externally	1 d	Yes
Nystatin vaginal tablet	Mycostatin	100,000 U intravaginally	1 d	No
Tioconazole 6.5% ointment	Vagistat-1, Monistat 1-day treatment	5 g intravaginally	1 d	Yes
Terconazole 0.4% cream	Terazol	5 g intravaginally	7 d	No
Terconazole 0.8% cream	Terazol-3	5 g intravaginally	3 d	No
Terconazole suppository	Terazol suppository	80 g intravaginally	3 d	No
Fluconazole 150 mg	Diflucan	One orally	1 day	No

Data from Refs.[9,17,18]

Bacterial vaginosis and pregnancy
The effect of bacterial vaginosis in pregnancy is not completely understood. BV has been associated with adverse pregnancy outcomes, including preterm labor and premature rupture of membranes, and infectious complications, such as chorioamnionitis and postpartum endometritis. Treatment of bacterial vaginosis before 20 weeks of gestation may reduce the risk for preterm delivery.[25] In women who have a history of previous preterm delivery, treatment with metronidazole has not been shown to affect the risk for subsequent preterm delivery, yet it may decrease the risk for preterm

Table 4
Predictive value of symptoms for bacterial vaginosis

Symptom	Sensitivity (%)	Specificity (%)	+LR (95% CI)	−LR (95% CI)	Reference
Yellow discharge	60	85	4.1 (2.4–7.1)	0.46 (0.35–0.62)	O'Dowd and West[22]
White discharge	37	31	0.55 (0.40–0.75)	2.0 (1.4–2.8)	O'Dowd and West[22]
Amsel criteria	92	77			Landers et al[23]

Abbreviation: LR, likelihood ratio.

premature rupture of membranes and low birth weight.[25] No clear treatment benefit has been demonstrated in asymptomatic women who are not at high risk for preterm delivery; thus routine screening and treatment in asymptomatic pregnant women is not recommended.[26] Symptomatic pregnant women who have BV should be treated with oral metronidazole. Treatment with clindamycin has not been shown to reduce the risk for preterm delivery.[25] Clindamycin gel given intravaginally at 16 to 20 weeks demonstrates an increased risk for low birth weight and neonatal infections; it should only be used in the first half of pregnancy.[9]

Bacterial vaginosis and other sexually transmitted infections

Bacterial vaginosis is commonly found in women who have other sexually transmitted diseases, including pelvic inflammatory disease (PID) and trichomonas.[23] Whether BV acts as a cofactor or a coinfection is unclear. In one study, after adjustment for confounding demographic and lifestyle factors, no overall increased risk for developing PID was seen in women who had BV.[27] Prophylactic treatment with metronidazole intravaginal gel in women who had asymptomatic BV has been shown to decrease the acquisition of *Chlamydia*.[28] Consistent condom use also seems to decrease the risk for bacterial vaginosis infection.[29]

Trichomonas Vaginalis

Trichomonas vaginalis is a single-celled flagellated protozoan organism that is sexually transmitted. In the NHANES IV survey (2001–2004), the overall prevalence in women aged 14 to 49 years old was 3.1%. Prevalence varied across different ethnic groups: white non-Hispanic 1.1%, Mexican American 1.8%, and African American 13.3%. These differences in prevalence remained after controlling for sociodemographic,

Box 1
Amsel criteria

Three out of four are necessary to diagnose bacterial vaginosis

Abnormal grayish homogenous discharge

Vaginal pH greater than 4.5

Positive amine test or "whiff test" ("fishy" odor with KOH applied to discharge)

More than 20% positive clue cells (epithelial cells surrounded by adherent coccobacilli) on microscopy

Data from Amsel R, Totten PA, Spiegel CA, et al. Non-specific vaginitis: diagnostic criteria and microbiological and epidemiologic associations. Am J Med 1983;74:14–22.

sexual, and behavioral variables.[30] Increased numbers of sexual partners, a recent new sexual partner, or early initiation of sexual activity (younger than age 16) was associated with an increased prevalence. Up to 86% of trichomonas infections may be asymptomatic and the duration of infection or carrier status is uncertain.[27] Because carriers may be asymptomatic and the duration of infection can be unknown, a current diagnosis may not predict the sexual partner who transmitted the infection. In addition, trichomonads can live for a limited length of time on moist surfaces and may be transmitted by fomites, such as towels or sexual toys.

Occasionally, asymptomatic women are diagnosed with trichomonas by routine Pap smear, which is reported to be 57% sensitive and 97% specific.[31] If symptomatic, trichomonas presents as vaginal itching, burning, vaginal discharge (frequently profuse, yellowish-green, and malodorous), or postcoital bleeding. Trichomonads often appear in motion on a vaginal secretion saline wet mount, "swimming" with the flagella in a jerking or tumbling action. The sensitivity of detecting trichomonads on saline wet mount is estimated at 62% with a specificity of 97% and a positive predictive value of 75%.[23] Culture is very sensitive (95%) and specific (greater than 95%),[23,32] but delays diagnosis and is not routinely performed. A trichomonas rapid antigen test increases sensitivity to 88% with 99% specificity, making it a valuable point-of-care diagnostic tool, but it lacks cost effectiveness compared with diagnosis by way of the standard wet prep test.[33]

Unlike bacterial vaginosis, asymptomatic trichomonas in nonpregnant women should be treated because of the risk for sexual transmission. The current recommended treatment is metronidazole 2 g as a single dose. Tinidazole also is also approved by the US Food and Drug Administration as a single-dose regimen of 2 g. Partners of infected women should be treated because men can carry *Trichomonas* asymptomatically and may reinfect the female partner unless treated. Because of a disulfiram-like reaction, including flushing, nausea, vomiting, thirst, palpitations, chest pain, vertigo, and hypotension, abstinence from alcohol is recommended for 24 hours after commencement of treatment with metronidazole and 72 hours after therapy with tinidazole.[9]

Trichomonas recurrences are frequently reinfections or secondary to a nonadherence to medical treatment. Some 2% to 5% of isolated trichomonads have low-level resistance to metronidazole; high-level resistance is rare.[9] Concurrent treatment of sexual partners is important to reduce reinfection. If reinfection or recurrence occurs, the recommended treatment is tinidazole 2 g once or metronidazole 500 mg twice daily for 7 days. For suspected metronidazole resistance, the CDC recommends in vitro culture and drug susceptibility testing, which can be obtained through the CDC (phone 770-448-4115), and treatment with larger doses of tinidazole, if needed.[9]

Trichomonas in pregnancy

Trichomonas infections have been associated with preterm delivery. Symptomatic infections during pregnancy can be treated with metronidazole. Because metronidazole crosses the placenta, some clinicians have recommended avoiding metronidazole in the first trimester to avoid possible teratogenicity. A meta-analysis found no relationship between metronidazole use in the first trimester and birth defects,[34] and the CDC no longer recommends avoiding metronidazole treatment of symptomatic trichomonas infections in early pregnancy.[9]

Asymptomatic pregnant women who have incidentally noted trichomonads, however, should not be treated.[9] In a randomized trial of metronidazole treatment of asymptomatic trichomonas, the treated group was three times more likely to go into preterm labor.[35] Women in a high-risk group for preterm labor who had positive fetal fibronectin testing empirically treated with metronidazole were 60% more likely to have a preterm delivery (risk ratio 1.6, 95% CI 1.05–2.4).[36] The severity of a woman's symptoms needs to be balanced against the risk that metronidazole therapy may increase preterm delivery.

Trichomonas and HIV

Trichomonas infection confers an increased risk for acquiring HIV. An analysis that adjusted for variables, including other sexually transmitted infections, hormonal contraception, behavioral factors, and demographics, determined that women who had trichomonas had more than double the risk for acquiring HIV (adjusted odds ratio 2.74 [95% CI 1.25–6.00]).[37] Treatment regimens for trichomonas in HIV-positive women are the same as for HIV-negative women. In women who have high-risk sexual behavior, reinfection rates may be higher. Drug resistance to metronidazole is more likely in patients who have had repeated treatments with metronidazole. HIV-positive women may require repeat screening after treatment, a longer course of treatment with metronidazole, or treatment with tinidazole.[9]

EVALUATION OF VAGINITIS

Because vaginal signs and symptoms are a frequent chief complaint in primary care, an efficient and cost-effective diagnostic strategy is desirable. Unfortunately, patient-reported symptoms and detected signs are not always helpful in determining the definitive cause of the vaginal complaints.[23,32] In addition, because Candida and G vaginalis exist normally in the vaginal flora, their presence on culture does not always determine infection. Many current clinical tests have limitations. For example, candidal hyphae may be found by KOH wet-mount in only approximately 35% to 50% of symptomatic women who have cultures positive for Candida.[15,16,38] The presence of trichomonads on saline wet-mount diagnoses trichomoniasis, but their absence does not eliminate the diagnosis.[14] Cervicitis caused by Neisseria gonorrhea or Chlamydia may present with vaginal symptoms. A sequence or battery of testing may thus be necessary to make a diagnosis (**Fig. 1**).

A review of the literature concluded that an initial office evaluation with a history and speculum examination, vaginal pH, wet-mount microscopy, and whiff test can correctly diagnose 60% of candida vaginitis, 70% of trichomonas vaginitis, and 90% of bacterial vaginosis.[32] Despite appropriate testing, up to 40% to 50% of women will not have a definitive diagnosis for their vaginal symptoms from this initial work-up.[39] The most cost-effective strategy for women not diagnosed at the initial office visit (by vaginal examination, vaginal pH, wet-mount microscopy, and whiff test) was vaginal pH testing, yeast culture, gonorrhea and chlamydia DNA genetic probes, and Gram stain and trichomonas culture only when the vaginal pH exceeded 4.9. The model also considered two empiric treatment strategies: (1) treatment guided by vaginal pH (single-dose fluconazole 150 mg when pH was less than 4.9 or metronidazole 2 g for pH greater than 4.9), or (2) treatment with both fluconazole and metronidazole. The two empiric treatment strategies had more adverse side effects than placebo (11% and 19% versus 6%, respectively), but resulted in shortened symptom duration, fewer referrals for continued nondiagnostic status, and decreased cost.[32] For non-pregnant, low-risk women, empiric treatment guided by pH may be considered. When no infection is found, other causes of vaginal itching, irritation, burning, or discharge must be considered, such as latex allergy to condoms, contact dermatitis, or atrophic vaginitis.

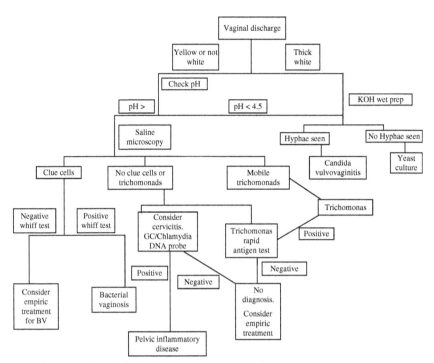

Fig. 1. Evaluation of vaginal discharge.

Cervicitis and Pelvic Inflammatory Disease

The sexually transmitted infections *Neisseria gonorrhea* and *Chlamydia trachomatis* are the two primary infectious agents for cervicitis, with chlamydial infections being the most prevalent. Other less common infectious causes are herpes simplex viruses, *Mycoplasma genitalium*, bacterial vaginosis, trichomonas, streptococcal infections (groups A and B), and rarely cytomegalovirus. In up to 50% of patients, clinical symptoms of cervicitis may not be noticeable. When symptomatic, clinical manifestations may include mucopurulent cervical discharge, cervical motion tenderness, cervical friability, postcoital bleeding, intermenstrual bleeding, dyspareunia, or concomitant external vaginal irritation and dysuria. Between 10% and 15% of gonorrhea and chlamydial infections cause concomitant urinary tract infections also. If the patient has further symptoms, such as fever and abdominal pain (especially in conjunction with cervical motion tenderness), then PID should be suspected and treated empirically. Chlamydial and gonorrheal infections may lead to scarring of the reproductive tract and subsequent infertility. Up to one half of women who test positive for gonorrhea may also have anorectal gonorrheal infections.[40]

According to CDC National Surveillance Data for Chlamydia, Gonorrhea, and Syphilis, 2006,[41] chlamydial infections are the leading cause of cervicitis with approximately 2.8 million new cases diagnosed each year, and rates of infection continue to increase. An increase of 5.6% occurred from 2005 to 2006 (from 329 to 348 cases per 100,000 persons); adolescents and young women make up the highest risk group. The CDC estimates that approximately 7% of women between the ages of 15 and 24 years of age are infected with *Chlamydia*. Racial disparities also exist, with the highest rates of disease occurring in African American females, followed by the American Indian/Alaskan Native females. The lowest rate of disease is noted in Asian/Pacific Islander females.[41]

The USPSTF published clinical guidelines in 2007 for sexually transmitted infection screening (available at www.preventiveservices.ahrq.gov). For chlamydia screening, all nonpregnant women younger than age 25 and women age 25 years and older who have high-risk behavior, such as having a new or multiple current sexual partners, inconsistent condom usage, engaging in sex under the influence of drugs or alcohol or for obtaining drugs or alcohol, should be screened. All pregnant women should be screened for chlamydia if they are less than 25 years old and those aged 25 years or older should be screened if they are considered to be at high risk. If the screening test is positive during pregnancy, the patient should be retested again in 3 weeks to ensure cure. Treating the patient's sexual partner at the time of diagnosis is also indicated. The CDC recommends screening all pregnant women for chlamydia but the American Academy of Family Practice (AAFP) and the ACOG advocate screening only pregnant women considered to be at high risk.[42]

Newer screening methods for gonorrhea and chlamydia have become less invasive. The preferred screening test is the Nucleic Acid Amplification Test (NAAT) because of its high sensitivity and specificity. Specimens from cervical swabs or urine may be used. If this test is unavailable, the DNA probe is an alternative. Screening for chlamydia in age-appropriate females at the time of their annual Pap smear should increase diagnostic yield and allow for facilitation of appropriate treatment. Azithromycin is an important single-dose regimen to improve compliance; however, several other treatment regimens for chlamydia exist (**Table 5**).

Gonorrhea is the second most common sexually transmitted infection, and the incidence of this infection also continues to increase in the United States. The CDC Trends in Reportable Sexually Transmitted Diseases in the United States, 2006, National Surveillance Data,[41] suggest that although numbers of reported gonorrhea infections are escalating, it still may be "substantially underdiagnosed and underreported, and approximately twice as many new infections are estimated to occur each year as are reported." Because the CDC Gonococcal Isolate Surveillance Project

Table 5
Treatment of chlamydia

	Nonpregnant	Pregnant
Drugs of choice	Azithromycin 1 g orally once or doxycycline 100 mg orally twice daily for 7 d	Azithromycin 1 g orally once or amoxicillin 500 mg orally three times daily for 7 d. Retest 3 wk after treatment to ensure cure of infection.
Alternative therapies	Erythromycin 500 mg orally four times daily for 7 d or erythromycin ethylsuccinate 800 mg orally four times a day for 7 d or ofloxacin 300 mg orally twice daily for 7 d or levofloxacin 500 mg orally once daily for 7 d. Because of high rates of recurrence, consider retesting in 4–6 months for nonpregnant patients.	Erythromycin base 500 mg orally four times a day for 7 d or erythromycin base 250 mg orally four times a day for 14 d or erythromycin ethylsuccinate 800 mg orally four times a day for 7 d or erythromycin ethylsuccinate 400 mg orally four times a day for 14 d. Retest 3 wk after treatment to ensure cure of infection.

Data from Centers for Disease Control and Prevention. Sexually Transmitted Disease Treatment Guidelines, 2006. MMWR Recomm Rep 2006 (RR-11);55:1–95. Available at: www.cdc.gov/STD/treatment.

2006 illustrated the widespread resistance to fluoroquinolones, the CDC no longer recommends fluoroquinolones for treatment of any gonorrheal infections.[43] Single class therapy is restricted to the cephalosporins (**Table 6**).

The CDC currently recommends screening all sexually active women at increased risk for gonorrhea. The USPSTF adds that women younger than 25 years of age are also at a high risk, paralleling their chlamydia screening guidelines. Like chlamydia, gonorrheal infections can cause PID with the potential for fallopian tube scarring, tubo-ovarian abscesses, chronic pelvic pain, ectopic pregnancies, and infertility. Additionally, the CDC recommends that any patient suspected of having gonorrhea or PID should undergo concurrent treatment of a coexistent chlamydial infection unless it has been ruled out. Sexual partners of patients who have gonorrhea should be treated at the same time, and expedited partner treatment is an option. If the first-trimester screening is positive for gonorrhea, a repeat screen for gonorrheal infections in the third trimester of pregnancy is recommended.[9]

For diagnosis of gonorrhea, the NAAT test is the most sensitive and specific test. Specimens from cervical swabs, self-collected vaginal swabs, rectal swabs, and urine are all appropriate for NAAT testing. For definitive diagnosis in populations with a low prevalence of disease, culture on Thayer-Martin media for gonorrhea is recommended. Cultures from endocervical specimens in asymptomatic women, however, may only yield 65% to 85% sensitivity.[44] Cephalosporins are the mainstay of treatment of gonorrhea (see **Table 6**).

Most women who have untreated gonorrhea and up to 40% of women who have untreated chlamydia may develop PID.[41] Gonorrhea and chlamydia may initiate a polymicrobial infection that includes Gram-positive and Gram-negative bacteria and anaerobes. Multiple antibiotic regimens exist for treatment, based on suspected

Table 6
Treatment of gonorrhea

	Nonpregnant	Pregnant
Drugs of choice	Ceftriaxone 125 mg IM once or cefixime 400 mg orally once	Ceftriaxone 125 mg IM once or cefixime 400 mg orally once or spectinomycin 2 g IM once (rarely used). If considered high risk, rescreen the patient in her third trimester
Alternative therapies	Ceftizoxime 500 mg IM once or cefoxitin 2 g IM once with probenecid 1 g orally once or cefotaxime 500 mg IM once or cefpodoxime 400 mg orally once or cefuroxime axetil 1 g orally once or spectinomycin 2 g IM once (rarely used). Because of high rates of recurrence, consider retesting in 4–6 months for nonpregnant patients	—

In addition to the regimens in this table, the clinician should always treat for coexistent chlamydia infection, unless ruled out. For severe, documented cephalosporin allergies, desensitization is recommended. If this is not possible, azithromycin 2 g orally once may be used; however, this is not routinely recommended because of concerns regarding macrolide resistance.

Data from CDC updated recommended treatment regimes for gonococcal infections and associated conditions – United States, April 2007. Available at: www.cdc.gov/STD/treatment.

organisms and patients' allergies (**Table 7**). If anaerobes are suspected, metronidazole should be added to the treatment regimen. If a patient can tolerate oral medications and is not severely ill, outpatient management with close follow-up is possible, because oral and intravenous antibiotic regimens have equal efficacy. Patients for

Table 7
Treatment of pelvic inflammatory disease

	Outpatient Therapy	Inpatient/Intravenous Therapy
Recommended regimens	Ceftriaxone 250 mg IM once plus doxycycline 100 mg twice daily for 14 d with/without metronidazole 500 mg orally twice daily for 14 d	Regimen A: Cefotetan 2 g IV every 12 h or cefoxitin 2 g IV every 6 h plus doxycycline 100 mg orally or IV every 12 h
	Cefoxitin 2 g IM once and probenecid 1 g orally once plus doxycycline 100 mg orally twice daily for 14 d with/without metronidazole 500 mg orally twice daily for 14 d	Regimen B: Clindamycin 900 mg IV every 8 h plus gentamicin loading dose (IV or IM) 2 mg/kg followed by maintenance dose 1.5 mg/kg every 8 h
	Third-generation cephalosporin (ceftizoxime or cefotaxime) parenteral plus doxycycline 100 mg orally twice daily with/without metronidazole 500 mg orally twice daily for 14 d	
Abbreviated therapy[a]	Ceftriaxone 250 mg IM once plus azithromycin 1 g orally once weekly for 2 wk	
Alternative regime	If NAAT for gonorrhea is positive, culture must be done for susceptibility. If not quinolone resistant: levofloxacin 500 mg orally once daily for 14 d or ofloxacin 400 mg orally twice daily for 14 d with/without metronidazole 500 mg orally twice daily for 14 d	Ampicillin/sulbactam 3 g IV every 6 h plus doxycycline 100 mg orally or IV every 12 h
Penicillin allergic patientss	Options for outpatient therapy are limited; consider inpatient therapy with clindamycin and gentamicin. If patient had a mild reaction to penicillin and no reaction to cephalosporins, consider treatment with ceftriaxone IM. If patient is at low risk for reaction, clinician may administer a test dose of ceftriaxone (1/10 of full dose) and observe for 2 h, if no reaction occurs, give full dose. If patient has history of life-threatening anaphylaxis reactions or IgE-mediated reactions, consults with infectious disease and allergy specialists are recommended.	

[a] Suggested abbreviated therapy from Savaris RF, et al. Comparing ceftriaxone plus azithromycin or doxycycline for pelvic inflammatory disease: a randomized controlled trial. Obstet Gynecol 2007;110:53–60.
Data from CDC Updated recommended regimes for Gonococcal infections and associated conditions—United States, April 2007. Available at: http://www.cdc.gov/STD/treatment.

whom a concern regarding nonadherence to medications exists or who are vomiting, pregnant, have tubo-ovarian abscesses, or severe abdominal pain with fever should be hospitalized. Outpatients who do not respond within 72 hours to oral antibiotics need reassessment and consideration for intravenous antibiotic management. Inpatients receiving intravenous antibiotic therapy should be transitioned to oral antibiotics as tolerated. Current CDC guidelines can be consulted for detailed recommendations at www.cdc.gov/STD/treatment.

Women who have chronic or recurrent cervicitis may require repeat screening for infections, assessment for any hypersensitivity reactions, or referral to a gynecologist. Patients who have chronic cervicitis who remain symptomatic even after antibiotic therapy may be infected with *M genitalium*.[45,46] Fortunately, *M genitalium* is responsive to single-dose therapies of azithromycin. Noninfectious hypersensitivity reactions may be provoked by foreign objects or substances inserted into the vagina, including various creams, douches, lubricants, spermicidal agents, latex condoms, diaphragms, pessaries, and contraceptive ring devices. Radiation therapy and inflammatory and autoimmune conditions, such as Behçet disease, may also cause chronic cervicitis. Screening, detection, and treatment of human papilloma virus (HPV) infections are beyond the scope of this article. New research focuses on investigating other causes for acute and chronic cervicitis, such as cytomegalovirus cervicitis, *M genitalium* infections, and herpes simplex virus infections. Because the burden of disease for sexually transmitted infections is high, research on vaccines to prevent infections is occurring. Future chlamydia vaccines may use influenza viruses as a delivery vector.[47]

SUMMARY

Many women seek care for vulvar, vaginal, or pelvic complaints. Primary care providers should possess a solid understanding of the differential diagnosis and treatment of gynecologic infections. Many infections in the reproductive tracts are sexually transmitted, whereas other common infections are attributable to an overgrowth of the normally present bacteria or yeast in vagina. Presenting symptoms and signs are helpful in determining the source of infection, but often a battery of tests must be performed to make a definitive diagnosis. Almost one half of the diagnoses of patients who have vaginal discharge remain inconclusive despite appropriate work-up and require empiric treatment or referral. Sexually transmitted infections, such as chlamydia or gonorrhea, may cause PID and affect future fertility. Multiple antibiotic regimens are available to treat sexually transmitted infections and are outlined in the CDC 2006 guidelines (www.cdc.gov/STD/treatment). Up-to-date knowledge regarding the diagnosis and treatment of gynecologic infections is crucial for family physicians.

REFERENCES

1. Armstrong G, Schillinger J, Markowitz L, et al. Incidence of herpes simplex virus type 2 infection in the United States. Am J Epidemiol 2001;153:912–20.
2. Fleming DT, McQuillan GM, Johnson RE, et al. Herpes simplex virus type 2 in the United States, 1976 to 1994. N Engl J Med 1997;337(16):1105–11.
3. Xu F, Sternberg MR, Kottiri BJ, et al. Trends in herpes simplex virus type 1 and type 2 seroprevalence in the United States. J Am Med Assoc 2006;296(8):964–73.
4. Ashley RL, Wald A. Genital herpes: review of the epidemic and potential use of type-specific serology. Clin Microbiol Rev 1999;12(1):1–8.

5. Corey L, Wald A, Patel R, et al. Once-daily valacyclovir to reduce the risk of transmission of genital herpes. N Engl J Med 2004;350(1):11–9.
6. Sacks SL. Famiciclovir suppression of asymptomatic and symptomatic recurrent anogenital herpes simplex virus shedding in women: a randomized, double-blind, double-dummy, placebo-controlled, parallel-group, single center trial. J Infect Dis 2004;189(8):1341–7.
7. ACOG practice bulletin. Management of herpes in pregnancy. Number 8, October 1999. Clinical management guidelines for obstetrician-gynecologists. Int J Gynaecol Obstet 2000;68(2):165–73.
8. U.S. Preventive Services Task Force (USPSTF). Screening for genital herpes: recommendation statement. Rockville (MD): Agency for Healthcare Research and Quality (AHRQ); 2005. p. 11.
9. Centers for Disease Control and Prevention. Sexually transmitted disease treatment guidelines, 2006. MMWR Recomm Rep 2006;55(RR-11):1–95.
10. Centers for Disease Control and Prevention. 2006 Syphilis surveillance report supplement. Available at: www.cdc.gov/std/Syphilis2006/Syphilis2006Complete.pdf. Accessed August 20, 2008.
11. Centers for Disease Control and Prevention website. Available at: www.cdc.gov/std/Trends2000/chancroid.htm. Accessed August 15, 2008.
12. Mabey D, Peeling RW. Lymphogranuloma venereum. Sex Transm Infect 2002;78:90–2.
13. Van Vranken M. Prevention and treatment of sexually transmitted diseases: an update. Am Fam Physician 2007;76(12):1827–32.
14. Anderson MR, Klink K, Cohrssen A. Evaluation of vaginal complaints. JAMA 2004;291(11):1368–78.
15. Eckert EO, Hawes SE, Stevens CE, et al. Vulvovaginal candidiasis: clinical manifestations, risk factors, management algorithm. Obstet Gynecol 1998;07:757–65.
16. Chandeying V, Skov S, Kempanmanus M, et al. Evaluation of two clinical protocols for the management of women with vaginal discharge in southern Thailand. Sex Transm Infect 1998;74:194–201.
17. Pharmacy Times. Available at: http://www.pharmacytimes.com/issues/articles/2006-06_3567.asp. Accessed July 4, 2008.
18. ACOG. ACOG practice bulletin. Vaginitis. Obstet Gynecol 2006;107(5):1195–206.
19. Sobel JD, Kapernick PS, Zervos M, et al. Treatment of complicated Candida vaginitis: comparison of single and sequential doses of fluconazole. Am J Obstet Gynecol 2001;185:363–9.
20. Sobel JD, Wiesenfeld HC, Martens M, et al. Maintenance fluconazole therapy for recurrent vulvovaginal candidiasis. N Engl J Med 2004;351:876–83.
21. Sobel JS, Chaim W, Nagapan V, et al. Treatment of vaginitis caused by Candida glabrata: use of topical boric acid and flucytosine. Am J Obstet Gynecol 2003;189:1297–300.
22. O'Dowd TC, West RR. Clinical prediction of Gardnerella vaginalis in general practice. J R Coll Gen Pract 1987;37:59–61.
23. Landers D, Wiesenfeld HC, Heine RP, et al. Predictive value of the clinical diagnosis of lower genital tract infection in women. Am J Obstet Gynecol 2004;190:1004–10.
24. Bradshaw CS, Morton AN, Hocking J, et al. High recurrence rates of bacterial vaginosis over the course of 12 months after oral metronidazole therapy and factors associated with recurrence. J Infect Dis 2006;193:1478–86.

25. McDonald HM, Brocklehurst P, Gordon A. Antibiotics for treating bacterial vaginosis in pregnancy. Cochrane Database Syst Rev 2007, (1). Art No.: CD000262. 10.1002/14651858.CD000262.pub3.
26. Carey JC, Klebanoff MA, Hauth JC, et al. Metronidazole to prevent preterm delivery in pregnant women with asymptomatic bacterial vaginosis. National institute of child health and human development network of maternal-fetal medicine units. N Engl J Med 2000;342:534–40.
27. Ness RB, Hillier SL, Kip KE, et al. Bacterial vaginosis and the risk of pelvic inflammatory disease. Obstet Gynecol 2004;104(4):761–9.
28. Schwebke JR, Desmond R. A randomized trial of metronidazole in asymptomatic bacterial vaginosis to prevent the acquisition of sexually transmitted diseases. Am J Obstet Gynecol 2007;196(6):517. e1–6.
29. Hutchinson KB, Kip KE, Ness RB. Condom use and its association with bacterial vaginosis and bacterial vaginosis-associated vaginal microflora. Epidemiology 2007;18(6):702–8.
30. Sutton M, Sternberg M, Koumans EH, et al. The prevalence of Trichomonas vaginalis infection among reproductive age women in the United States, 2001–2004. Clin Infect Dis 2007;45:1319–26.
31. Wiese W, Patel ST, Patel SC, et al. A meta-analysis of the Papanicolaou smear and wet mount for the diagnosis of vaginal trichomoniasis. Am J Med 2000; 108:301–8.
32. Carr PL, Rothberg MB, Friedman RH, et al. "Shotgun" versus sequential testing: cost-effectiveness of diagnostic strategies for vaginitis. J Gen Intern Med 2005; 20:793–9.
33. Heppert JS, Batteiger BE, Braslins P, et al. Use of an immunochromatographic assay for rapid detection of trichomonas vaginalis in vaginal specimens. J Clin Microbiol 2005;43:684–7.
34. Caro-Paton T, Carvajal A, Martin de Diego I, et al. Is metronidazole teratogenic? A meta-analysis. Br J Clin Pharmacol 1997;44(2):179–82.
35. Klebanoff MA, Carey JC, Hauth JC, et al. Failure of metronidazole to prevent preterm delivery among pregnant women with asymptomatic Trichomonas vaginalis infection. N Engl J Med 2001;345(7):487–93.
36. Shennan A, Crawshaw S, Briley A, et al. A randomized controlled trial of metronidazole for the prevention of preterm birth in women positive for cervicovaginal fetal fibronectin: the PREMET study. BJOG 2006;113(1):65–74.
37. Van der Pol B, Kwok C, Pierre-Louis B, et al. Trichomonas vaginalis infection and human immunodeficiency virus acquisition in African women. J Infect Dis 2008; 197(4):548–54.
38. Abbott J. Clinical and microscopic diagnosis of vaginal yeast infection: a prospective analysis. Ann Emerg Med 1995;25:587–91.
39. Schaaf MV, Perez-Stable EJ, Borchardt K. The limited value of symptoms and signs in the diagnosis of vaginal infections. Arch Intern Med 1990;150: 1929–33.
40. Stansfield V. Diagnosis and management of anorectal gonorrhea in women. Br J Vener Dis 1980;56:319–21.
41. Center for Disease Control. Trends in reportable sexually transmitted diseases in the United States, 2006. CDC Available at: www.cdc.gov/std/stats/trends2006. htm Accessed August 4, 2008.
42. Meyers D, Gregory K, Nelson H, et al. USPSTF recommendations for STI screening. Am Fam Physician 2008;77(6):819–24.

43. Centers for Disease Control. Update to CDC's sexually transmitted disease treatment guidelines, 2006: fluoroquinolones no longer recommended for treatment of gonococcal infections. MMWR Recomm Rep 2007;56(14):332–6. Available at: http://www.cdc.gov/mmwr/preview/mmwrhtml/mm5614a3.htm. Accessed August 4, 2008.
44. Schink JC, Keith LG. Problems in the culture diagnosis of gonorrhea. J Reprod Med 1985;30:244–9.
45. Jensen JS. Mycoplasma genitalium: the aetiologial agent of urethritis and other sexually transmitted diseases. J Eur Acad Dermatol Venereol 2004;18(1):1–11.
46. Angarius C, Lore B, Jensen JS. Mycoplasma genitalium: prevalence, clinical significance, and transmission. Sex Transm Infect 2005;81(6):458–62.
47. He Q, Martinez-Sobrido L, Edo FO, et al. Live-attenuated influenza viruses as delivery vectors for chlamydia vaccines. Immunology 2007;122(2):28–37 [Epub 2007 Apr 23].

Urinary Problems in Women

Linda French, MD[a,*], Kevin Phelps, DO[a],
Nageswar Rao Pothula, MD, MHA[a], Saudia Mushkbar, MD[b]

KEYWORDS

- Women • Urinary symptoms • Urinary incontinence
- Urinary tract infection • Irritable bladder • Overactive bladder
- Interstitial cystitis • Painful bladder syndrome

Women who have symptoms related to the genitourinary system present daily in a typical family medicine practice. The most common complaints are dysuria, increased urinary frequency, and incontinence. In the vast majority of cases the underlying problem is either urinary tract infection (UTI), urinary incontinence (UI) without infection, or bladder pain without infection that may be termed painful bladder syndrome/interstitial cystitis (PBS/IC). Other pathologic conditions related to the urinary system are not emphasized in this article, because they have little predilection for women or because they occur much less commonly.

URINARY TRACT INFECTION

The most common urinary problem in women is the UTI. UTI is defined as the presence of microbial pathogens in the urinary tract with associated symptoms and usually refers to cystitis unless otherwise specified. The most common symptoms of UTI are dysuria and increased urinary frequency. Fever and flank pain suggest infection of the upper urinary tract, specifically pyelonephritis. Structural or functional abnormalities of the urinary tract confer an increased risk for pyelonephritis, which may lead to renal damage and increased morbidity, especially renal abscess and urosepsis. Asymptomatic bacteriuria refers to the asymptomatic presence of pathogens in the urine. Recurrent UTI is defined as at least two episodes within a 6-month period or three episodes within a 12-month period.

Epidemiology and Economic Impact

UTI is the most frequently diagnosed bacterial infection in adult women according to National Ambulatory Medial Care Survey data.[1] The direct costs associated with community-acquired UTI are estimated at about $2 billion annually in the United States.[2]

[a] Department of Family Medicine, University of Toledo, College of Medicine, 3000 Arlington Avenue, Toledo, OH 43614, USA
[b] Neighborhood Health Clinic, Fort Wayne, IN, USA
* Corresponding author.
E-mail address: linda.french@utoledo.edu (L. French).

Prim Care Clin Office Pract 36 (2009) 53–71
doi:10.1016/j.pop.2008.10.003
0095-4543/08/$ – see front matter © 2009 Elsevier Inc. All rights reserved.

primarycare.theclinics.com

More than one half of women will receive antibiotic therapy for UTI at some time in their lives,[3] with a reported incidence of 0.5 to 0.7 per person-years in premenopausal women.[4] True population incidence rates are impossible to obtain, however, because a UTI is often a self-limited process that is not diagnosed or treated by health care providers, because there is not a consensus on what colony count constitutes a positive culture, and because diagnosis in the ambulatory setting may not always be verified by culture. Progression of UTI to pyelonephritis and sepsis is rare in otherwise healthy nonpregnant adult women.

Pathogenesis and Microbiology

Uropathogens typically gain access to the urinary system through ascending migration through the urethra from the vaginal introitus contaminated by fecal flora. The most common pathogen in uncomplicated UTI in women is *Escherichia coli*, which accounts for approximately 80% of cases. Specific strains of *E coli* seem to be especially pathogenic.[5] The fimbriae or pili of *E coli* facilitate adherence to the uroepithelium. Virulent strains with the adhesion molecule FimH attach to the uroepithelial cells through specific receptors. The second most common pathogen is *Staphylococcus saprophyticus*, which accounts for 5% to 15% of cases.[6,7] Other less common uropathogens in uncomplicated UTI in women include enterococci and Gram-negative rods, including *Klebsiella*, *Serratia*, *Enterobacter*, *Proteus*, and *Pseudomonas*.

Risk Factors

Among otherwise healthy women of reproductive age, risk factors are largely related to disruption of the normal vaginal flora, which permits the proliferation of fecal flora. These factors include spermicides, barrier contraceptives, coital frequency, new sexual partner, and recent use of antibiotics.[3,4,8] Additionally, nonoxynol-9 is known to enhance adherence of *E coli* to epithelial cells.[9] Lewis blood group nonsecretors, who compose approximately 25% of the population, have an increased risk for recurrent UTIs.[10] This susceptibility is believed to be related to cellular change that facilitates adherence of bacterial fimbriae.

Populations at increased risk for pyelonephritis include women who have weakened immune systems, including those who have diabetes, older women, and those who have underlying urologic or neurologic disorders. Pregnant women are also at increase risk for pyelonephritis associated with the relative ureteral obstruction during gestation. Risk factors for UTI in postmenopausal women include recurrent UTI, bladder prolapse or cystocele, and increased postvoid residual.[11] Women who have urinary incontinence have an increased risk for UTI and experience increased incontinence during an acute episode.[12] The high pH of the vagina without estrogen allows for a vaginal flora in which uropathogens may predominate.

Clinical Presentation

The most helpful combination of factors on history and physical examination is dysuria without vaginal discharge or irritation, which has a positive predictive value of 77% for a positive urine culture.[13] Other individual findings that increase the likelihood of a positive urine culture include urinary frequency, hematuria, back pain, and fever. Women who have recurrent culture-proven UTIs have a good ability to self-diagnose an acute episode.[13] Findings of fever, flank pain, and costovertebral tenderness suggest pyelonephritis.

Diagnostic Testing

Dipstick urinalysis that shows presence of either leukocyte esterase or nitrites is highly predictive of a positive urine culture, whereas absence of both findings markedly reduces the likelihood.[14] A negative dipstick urinalysis is sufficient to rule out UTI in most cases for otherwise healthy women of reproductive age. The use of dipstick urinalysis improves physicians' diagnostic accuracy and can reduce antibiotic prescribing compared with history and physical examination alone.[15,16]

Urine culture with a colony count of at least 10^5 colony forming units (cfu) has traditionally been considered to be the gold standard for the diagnosis of UTI. Culture is unnecessary in women who have typical symptoms and a positive dipstick urinalysis unless there is a lack of response to therapy, recurrent infection, complicating factors, such as diabetes or anatomic abnormalities, or a suspicion of pyelonephritis.[17] For symptomatic women, a colony count of more than 10^2 cfu of a single species known to be a uropathogen is generally considered to be positive because up to one-half of symptomatic women whose urine cultures grow uropathogens have colony counts less than 10^5 cfu.[18]

Imaging studies have low yield in otherwise healthy women who have uncomplicated UTIs.[19] Likewise, a single episode of pyelonephritis is not associated with clinically significant risk for anatomic abnormality.[20] Imaging with renal ultrasound, intravenous pyelogram, or voiding cystourethrogram is indicated in cases of recurrent pyelonephritis.

Treatment

A list of commonly prescribed antibiotic regimens for uncomplicated UTI in women can be found in **Table 1**. All regimens have cure rates greater than 90% unless there is a high prevalence of resistance in the local community. In most United States communities a short course of any generic antibiotic can be obtained for $4. The Infectious Diseases Society of America (IDSA) published guidelines for treatment of uncomplicated UTI and acute pyelonephritis in 1999.[21] The drug of choice per those guidelines is a 3-day course of trimethoprim-sulfamethoxazole (TMP-SMZ). British guidelines recommend trimethoprim alone as first choice.[22] Alternative therapies are 3-day courses of trimethoprim alone or ofloxacin. One-day treatments are less effective and longer treatments are associated with increased risk for adverse effects without clinically meaningful improvement in effectiveness. Other fluoroquinolones are not recommended because of

Table 1		
Commonly used therapies for urinary tract infection in women		
Drug	**Dosing**	**Duration of Treatment**
First line		
Trimethoprim-sulfamethoxazole	80 mg/400 mg twice daily	3 d
Trimethoprim alone	100 mg twice daily	3 d
Second line		
Cephalexin	500 mg 3 times daily	3 d 7–10 d in pregnancy
Ciprofloxacin	500 mg twice daily	3 d
Nitrofurantoin macrocrystals	100 mg twice daily	5 d 7–10 d in pregnancy
Ofloxacin	200 mg twice daily	3 d

Data from Car J. Urinary tract infections in women: diagnosis and management in primary care. BMJ 2006;332(7533):94–7; and Warren JW, Abrutyn E, Hebel JR, et al. Guidelines for antimicrobial treatment of uncomplicated acute bacterial cystitis and acute pyelonephritis in women. Infectious Diseases Society of America (IDSA). Clin Infect Dis 1999;29(4):745–58.

concerns about promoting drug resistance. In fact, increasing rates of resistance to ciprofloxacin have been noted in Israel and Canada.[23,24]

IDSA did not include cephalosporins among their recommendations for first-line therapy because of concerns about disruption of the vaginal flora. Cephalexin 500 mg twice daily for 7 to 10 days is recommended for pregnant women.[17] It can also be used three times daily for 3 days as a second-line therapy.

Nitrofurantoin 100 mg twice daily for 7 to 10 days is another first-line therapy for pregnant women.[17] Nitrofurantoin has been used to treat UTIs for more than 50 years with no significant trend toward development of resistance. It achieves high concentration in urine, but not in renal tissue. It is especially effective against E coli and S saprophyticus but not other less-frequent uropathogens. Recently a 5-day course of nitrofurantoin has been shown to be as effective as a 7-day course.[25] A 3-day course has been shown to be less effective with a cure rate of only 70% to 80%.[26]

In vitro resistance to TMP-SMZ has been documented in many communities in the United States with rates as high as 22%.[27,28] Laboratory data are not likely to be representative of primary care practice where empiric therapy is the rule, however, and cultures are ordered in specific contexts likely to be associated with increased resistance, such as lack of therapeutic response and recurrent infections. In vitro sensitivities may also underestimate the clinical effectiveness of the high concentration of antibiotics achieved in the urine. Oral treatment for 7 to 14 days in the ambulatory setting using drugs listed in **Table 1** (except nitrofurantoin) may be given for women presumed to have acute pyelonephritis without complicating factors.[21] An initial dose of gentamicin or ceftriaxone followed by oral therapy has been advocated for women presenting to an emergency department, although randomized controlled trials to substantiate superiority of this approach are lacking.[29]

Prevention and Treatment of Recurrent Urinary Tract Infections

Approximately 25% of young women who have UTI will have a recurrence within 6 months.[3] Urine cultures should be performed when women have recurrent symptoms within 6 months to confirm the presence of UTI and to test for sensitivities to antibiotics. Cranberry juice or tablets containing proanthocyanidin can reduce the rate of recurrences of UTI by one half, exercising their effect by inhibiting adherence of E coli.[30] Proanthocyanidin is not an effective treatment of UTI once established, however. In postmenopausal women, vaginal estrogens reduce the number of recurrent UTIs by decreasing the vaginal pH and permitting a vaginal flora in which uropathogens are less likely to dominate.[11] There is no evidence of effectiveness for preventive measures, including voiding after sexual intercourse, lactobacillus drinks, and direction of perineal wiping, although this advice is commonly given.[17]

Women who have three or more recurrences annually may be offered the option of self-treatment of recurrences. Postcoital use of antibiotic prophylaxis is effective for women who have recurrences with a temporal relationship to intercourse.[31] Continuous antibiotic prophylaxis in a single bedtime dose is also accepted practice for women who have frequent recurrences. Antibiotics that have been shown to reduce the number of recurrences to 0.3 or fewer per year are TMP-SMZ 40 mg/200 mg, TMP 100 mg, norfloxacin 200 mg, and nitrofurantoin macrocrystals 50 to 100 mg.[32]

URINARY INCONTINENCE

UI is the involuntary loss of urine, a condition commonly seen in women in primary care practices.[33,34] It is associated with poor self-esteem, impaired quality of life, social isolation, and depression.[34–36] Although UI is common, several studies have shown that a relatively small proportion of patients discuss the condition with their physicians.[37–41] Overactive bladder is an overlapping condition characterized by one or more symptoms of urgency, frequency (greater than eight urinations per 24 hours), nocturia, and incontinence.

Epidemiology and Economic Impact

UI, defined as any leakage or involuntary loss of urine during the preceding 30 days, had a prevalence of 37% in one study with 82% of responders being female.[42] Another study found an overall prevalence of UI of 25% among community-dwelling women, aged 20 years or older.[43] Prevalence increases with age with 12% of women older than 65 years reporting daily incontinence.[36,44] An estimated 17 million community-dwelling adults in the United States in 2000 had daily UI, and an additional 33 million suffered from the overlapping condition, overactive bladder. Risk factors for UI in women are highlighted in **Box 1**. UI has a substantial economic impact on individual women and society with an estimated direct cost in excess of $12 billion.[45] Women who have severe UI spend nearly $900 annually for treatment.[46]

Box 1
Risk factors for urinary incontinence
Irreversible
Age
Race (non-Hispanic white women)
Less than high school education
Family history
Childhood enuresis
Multiparity
Forceps delivery
Hysterectomy
Surgery for pelvic organ prolapse
Reversible
Body mass index >30
Smoking
High caffeine intake
Participation in high-impact sports, such as running
Diabetes
Depression
Central nervous system disorders
Recurrent urinary tract infections
Constipation
Drugs (oral estrogen, diuretics, antipsychotics, benzodiazepines, alpha adrenergic agonists)
Pelvic organ prolapse
Environmental barriers
Data from Refs.[102–108]

Pathophysiology

Voiding is under parasympathetic control and occurs when the detrusor muscle contracts and the urethral sphincter tone relaxes, thus resulting in the bladder pressure exceeding the urethral pressure. In contrast, urine storage is under sympathetic control and occurs when the urethral pressure exceeds the bladder pressure. The brain also performs an important role, and the decision to void is normally under voluntary control.[47]

Innervation of the bladder is complex, yet two general concepts can help in the management of UI. The first concept is the effect of neurologic control of bladder function by the upper motor neuron (UMN) and lower motor neuron (LMN). Stroke, spinal cord injury, and multiple sclerosis cause UMN lesions and result in the loss of inhibition of reflexes leading to spasticity. In contrast, LMN lesions, such as those caused by diabetic neuropathy, interrupt the reflex arc leading to flaccidity. The term neurogenic bladder is ambiguous and should be avoided. The second concept relates to autonomic innervation and can be remembered with the simple rule that the sympathetic response favors storage of urine. Alpha-adrenergic medications tend to increase urethral pressure and relax the detrusor, whereas adrenergic blockers have the opposite effect. Cholinergic agonists tend to relax the sphincter, and anticholinergics tend to increase its pressure. Understanding this balance facilitates understanding of drug therapy and unintended adverse effects.[48]

Classification of Urinary Incontinence

UI can be classified as stress, urge, functional, overflow, and mixed. The International Continence Society has defined stress UI as a constellation of signs or symptoms of involuntary leakage of urine on effort or exertion, or on sneezing or coughing.[49] Stress incontinence occurs when intra-abdominal pressure overcomes the sphincter closure mechanism. In cases of stress incontinence, there is lack of anatomic support at the urethra-vesical junction (or bladder neck), which causes urethral hypermobility. When intra-abdominal pressure increases, the bladder neck is displaced outside the abdominal cavity allowing an increase in bladder pressure that overcomes urethral pressure resulting in loss of urine. Intrinsic urethral sphincter deficiency leads to the same result.[50]

Urge incontinence is an involuntary leakage of urine resulting from detrusor overactivity, usually in relatively large amounts, and accompanied or immediately preceded by a sense of urgency to void. Some cases of overactive bladder can be attributed to specific conditions, such as acute or chronic infection, bladder cancer, or bladder stones, but most cases result from an idiopathic inability to suppress detrusor contractions.

Functional incontinence results from impairment of cognitive function or mobility with either loss of voluntary control or the ability to act on the urge to void. Overflow incontinence results in urine loss associated with overdistension of the bladder. Patients may present with constant dribbling or symptoms suggesting stress or urge incontinence. Overdistension is typically caused by an underactive detrusor mechanism or bladder outlet obstruction. An underactive bladder may be caused by medications, including anticholinergic agents, or conditions, such as diabetic neuropathy, cauda equina syndrome, and radical pelvic surgery. Outlet obstruction in women is usually a result of urethral occlusion from pelvic organ prolapse or previous continence surgery.

In many patients, a combination of factors contributes to incontinence. This combination may result in a mixed picture, most commonly a combination of stress and urge incontinence. Patients can have both stress and urge incontinence with the same episode, whereas others can experience discrete episodes of stress and urge incontinence.[51] Another form of mixed incontinence occurs when the overactive bladder syndrome is coupled with functional limitations in mobility leading to loss of urine.

Clinical Presentation

Women who may be reluctant to initiate a discussion about their concerns of incontinence can be encouraged to do so by direct inquiry at the time of health maintenance or other routine visits; this can be incorporated into the genitourinary review of systems. Further evaluation is warranted for women who judge that the impact of their UI is sufficient to warrant treatment. In these cases, the next step is to identify the type of UI and associated symptoms.

An accurate urinary history is the cornerstone of evaluation, beginning with an assessment of reversible risk factors (see **Box 1**). Several questionnaires have been developed with variable diagnostic usefulness.[52] The accuracy of a three-question screen (Brief 3IQ) compared favorably with an extended evaluation in a multicenter, prospective study to distinguish between urge and stress incontinence (**Fig. 1**).[53] A voiding diary may also be helpful, whereby the patient records the times of voiding, incontinence episodes, circumstances of incontinence episodes (such as whether it was associated with cough or accompanied by urge), and an estimated amount of urine lost. Physical examination should include a gynecologic examination to identify prolapse or mass. Neurologic examination of the perineum may be performed if indicated.[51]

Diagnostic Testing

In a cooperative patient, a cough stress test may be used in the office setting. This technique is best performed when the patient has not recently voided and is in a standing position over a pad with a relaxed perineum. The patient is asked to give a single vigorous cough and the physician or nurse observes directly whether a UI episode occurs. Instantaneous leakage with cough suggests stress incontinence.[51] If leakage is delayed, it suggests a mixed incontinence picture of stress-induced overactive bladder.

The need to determine post-void residual (PVR) volume in a primary care practice is controversial because parameters for interpreting the results are neither standardized

1. During the last 3 months, have you leaked urine (even a small amount)?

☐ Yes   ☐ No
                    ↓
          Questionnaire completed.

2. During the last 3 months, did you leak urine:
(Check all that apply.)

☐ a. When you were performing some physical activity, such as coughing, sneezing, lifting, or exercise?
☐ b. When you had the urge or the feeling that you needed to empty your bladder, but you could not get to the toilet fast enough?
☐ c. Without physical activity and without a sense of urgency?

3. During the last 3 months, did you leak urine *most often*:
(Check only one.)

☐ a. When you were performing some physical activity, such as coughing, sneezing, lifting, or exercise?
☐ b. When you had the urge or the feeling that you needed to empty your bladder, but you could not get to the toilet fast enough?
☐ c. Without physical activity and without a sense of urgency?
☐ d. About equally as often with physical activity as with a sense of urgency?

Definitions of type of urinary incontinence are based on responses to question 3:

Response to Question 3	Type of Incontinence
a. Most often with physical activity	Stress only or stress predominant
b. Most often with the urge to empty the bladder	Urge only or urge predominant
c. Without physical activity or sense of urgency	Other cause only or other cause predominant
d. About equally with physical activity and sense of urgency	Mixed

Fig. 1. Incontinence questionnaire (3IQ). (*From* Brown JS, Bradley CS, Subak LL, et al. The sensitivity and specificity of a simple test to distinguish between urge and stress urinary incontinence. Ann Intern Med 2006;144(10):716; with permission.)

nor well tested; recommendations to determine PVR are based on expert opinion rather than evidence.[54,55] PVR should be considered in patients at risk for urinary retention, however, such as women who have had previous anti-incontinence surgery, those who have significant pelvic organ prolapse or spinal cord injury, or those who are taking medications that can suppress detrusor contractility or increase sphincter tone. A PVR volume can be measured either by direct bladder catheterization after the patient has urinated or by pelvic ultrasonography. In general, a PVR of less than 50 ml is considered adequate emptying and greater than 200 ml is inadequate, whereas at intermediate volumes the test result is equivocal and should be repeated.[56]

Although simple or complex urodynamic studies may be performed to make the definitive diagnosis of detrusor instability or detrusor hyperreflexia, most patients may be treated without undergoing invasive testing.[57] Although they are considered to be the gold standard for diagnosing UI, urodynamics studies are invasive, expensive, require special training and equipment, and have not been found to positively affect outcomes. Urodynamic testing is most useful for preoperative evaluation of stress UI or outlet obstruction.[58]

If the type of incontinence remains unclear after completing an initial assessment, a referral to a urologist or urogynecologist should be considered. Other reasons for referral include lack of a response to an adequate therapeutic trial, patient's decision to pursue further investigations or surgical options, history of previous anti-incontinence or radical pelvic surgery, or the presence of symptomatic pelvic prolapse.

Treatment

Stress incontinence

In general, treatment of stress incontinence emphasizes strategies to decrease sudden increases in abdominal pressure or increase the pressure in the urethral sphincter. Lifestyle modifications that can improve stress incontinence include weight loss, smoking cessation, and reduction of caffeine intake.[59,60] Weight loss of 5% to 10% has an efficacy similar to that of other nonsurgical treatments and should be considered as a first-line therapy for UI in obese women.[61]

Pelvic floor muscle exercises, also known as Kegel exercises, are intended to increase the resting tension, contractile force, and recruitment speed of the voluntary sphincter component of the pelvic diaphragm. These exercises focus on squeezing the pubococcygeus muscles and holding force for several seconds. A usual regimen is three sets of 8 to 12 slow velocity contractions sustained for 6 to 8 seconds each, at least three times a week for at least 15 weeks.[62] A 2006 Cochrane systematic review suggests that pelvic floor muscle exercises be included in first-line conservative management programs for women who have stress, urge, or mixed urinary incontinence.[63] Long-term outcomes have been disappointing, however.[64] Self-administered behavioral interventions, including pelvic floor muscle training with biofeedback and bladder training, have shown some effectiveness in combination for women who have stress UI.[65]

Pharmacotherapy has a limited role in the treatment of stress incontinence. Duloxetine has shown modest reduction in symptoms of both stress and mixed urinary incontinence in randomized controlled trials.[66,67] Traditionally, alpha agonists and estrogens have been used to treat stress incontinence. In one uncontrolled case series, estrogen therapy was associated with an improvement in stress incontinence symptoms. In later large randomized trials, however, women assigned to receive estrogen were more likely to experience the onset of UI or a worsening of baseline symptoms.[68] Alpha agonists, such as norephedrine, have shown only modest effect in small trials.[69]

Pessaries and other mechanical devices to selectively support the bladder neck have been marketed for treating women who have UI with little evidence of their effectiveness. Recently, use of a self-adjusting incontinence pessary was shown to significantly reduce UI, was easy for women to use, and had a 76% continuation rate at 1 year.[70] Surgical intervention is indicated when conservative measures have failed and the patient wishes further treatment to achieve continence. Retropubic urethropexy procedures have long-term success rates consistently reported in the 80% to 96% range and are clearly superior to other procedures.[71] The use of tension-free tape has become popular and allows for a less invasive procedure. This procedure uses a meshlike tape that is placed under the urethra like a sling to keep it in its normal position. The tape is inserted through small incisions in the lower abdomen and vaginal wall, and no sutures are required to hold the tape in place. A substantial proportion of women still have some degree of urinary incontinence 4 to 8 years after surgery, but in most cases, the severity of UI is not bothersome.[65,72,73]

A minimally invasive approach to treatment of UI is by way of periurethral injection. The Food and Drug Administration (FDA) has approved two injectable agents for this purpose, glutaraldehyde cross-linked bovine collagen (Contigen Bard Collagen Implant, C.R. Bard, Inc., Covington, Georgia), and carbon-coated beads (Durasphere, Advanced Uroscience, Inc., St. Paul, Minnesota). Both agents typically require multiple treatment sessions to achieve cure. Long-term outcomes after periurethral injections warrant further and more rigorous study.

Urge and mixed incontinence

Nonpharmacologic therapy is recommended for patients who have overactive bladder syndrome and is the foundation of treatment of this condition. Pelvic floor muscle training and bladder training have been proved to be effective strategies and in motivated patients can be more effective than medication.[74] Bladder training is based on keeping the bladder volume low by encouraging frequent voiding and voluntary effort to inhibit detrusor contraction. The patient is instructed to void at scheduled intervals regardless of urge or whether or not she has just been incontinent. She is instructed to suppress urges between scheduled voids using relaxation techniques. Timed voluntary voiding begins with the shortest interval between voids based on a voiding diary or every 2 hours. Once the woman has achieved 2 days without incontinence, the time between scheduled voids is increased by 30 minutes until she is able to void every 3 to 4 hours. Although not proved, it may be reasonable to eliminate alcoholic beverages, carbonated beverages (with or without caffeine), coffee or tea (with or without caffeine), tomatoes, spicy foods, artificial sweetener, chocolate, corn syrup, sugar, or honey to see if these dietary modifications are helpful in treating incontinence.

The anticholinergics tolterodine and oxybutynin are well established in the management of urge incontinence and overactive bladder syndrome. Trospium, a newer agent, is less able to cross the blood–brain barrier into the central nervous system. This feature has not been shown to minimize centrally mediated side effects, including dizziness, drowsiness, and cognitive impairment, as initially suggested.[75] It is better tolerated than immediate-release oxybutynin causing a lower incidence of dry mouth.[75–77]

Solifenacin and darifenacin are more selective for the bladder than older agents. Trials have shown that these newer agents decrease the frequency of incontinence episodes, the number of voids per day, and the number and severity of urgency episodes compared with placebo.[78] Head-to-head trials comparing the efficacy and tolerability of newer options to older medications are lacking.

Unconventional approaches to the treatment of UI include neuromodulation, botulinum toxin injection, and acupuncture. Small studies suggest that sacral neuromodulation may be an effective therapy for UI with a positive effect on quality of life.[65,79] A small case series suggests that intradetrusor botulinum-A toxin injections may be an effective option in patients who have severe overactive bladder resistant to conventional treatments.[80] A randomized controlled trial of acupuncture four times weekly showed significant improvements in bladder capacity, urgency, frequency, and quality-of-life scores in treated women as compared with women who received sham treatments.[81]

PAINFUL BLADDER SYNDROME/INTERSTITIAL CYSTITIS

Urinary symptoms suggestive of cystitis may occur in the absence of an identifiable infection. This phenomenon eventually became known as interstitial cystitis (IC). The traditional definition of IC is a chronic sterile inflammatory disease of the bladder. On the other hand, painful bladder syndrome (PBS) is defined as a "complaint of suprapubic pain related to bladder filling, accompanied by other symptoms such as increased day- and nighttime frequency, in the absence of proven urinary infection or other obvious pathology."[82] Because these two definitions overlap, the International Continence Society prefers to use the term painful bladder syndrome/interstitial cystitis (PBS/IC) to describe this constellation of symptoms. There is not universal consensus on this terminology, however.

Epidemiology and Economic Impact

Prevalence studies have been difficult to perform because of an evolving understanding of the disease processes involved in PBS/IC. A current estimate is that approximately 1 in 500 adult women in the United States have IC.[83] Experts believe that the disease is markedly underdiagnosed and that most recognized cases represent the severe or advanced end of the spectrum of disease.[84] Diagnosis is often 4 to 7 years after symptom onset and after consulting multiple physicians.[85] The medical costs associated with PBS/IC are high. In a managed care population studied from 1998 to 2003, the average health care expenditure was nearly $4000 higher among patients who had a diagnosis of IC than for age-matched controls, primarily because of costs of outpatient services and medications.[86]

Pathophysiology

Our understanding of the pathophysiology of PBS/IC has evolved rapidly over the last decade, promising important advances in diagnosis and treatment. Central to this evolution has been a growing recognition of the importance of the role of the bladder's epithelium, or urothelium, in the protection of the bladder.[87] The term lower urinary epithelial dysfunction has been proposed to replace IC. This term is inclusive, applicable also to men in whom the same pathophysiology results in chronic prostatic pain and chronic noninfectious urethritis of both sexes.[87]

Bladder mucous is produced by the urothelium and is composed of glucosaminoglycans and proteoglycans, which provide a protective coating. Disruption of this barrier seems to be the central feature of the pathophysiology of classical interstitial cystitis leading to a permeability defect in the epithelium.[87] Toxins in the urine are then able to penetrate the bladder wall. A lack of protective mucous in the bladder allows an increase in potassium concentration from normal level of about 4 MEq/L to more than 24 mEq/L, which is sufficient to depolarize nerves and muscle fibers.

Numerous pathways have been proposed to lead to a functional defect in the urothelium. Recently, research has shown that an abundant protein in the urine, Tamm-Horsfall protein, binds toxic cations, including potassium. A primary defect in the quantity or function of this protein could be an initiating factor in some individuals who have PBS/IC. Patients who have PBS/IC often have associated allergic and immunologic disorders. Some patients may have autoimmune mechanisms involved in their PBS/IC, but causative links have not been established.

A consistent finding in patients who have IC is an increase in mast cell numbers and activation.[88] Mast cell degranulation releases histamine, cytokines, and other inflammatory mediators. Mast cell activation by urine solutes can lead to a vicious cycle of afferent nerve activation and further mast cell stimulation.[89] Neural up-regulation then contributes to the chronicity of bladder pain and urinary urgency and frequency.[89]

Neurogenic inflammation may be the primary disorder in some patients who have bladder pain whose bladders are normal in appearance and have good capacity.[89] IC shares many features with other chronic nonmalignant visceral pain syndromes. Different insults can lead to chronic visceral pain, and multiple pain mechanisms may coexist in one individual. The diffuse painful sensation in the pelvis that is often observed in PBS/IC can be explained by extensive convergence of visceral afferent input on the spinal cord with overlap of projections over adjacent visceral organs.[90]

Clinical Presentation

Two consensus groups that met in 2003 and 2004 recommended making the diagnosis of PBS/IC based on typical signs and symptoms and the exclusion of obvious or confusable diseases, especially infections and carcinoma.[91,92] Both groups agreed that the diagnostic criteria published in 1988 by National Institutes of Diabetes and Digestive and Kidney Disease (NIDDK) should be superseded. The NIDDK criteria require the presence of "classic" findings on cystoscopy of granulation tissue, or glomerulations, and/or Hunner patches. These findings were developed for research purposes rather than for clinical diagnostic purposes and are now believed to represent severe and advanced disease.[91]

The typical symptoms of PBS/IC are pelvic pain and urinary urgency or frequency. Pain or pressure discomfort is required to make the diagnosis.[93] Diagnosis is aided by the use of a validated questionnaire. The most useful tool seems to be the Pelvic Pain and Urgency/Frequency Patient Symptom (PUF) Scale (**Fig. 2**). Scoring ranges from 1 to 35 with a score of 15 considered sufficient for a trial of therapy.

Pain with PBS/IC is most often localized to the suprapubic, pubic, vaginal, and genital areas, but can be located anywhere from the waist to the upper thighs, front or back. Dyspareunia is common both within the introitus and vagina, and with deep penetration. Chronic pelvic pain is often the dominant feature. In one recent study, 80% of women who had chronic pelvic pain had a positive potassium stress test (described later) suggestive of a diagnosis of IC.[94]

Urinary frequency is defined as at least eight voids within 24 hours. Many women may not realize that they are voiding that frequently, so a voiding diary can help to accurately determine frequency. Low-volume and frequent voids up to 25 times daily may not be unusual. Symptom flares may be associated with seasonal allergies, the premenstrual phase of cycles, sexual activity, and physical or emotional stress. Most women diagnosed with IC by NIDDK criteria report worse pain after consumption of certain foods or beverages, most commonly coffee, tea, soda, alcoholic beverages, citrus fruits and juices, artificial sweeteners, and hot peppers.[95] The most common physical findings are suprapubic tenderness and anterior vaginal wall tenderness.[96] Physical examination may reveal pelvic floor muscle spasms, detected as tender ridges at the 5 and 7 o'clock positions.[97]

Patient's name:_____ Today's date: _____

Please circle the answer that best describes how you feel for each question.

		0	1	2	3	4	SYMPTOM SCORE	BOTHER SCORE
1	How many times do you go to the bathroom during the day?	3–6	7–10	11–14	15–19	20+		
2	a. How many times do you go to the bathroom at night?	0	1	2	3	4+		
	b. If you get up at night to go to the bathroom, does it bother you?	Never bothers	Occasionally	Usually	Always			
3	Are you currently sexually active. YES _____ NO_____							
4	a. If you are sexually active, do you now or have you ever had pain or symptoms during or after sexual activity?	Never	Occasionally	Usually	Always			
	b. If you have pain, does it make you avoid sexual activity?	Never	Occasionally	Usually	Always			
5	Do you have pain associated with your bladder or in your pelvis (vagina, labia, lower abdomen, urethra, perineum, penis, testes or scrotum)?	Never	Occasionally	Usually	Always			
6	a. If you have pain, is it usually		Mild	Moderate	Severe			
	b. Does your pain bother you?	Never	Occasionally	Usually	Always			
7	Do you still have urgency after you go to the bathroom?	Never	Occasionally	Usually	Always			
8	a. If you have urgency, is it usually		Mild	Moderate	Severe			
	b. Does your urgency bother you?	Never	Occasionally	Usually	Always			
	SYMPTOM SCORE (1, 2a, 4a, 5, 6a, 7, 8a)							
	BOTHER SCORE (2b, 4b, 6b, 8b)							
	TOTAL SCORE (Symptom Score + Bother Score) =							

Total score ranges are from 1 to 35. A total score of 10–14 = 74% likelihood of positive PST; 15–19 = 76%; 20+ = 91% potassium positive

Fig. 2. The Pelvic Pain and Urgency/Frequency Patient Symptom (PUF) scale. (*Courtesy of* C. Lowell Parsons, MD, University of California, San Diego, CA.)

Diagnostic Testing

Cystoscopy with hydrodistention

The value of cystoscopy with hydrodistention in the diagnosis and management of BPS/IC is currently debated. In the diagnostic evaluation, cystoscopy is indicated principally to rule out other intravesical pathology, including bladder cancer, especially when gross or microscopic hematuria is present. Cystoscopy is unremarkable in nearly one half of patients who have symptoms consistent with PBS/IC. The presence of glomerulations and severely reduced bladder volume indicate severe disease. A Hunner patch or ulcer is associated with the most severe cases and is not a true ulcer. It is a distinctive inflammatory lesion with a deep rupture through the mucosa and submucosa visible on hydrodistention of the bladder. It appears as a reddened area with blood vessels radiating from a central scar covered by a coagulum and petechial oozing of blood from the margins.[93]

Assessment of bladder capacity can be useful for prognosis and treatment selection. Normal adult bladder capacity is approximately 1150 mL, with an average capacity of approximately one half of normal in patients who have classic IC. Hydrodistention has also been used as a treatment modality, but long-term efficacy has not been demonstrated. Biopsies are not routinely performed during cystoscopy at present, but may become more useful to direct therapy in the future, as specific pathologic abnormalities become more thoroughly understood.

Potassium sensitivity test and intravesical anesthesia challenge

A solution of potassium (40 mEq KCl in 40 mL water) can be instilled into the bladder constituting a potassium sensitivity test (PST). A positive result is defined as an increase in reported pain providing evidence that the urothelium is permeable. False negative results may be attributable to severe or advanced disease incapable of increase in pain, or recent treatments, including narcotic medications. An anesthetic bladder challenge may be used following PST or separately from PST. An anesthetic solution instilled into the bladder that provides a pain relief response differentiates pain of bladder origin from other sources of pelvic pain.

Therapy

Multimodal medical treatment

Many therapies have been reported to provide symptomatic relief for patients with PBS/IC with scant evidence of effectiveness based on randomized controlled trials. A promising approach known as multimodal medical treatment has been proposed by some experts to be the first-line approach to PBS/IC.[97] It consists of three components to address different aspects of the pathologic process (**Box 2**). Randomized, controlled trials of this approach are lacking to date.

Other pharmacologic and herbal therapies

Cyclosporine and prednisone have been used in uncontrolled trials to treat PBS/IC with observed benefits. The rationale for their use is that many women have autoantibodies to the uroepithelium and other autoimmune disorders. Many other oral

---

Box 2
Multimodal treatment of painful bladder syndrome/interstitial cystitis

To restore epithelial function

Oral pentosan polysulfate sodium (PPS) 300–400 mg daily in two or three divided doses, only FDA-approved treatment

And/or intravesical heparin 40,000 IU in 10 mL water (buffered lidocaine can be added), usually used three times a week for 2 weeks, but in severe cases women can learn to self-administer and use up to three times daily

To prevent mast cell activation

Hydroxyzine 10–25 mg at bedtime, can be gradually increased up to 100 mg if needed

To inhibit neural activation

Tricyclic antidepressant, amitriptyline or nortriptyline 10–25 mg at bedtime, can be increased gradually up to 75–100 mg if needed

Consider gabapentin or topiramate if anticholinergic effects of tricyclics are problematic

From Moldwin RM, Evans RJ, Stanford EJ, et al. Rational approaches to the treatment of patients with interstitial cystitis. Urology 2007;69(4 Suppl):73–81; with permission.

medications have been used that do not address the pathophysiologic process directly, including cimetidine,[98] alpha-blockers, benzodiazepines, other muscle relaxants, such as cyclobenzaprine, and narcotics. Herbal therapies with beneficial effects in uncontrolled trials include chondroitin, the bioflavonoid quercetin, and aloe vera. Chondroitin and quercetin act synergistically to inhibit mast cell activation.[88]

Intravesical instillations and procedures
Pentosan 100 mg dissolved in water can be used in three instillations per week for 2 to 3 weeks, or up to three times daily by self-administration for severe cases. Pentosan can be used simultaneously by both oral and intravesical routes.[99] Dimethylsulfoxide is also approved by the FDA for intravesical treatment of IC. The usual regimen is weekly instillations for 6 to 8 weeks followed by maintenance treatment every 2 weeks for 3 to 12 months, used at concentration of 50%, but some authors recommend a concentration of 25%.[82]

Hyaluronic acid is used in Europe and Canada, but is not FDA approved in the United States. Uncontrolled studies have shown significant decrease in pain and increase in voiding volume.[100] Bacille Calmette-Guerin is under investigation currently, but early results suggest that it is probably not a viable option with a relatively poor risk-benefit ratio.

Nonpharmacologic therapies
Nonpharmacologic therapies for the treatment of IC include sacral or pudendal nerve stimulation, dietary modification, physical therapy (for pelvic floor dysfunction), and behavior modification. Promising among these is pudendal nerve stimulation; a recent randomized controlled trial demonstrated excellent results versus sacral nerve stimulation with an overall mean symptom reduction of 59%.[101] Cystectomy with urinary diversion is reserved for severe refractory cases.

The last decade has provided important advances in our understanding of the pathophysiology of PBS/IC, yet many questions remain. Current basic and clinical research is ongoing. A current European study aims to address issues regarding the value of cystoscopy and biopsies in the management of PBS/IC. Several potential urinary biomarkers are also being tested for use in the diagnostic or therapeutic evaluation of PBS/IC. Randomized controlled trials of therapy for PBS/IC are needed.

REFERENCES

1. Schappert SM. Ambulatory care visits to physician offices, hospital outpatient department, and emergency departments: United States, 1997. Vital Health Stat 1999;13:1–39, i–iv.
2. Rosenberg M. Pharmacoeconomics of treating uncomplicated urinary tract infections. Int J Antimicrob Agents 1999;11(3–4):247–51 [discussion 261–4].
3. Foxman B, Barlow R, D'Arcy H, et al. Urinary tract infection: self-reported incidence and associated costs. Ann Epidemiol 2000;10(8):509–15.
4. Hooton TM, Scholes D, Hughes JP, et al. A prospective study of risk factors for symptomatic urinary tract infection in young women. N Engl J Med 1996;335(7):468–74.
5. Moreno E, Andreu A, Perez T, et al. Relationship between Escherichia coli strains causing urinary tract infection in women and the dominant faecal flora of the same hosts. Epidemiol Infect 2006;134(5):1015–23.
6. Ronald A. The etiology of urinary tract infection: traditional and emerging pathogens. Am J Med 2002;113(Suppl 1A):14S–9S.

7. Gupta K, Scholes D, Stamm WE. Increasing prevalence of antimicrobial resistance among uropathogens causing acute uncomplicated cystitis in women. JAMA 1999;281(8):736–8.

8. Scholes D, Hooton TM, Roberts PL, et al. Risk factors for recurrent urinary tract infection in young women. J Infect Dis 2000;182(4):1177–82.

9. Hooton TM, Hillier S, Johnson C, et al. Escherichia coli bacteriuria and contraceptive method. JAMA 1991;265(1):64–9.

10. Sheinfeld J, Schaeffer AJ, Cordon-Cardo C, et al. Association of the Lewis blood-group phenotype with recurrent urinary tract infections in women. N Engl J Med 1989;320(12):773–7.

11. Perrotta C, Aznar M, Mejia R, et al. Oestrogens for preventing recurrent urinary tract infection in postmenopausal women. Cochrane Database of Systematic Reviews (Online) 2008;(2):CD005131.

12. Moore EE, Jackson SL, Boyko EJ, et al. Urinary incontinence and urinary tract infection: temporal relationships in postmenopausal women. Obstet Gynecol 2008;111(2 Pt 1):317–23.

13. Bent S, Nallamothu BK, Simel DL, et al. Does this woman have an acute uncomplicated urinary tract infection? JAMA 2002;287(20):2701–10.

14. Hurlbut TA 3rd, Littenberg B. The diagnostic accuracy of rapid dipstick tests to predict urinary tract infection. Am J Clin Pathol 1991;96(5):582–8.

15. Sultana RV, Zalstein S, Cameron P, et al. Dipstick urinalysis and the accuracy of the clinical diagnosis of urinary tract infection. J Emerg Med 2001;20(1):13–9.

16. Fenwick EA, Briggs AH, Hawke CI. Management of urinary tract infection in general practice: a cost-effectiveness analysis. Br J Gen Pract 2000;50(457):635–9.

17. Car J. Urinary tract infections in women: diagnosis and management in primary care. BMJ 2006;332(7533):94–7.

18. Kunin CM, White LV, Hua TH. A reassessment of the importance of "low-count" bacteriuria in young women with acute urinary symptoms. Ann Intern Med 1993;119(6):454–60.

19. Papanicolaou N, Pfister RC. Acute renal infections. Radiol Clin North Am 1996;34(5):965–95.

20. Johnson JR, Vincent LM, Wang K, et al. Renal ultrasonographic correlates of acute pyelonephritis. Clin Infect Dis 1992;14(1):15–22.

21. Warren JW, Abrutyn E, Hebel JR, et al. Guidelines for antimicrobial treatment of uncomplicated acute bacterial cystitis and acute pyelonephritis in women. Infectious Diseases Society of America (IDSA). Clin Infect Dis 1999;29(4):745–58.

22. Anderson VR, Perry CM. Pentosan polysulfate: a review of its use in the relief of bladder pain or discomfort in interstitial cystitis. Drugs 2006;66(6):821–35.

23. Kahan NR, Chinitz DP, Waitman D, et al. Empiric treatment of uncomplicated urinary tract infection with fluoroquinolones in older women in Israel: another lost treatment option? Ann Pharmacother 2006;40(12):2223–7.

24. Nicolle L, Anderson PAM, Conly J. Uncomplicated urinary tract infection in women. Current practice and the effect of antibiotic resistance on empiric treatment. Can Fam Physician 2006;52:612–8.

25. Gupta K, Hooton TM, Roberts PL, et al. Short-course nitrofurantoin for the treatment of acute uncomplicated cystitis in women. Arch Intern Med 2007;167(20):2207–12.

26. Hooton TM, Winter C, Tiu F, et al. Randomized comparative trial and cost analysis of 3-day antimicrobial regimens for treatment of acute cystitis in women. JAMA 1995;273(1):41–5.

27. Gupta K, Hooton TM, Stamm WE. Increasing antimicrobial resistance and the management of uncomplicated community-acquired urinary tract infections. Ann Intern Med 2001;135(1):41–50.
28. Manges AR, Johnson JR, Foxman B, et al. Widespread distribution of urinary tract infections caused by a multidrug-resistant Escherichia coli clonal group. N Engl J Med 2001;345(14):1007–13.
29. Pinson AG, Philbrick JT, Lindbeck GH, et al. ED management of acute pyelonephritis in women: a cohort study. Am J Emerg Med 1994;12(3):271–8.
30. Lowe FC, Fagelman E. Cranberry juice and urinary tract infections: what is the evidence? Urology 2001;57(3):407–13.
31. Stapleton A, Latham RH, Johnson C, et al. Postcoital antimicrobial prophylaxis for recurrent urinary tract infection. A randomized, double-blind, placebo-controlled trial. JAMA 1990;264(6):703–6.
32. Stapleton A. Urinary tract infections in patients with diabetes. Am J Med 2002; 113(Suppl 1A):80S–4S.
33. Dean NM, Ellis G, Wilson PD, et al. Laparoscopic colposuspension for urinary incontinence in women. Cochrane Database Syst Rev 2006;(3):CD002239.
34. Moehrer B, Hextall A, Jackson S. Oestrogens for urinary incontinence in women. Cochrane Database Syst Rev 2003;(2):CD001405.
35. Gibbs CF, Johnson TM 2nd, Ouslander JG, et al. Office management of geriatric urinary incontinence. Am J Med 2007;120(3):211–20.
36. Nygaard I, Turvey C, Burns TL, et al. Urinary incontinence and depression in middle-aged United States women. Obstet Gynecol 2003;101(1):149–56.
37. Melville JL, Newton K, Fan MY, et al. Health care discussions and treatment for urinary incontinence in U.S. women. Am J Obstet Gynecol 2006;194(3):729–37.
38. Hannestad YS, Rortveit G, Hunskaar S. Help-seeking and associated factors in female urinary incontinence. The Norwegian EPINCONT Study. Epidemiology of Incontinence in the County of Nord-Trondelag. Scand J Prim Health Care 2002;20(2):102–7.
39. Ricci JA, Baggish JS, Hunt TL, et al. Coping strategies and health care-seeking behavior in a US national sample of adults with symptoms suggestive of overactive bladder. Clin Ther 2001;23(8):1245–59.
40. Roberts RO, Jacobsen SJ, Rhodes T, et al. Urinary incontinence in a community-based cohort: prevalence and healthcare-seeking. J Am Geriatr Soc 1998;46(4): 467–72.
41. Stoddart H, Donovan J, Whitley E, et al. Urinary incontinence in older people in the community: a neglected problem? Br J Gen Pract 2001;51(468):548–52.
42. Kinchen K, Bump R, JR.Gobier. Prevalence and frequency of stress urinary incontinence among community- dwelling women. Eur Urol 2002;1(1):85.
43. Hunskaar S, Burgio K, Diokno A, et al. Epidemiology and natural history of urinary incontinence. In: Abrams P, et al, editors. Incontinence: 2nd International Consultation on Incontinence, July 1–3, 2001. Plymouth (UK): Health Publication Ltd.; 2002. p. 165–201.
44. Thom D. Variation in estimates of urinary incontinence prevalence in the community: effects of differences in definition, population characteristics, and study type. J Am Geriatr Soc 1998;46(4):473–80.
45. Wilson L, Brown JS, Shin GP, et al. Annual direct cost of urinary incontinence. Obstet Gynecol 2001;98(3):398–406.
46. Subak LL, Brown JS, Kraus SR, et al. The "costs" of urinary incontinence for women. Obstet Gynecol 2006;107(4):908–16.
47. Holroyd-Leduc JM, Straus SE. Management of urinary incontinence in women: clinical applications. JAMA 2004;291(8):996–9.

48. Barker LR, Burton JR, Zieve PD. Principles of ambulatory medicine. 6th edition. Philadelphia: Lippincott Williams & Wilkins; 2003.
49. Abrams P, Cardozo L, Fall M, et al. The standardisation of terminology of lower urinary tract function: report from the standardisation sub-committee of the International Continence Society. Neurourol Urodyn 2002;21(2):167–78.
50. Culligan PJ, Heit M. Urinary incontinence in women: evaluation and management. Am Fam Physician 2000;62(11):2433–44, 2447, 2452.
51. Holroyd-Leduc JM, Tannenbaum C, Thorpe KE, et al. What type of urinary incontinence does this woman have? JAMA 2008;299(12):1446–56.
52. Bradley CS, Rovner ES, Morgan MA, et al. A new questionnaire for urinary incontinence diagnosis in women: development and testing. Am J Obstet Gynecol 2005;192(1):66–73.
53. Brown JS, Bradley CS, Subak LL, et al. The sensitivity and specificity of a simple test to distinguish between urge and stress urinary incontinence. Ann Intern Med 2006;144(10):715–23.
54. Urinary incontinence in women. Obstet Gynecol 2005;105(6):1533–45.
55. Nice. The management of urinary incontinence in women. Available at: www.nice.org.uk/Guidance/CG40; 2006 [cited]. Accessed August 27, 2008.
56. Fantl J, Newman D, Colling J. Urinary incontinence in adults: acute and chronic management. 1996: Rockville, MD.
57. McKertich K. Urinary incontinence—assessment in women: stress, urge or both? Aust Fam Physician 2008;37(3):112–7.
58. Weidner AC, Myers ER, Visco AG, et al. Which women with stress incontinence require urodynamic evaluation? Am J Obstet Gynecol 2001;184(2):20–7.
59. Nygaard IE, Heit M. Stress urinary incontinence. Obstet Gynecol 2004;104(3):607–20.
60. Hannestad YS, Rortveit G, Daltveit AK, et al. Are smoking and other lifestyle factors associated with female urinary incontinence? The Norwegian EPINCONT Study. BJOG 2003;110(3):247–54.
61. Subak LL, Whitcomb E, Shen H, et al. Weight loss: a novel and effective treatment for urinary incontinence. J Urol 2005;174(1):190–5.
62. Wilson P, Bo K, Hay-Smith J. Conservative treatment in women. In: Abrams P, et al, editors. Incontinence. Plymouth UK: Health Publication Ltd; 2002. p. 823–6.
63. Hay-Smith EJ, Dumoulin C. Pelvic floor muscle training versus no treatment, or inactive control treatments, for urinary incontinence in women. Cochrane Database Syst Rev 2006;(1):CD005654.
64. Bo K, Kvarstein B, Nygaard I. Lower urinary tract symptoms and pelvic floor muscle exercise adherence after 15 years. Obstet Gynecol 2005;105(5 Pt 1):999–1005.
65. Shamliyan T, Wyman J, Bliss DZ, et al. Prevention of urinary and fecal incontinence in adults. Evid Rep Technol Assess 2007;161:27–35.
66. Norton PA, Zinner NR, Yalcin I, et al. Duloxetine versus placebo in the treatment of stress urinary incontinence. Am J Obstet Gynecol 2002;187(1):40–8.
67. Bump RC, Norton PA, Zinner NR, et al. Mixed urinary incontinence symptoms: urodynamic findings, incontinence severity, and treatment response. Obstet Gynecol 2003;102(1):76–83.
68. Grady D, Brown JS, Vittinghoff E, et al. Postmenopausal hormones and incontinence: the Heart and Estrogen/Progestin Replacement Study. Obstet Gynecol 2001;97(1):116–20.
69. Nygaard IE, Kreder KJ. Pharmacologic therapy of lower urinary tract dysfunction. Clin Obstet Gynecol 2004;47(1):83–92.

70. Farrell SA, Baydock S, Amir B, et al. Effectiveness of a new self-positioning pessary for the management of urinary incontinence in women. Am J Obstet Gynecol 2007; 196(5):474 e1–8.

71. Leach GE, Dmochowski RR, Appell RA, et al. Female stress urinary incontinence clinical guidelines panel summary report on surgical management of female stress urinary incontinence. The American Urological Association. J Urol 1997; 158(3 Pt 1):875–80.

72. Jelovsek JE, Barber MD, Karram MM, et al. Randomised trial of laparoscopic Burch colposuspension versus tension-free vaginal tape: long-term follow up. BJOG 2008;115(2):219–25 [discussion 225].

73. Liapis A, Bakas P, Creatsas G. Long-term efficacy of tension-free vaginal tape in the management of stress urinary incontinence in women: efficacy at 5- and 7-year follow-up. Int Urogynecol J Pelvic Floor Dysfunct 2008;19(11): 1509–12.

74. Robert M, Ross S, Farrel SA, et al. Conservative management of urinary incontinence. J Obstet Gynaecol Can 2006;28(12):1113–25.

75. Halaska M, Ralph G, Wiedemann A, et al. Controlled, double-blind, multicentre clinical trial to investigate long-term tolerability and efficacy of trospium chloride in patients with detrusor instability. World J Urol 2003;20(6):392–9.

76. Madersbacher H, Stohrer M, Richter R, et al. Trospium chloride versus oxybutynin: a randomized, double-blind, multicentre trial in the treatment of detrusor hyper-reflexia. Br J Urol 1995;75(4):452–6.

77. Haab F, Halasaka M, Klaver M. Favorable efficacy and tolerability with long-term solifenacin treatment support high patient persistence. In: Annual Meeting of the International Continence Society. 2004, August 25–27. Paris France.

78. Epstein BJ, Gums JG, Molina E. Newer agents for the management of overactive bladder. Am Fam Physician 2006;74(12):2061–8.

79. Cappellano F, Bertapelle P, Spinelli M, et al. Quality of life assessment in patients who undergo sacral neuromodulation implantation for urge incontinence: an additional tool for evaluating outcome. J Urol 2001;166(6):2277–80.

80. Schmid DM, Sauermann P, Werner M, et al. Experience with 100 cases treated with botulinum-A toxin injections in the detrusor muscle for idiopathic overactive bladder syndrome refractory to anticholinergics. J Urol 2006;176(1):177–85.

81. Emmons SL, Otto L. Acupuncture for overactive bladder: a randomized controlled trial. Obstet Gynecol 2005;106(1):138–43.

82. Kelada E, Jones A. Interstitial cystitis. Arch Gynecol Obstet 2007;275(4): 223–9.

83. van de Merwe JP, Nordling J, Bouchelouche P, et al. Diagnostic criteria, classification, and nomenclature for painful bladder syndrome/interstitial cystitis: an ESSIC proposal. Eur Urol 2008;53(1):60–7.

84. Clemens JQ, Meenan RT, Rosetti MC, et al. Prevalence and incidence of interstitial cystitis in a managed care population. J Urol 2005;173(1):98–102 [discussion 102].

85. Parsons JK, Kurth K, Sant GR. Epidemiologic issues in interstitial cystitis. Urology 2007;69(4 Suppl):5–8.

86. Driscoll A, Teichman JM. How do patients with interstitial cystitis present? J Urol 2001;166(6):2118–20.

87. Clemens JQ, Meenan RT, O'Keeffe R, et al. Costs of interstitial cystitis in a managed care population. Urology 2008;71(5):776–80 [discussion 780–1].

88. Parsons CL. The role of the urinary epithelium in the pathogenesis of interstitial cystitis/prostatitis/urethritis. Urology 2007;69(4 Suppl):9–16.

89. Sant GR, Kempuraj D, Marchand JE, et al. The mast cell in interstitial cystitis: role in pathophysiology and pathogenesis. Urology 2007;69(4 Suppl):34–40.
90. Nazif O, Teichman JMH, Gebhart GF. Neural upregulation in interstitial cystitis. Urology 2007;69(4 Suppl):24–33.
91. Wesselmann U. Interstitial cystitis: a chronic visceral pain syndrome. Urology 2001;57(6 Suppl 1):32–9.
92. Evans RJ, Sant GR. Current diagnosis of interstitial cystitis: an evolving paradigm. Urology 2007;69(4 Suppl):64–72.
93. van de Merwe JP. Interstitial cystitis and systemic autoimmune diseases. Nature Clinical Practice. Urology 2007;4(9):484–91.
94. Parsons CL, Dell J, Stanford EJ, et al. The prevalence of interstitial cystitis in gynecologic patients with pelvic pain, as detected by intravesical potassium sensitivity. Am J Obstet Gynecol 2002;187(5):1395–400.
95. Shorter B, Lesser M, Moldwin RM, et al. Effect of comestibles on symptoms of interstitial cystitis. J Urol 2007;178(1):145–52.
96. Teichman JMH, Parsons CL. Contemporary clinical presentation of interstitial cystitis. Urology 2007;69(4 Suppl):41–7.
97. Moldwin RM, Evans RJ, Stanford EJ, et al. Rational approaches to the treatment of patients with interstitial cystitis. Urology 2007;69(4 Suppl):73–81.
98. Thilagarajah R, Witherow RO, Walker MM. Oral cimetidine gives effective symptom relief in painful bladder disease: a prospective, randomized, double-blind placebo-controlled trial. BJU Int 2001;87(3):207–12.
99. Davis EL, El Khoudary SR, Talbott EO, et al. Safety and efficacy of the use of intravesical and oral pentosan polysulfate sodium for interstitial cystitis: a randomized double-blind clinical trial. J Urol 2008;179(1):177–85.
100. Porru D, Cervigni M, Nasta L, et al. Results of endovesical hyaluronic acid/chondroitin sulfate in the treatment of interstitial cystitis/painful bladder syndrome. Rev Recent Clin Trials 2008;3(2):126–9.
101. Peters KM, Feber KM, Bennett RC. A prospective, single-blind, randomized crossover trial of sacral vs pudendal nerve stimulation for interstitial cystitis. BJU Int 2007;100(4):835–9.
102. Anger JT, Saigal CS, Litwin MS. The prevalence of urinary incontinence among community dwelling adult women: results from the National Health and Nutrition Examination Survey. J Urol 2006;175(2):601–4.
103. Kuh D, Cardozo L, Hardy R. Urinary incontinence in middle aged women: childhood enuresis and other lifetime risk factors in a British prospective cohort. J Epidemiol Community Health 1999;53(8):453–8.
104. Parazzini F, Chiaffarino F, Lavezzari M, et al. Risk factors for stress, urge or mixed urinary incontinence in Italy. BJOG 2003;110(10):927–33.
105. Bump RC, McClish DK. Cigarette smoking and urinary incontinence in women. Am J Obstet Gynecol 1992;167(5):1213–8.
106. Larsen WI, Yavorek TA. Pelvic organ prolapse and urinary incontinence in nulliparous women at the United States Military Academy. Int Urogynecol J Pelvic Floor Dysfunct 2006;17(3):208–10.
107. Jackson SL, Scholes D, Boyko EJ, et al. Urinary incontinence and diabetes in postmenopausal women. Diabetes Care 2005;28(7):1730–8.
108. Zorn BH, Montgomery H, Pieper K, et al. Urinary incontinence and depression. J Urol 1999;162(1):82–4.

Cardiovascular Disease in Women

Alan M. Weiss, MD, MBA

KEYWORDS

- Cardiovascular disease • Women • Risk • Hypertension
- Hypercholesterolemia • Diabetes

The most important health issue facing women is cardiovascular disease (CVD). CVD has been the leading cause of death in US women every year since 1900 with the exception of 1918, when the United States was overwhelmed by the influenza pandemic. Heart disease and stroke are currently the first and third leading causes, respectively, of death among American women. Together, they account for 41.3% of all deaths in US women.[1] Mortality from CVD and cerebrovascular disease affects nearly half a million women annually, to a greater degree than the next five leading causes of death combined and more than all cancers combined.[2] These statistics equate to a woman dying from CVD in the United States every minute of every day throughout the entire year.

CVD represents a significant financial burden to the US health care system. More than 2.5 million US women are hospitalized for cardiovascular illness each year.[3] In 2001, the cost of hospitalization for CVD among Medicare beneficiaries exceeded $29 billion. In 2005, the costs from heart disease and stroke in the United States were projected to exceed $394 billion: $242 billion attributed to direct health care expenditures and $152 billion for lost productivity resulting from death and disability. That year, nearly $60 billion in health care expenditure was attributed to hypertension alone.[4]

CVD consists of a myriad of thromboembolic diseases, including coronary artery disease (CAD; eg, angina, heart attacks), cerebrovascular disease (eg, strokes, transient ischemic attacks [TIAs]), and congestive heart failure (CHF). The goals of this article are to discuss women's awareness of CVD in addition to its prevalence, incidence, and risk factors, all centered on a discussion of the prevention, diagnosis, and treatment of CVD.

LACK OF AWARENESS

Despite the importance of early recognition and treatment of CVD, women commonly underestimate its dangerous potential. In 1997, a survey by the American Heart Association (AHA) found that only 7% of women considered CVD to be their biggest

Cleveland Clinic Main Campus, Mail Code A91, 9500 Euclid Avenue, Cleveland, OH 44195, USA
E-mail address: weissa1@ccf.org

Prim Care Clin Office Pract 36 (2009) 73–102
doi:10.1016/j.pop.2008.10.012
0095-4543/08/$ – see front matter © 2009 Elsevier Inc. All rights reserved.

mortality and health risk. Less than one third of women claimed awareness that CVD was the greatest killer of US women, because[5] most women surveyed thought that their greatest threat was breast cancer.[4] The truth is that although 1 of every 26 US women dies from breast cancer, CVD kills nearly 1 of every 2 women and 12 times as many women each year as breast cancer.[6]

The AHA survey also examined women's knowledge about CVD and inherent risk factors, in addition to their perception of their own personal risk. The results showed a significant paradox between knowledge and perception, because 40% of women consider themselves "well informed" about heart disease, yet only 13% considered it to be their greatest health risk. Although women thought that they were moderately informed about CVD, specific heart disease risk factors were identified by less than one third of respondents. A larger percentage of "don't know" responses with regard to perception of risk factors came from African-American, Hispanic, and older women. Women in these subgroups were also less likely to answer specific questions about CVD risk and prevention correctly. This result was particularly worrisome, because women in these groups also have a greater prevalence of risk factors for CVD, and are therefore at a higher risk for mortality from heart disease, stroke, and other forms of CVD. African-American women have the highest CVD mortality rate among ethnic minority groups;[6] by not recognizing their risks, they are less likely to take preventive measures and seek treatment.

Based on these sobering statistics, the AHA launched several efforts to raise awareness of the threat of CVD to women and to improve lifestyle behaviors. The AHA's belief was that effective health education efforts should be inherent as a first step in CVD prevention strategies.[7] Campaigns, such as "Go Red for Woman" (www.goredforwomen.org), have set as their goal a 25% reduction in coronary heart disease (CHD) and stroke risk by the year 2010. A follow-up survey in 2003[7] demonstrated a significant improvement in women's knowledge and perception of CVD (**Fig. 1**). By 2003, 46% of women surveyed spontaneously identified heart disease as the leading cause of death in US women, compared with 30% in 1997. The percentage of women citing cancer as leading cause of death correspondingly decreased. African-American, Hispanic, and younger women continued to have a lower awareness of heart disease as their leading cause of death compared with white and older women. Despite the increase in knowledge of heart disease as the primary cause of mortality, the perception of personal mortality risk remained relatively small and only increased from 7% in 1997 to 13% in 2003. Identification of personal risk factors, including smoking, lack of exercise, and high cholesterol, improved but still remained relatively low. Women at the highest risk for heart disease, including African Americans and Hispanics, had the smallest improvement in risk factor identification.[7]

The disconnection between women's awareness of CVD and their perceptions of CVD risk may result from impaired physician-patient communication. Certainly, preventive strategies can be initiated and monitored by health care providers, but the AHA survey also revealed a lack of communication in this regard between women and their physicians. Most women felt comfortable in talking with their physician about preventive health, but 70% of women stated that their physician had never discussed CVD with them.[5] This lack of communication represents a lost opportunity to address preventive strategies and to provide counseling on lifestyle modification.

PREVALENCE AND INCIDENCE

CVD affects 42.1 million American women, or 36.6% of the adult female population (**Fig. 2**). CAD affects 7.2 million American women. The prevalence of CVD increases

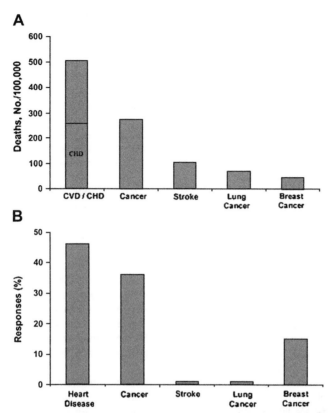

Fig.1. Actual leading cause of death for women (*A*) versus perceived leading causes of death for women (*B*). (*Data from* Mosca L, Ferris A, Fabunmi R, et al. Tracking women's awareness of heart disease. Circulation 2004;109:575.)

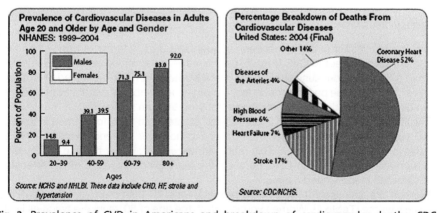

Fig. 2. Prevalence of CVD in Americans and breakdown of cardiovascular deaths. CDC, Centers for Disease Control and Prevention, HF, heart failure; NCHS, National Center for Health Statistics; NHANES, National Health and Nutrition Examination Survey; NHLBI, National Heart, Lung, and Blood Institute. (*From* the National Center for Health Statistics, Centers for Disease Control, Atlanta, GA; and the the National Heart, Lung and Blood Institue, National Institute of Health, Bethesda, MD.)

as women age and affects 36.2% of women aged 45 to 54 years, 52.9% of women aged 55 to 64 years, and more than 68.5% of women aged 65 years and older. Three million women have a history of having had a myocardial infarction, and 3.3 million have had a stroke. Nearly 365,000 American women have heart attacks each year; 83,000 are younger than the age of 65 years, and 9000 are younger than the age of 45 years, with an average age of 70.4 years. Four million women have angina, with approximately 10% being hospitalized each year. CHF affects 2.7 million women and kills nearly 162,000.[8]

The incidence of CVD is age related. In persons younger than the age of 75 years, more CVD events occur in men because of CHD than in women, whereas more CHF events occur in women than in men.[5] Annual rates of the first major cardiovascular event for women track those of men but are delayed by 10 years.[9] The average annual rates of first major cardiovascular events increase from 7 per 1000 men at the age of 35 to 44 years to 68 per 1000 men at the age of 85 to 94 years. The gap narrows with advancing age.

Most deaths attributable to heart disease among adult women occur in the elderly. This situation may arise not only because of the increasing number and severity of medical problems in elderly women but because of their living situations. Elderly women have increased social vulnerability; they are more likely to live alone, live in poverty, have physical disabilities, and lack social support. Because elderly woman often outlive their spouses, they are more likely to be widowed. Socially isolated women have a two- to threefold increased risk for death from heart disease.[8] Living alone has also been linked to being economically disadvantaged, leading to additional barriers to health care services, such as finding rides to appointments and attaining medications.[2]

Some elderly women have a limited ability to leave their homes, which may deter them from regular physician appointments for acute medical problems and preventive services. Self-care limitations, those conditions that last for 6 months or more and make it difficult to attend to personal needs, such as dressing and bathing, may also affect an elderly woman's ability to eat regularly and take prescriptions. In the United States in 1990, 19.8% of elderly women had a mobility or a self-care limitation.[2]

WOMEN VERSUS MEN

There is a significant disparity between women and men in terms of prevalence and treatment with respect to CVD (**Fig. 3**). CVD is no longer considered to be exclusively a "man's disease," because since 1983, more women than men have died of CVD every year.[10,11] Over the past few decades, although the number of deaths from CVD has been declining, the decline has been less for women than for men.

The lifetime risk for CVD is 2 in 3 for men and greater than 1 in 2 for women at the age of 40 years. At an age younger than 55 years, however, the incidence of CHD in women is one third that of men. This ratio normalizes to 1:1 after the age of 75 years. The increasing incidence in CHD parallels the increasing incidence of hypertension and diabetes in the United States.[12]

Women are less likely to be treated properly for CVD than men, and their survival rates are worse (**Table 1**). Women younger than the age of 50 years are twice as likely to die of a heart attack as men the same age.[13] Women are more likely to die within 1 year after a heart attack, are more likely to die after open heart surgery, and are more likely to have a second heart attack within 6 years of their first event. Silent myocardial infarctions, in which blood flow is reduced but a patient exhibits no symptoms, are also more common in women.[14] Per the Framingham Heart Study, a 44-year

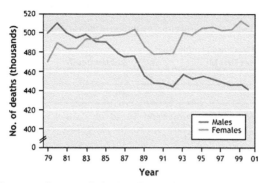

Fig. 3. Cardiovascular mortality trends by gender in the United States. (*From* the National Center for Health Statistics, Centers for Disease Control, Atlanta, GA; and the the National Heart, Lung and Blood Institue, National Institute of Health, Bethesda, MD.)

follow-up study, two thirds of sudden deaths in women occurred in women without any history of symptoms, whereas only 50% of men were similarly affected (**Table 2**).[15]

Several theories have been proposed to explain these gender disparities. Women often present with CVD at an older age than men, and the disease can present in more subtle ways. Women live longer, on average, and have a longer time to develop associated risk factors. Women also wait longer, on average, after developing symptoms of CVD before seeking help, leading to worse outcomes as a result.[16] The combination of older age at presentation, longer delays in seeking medical treatment, and lower intensity of treatments after hospitalization contributes to poorer outcomes in women.[17] Women with an acute myocardial infarction, for example, are less likely to undergo primary angioplasty within 2 hours and are treated less aggressively than men.[16] Women undergo 33% of angioplasties, stents, and bypass surgery; 28% of surgery for implantable defibrillators; and 36% of open heart surgery[18] in the United States. Angioplasty outcomes are equivalent between men and women, yet women have procedural morbidity and mortality three times those of men. Thrombolytics, which need to be given within 12 hours after a myocardial infarction, are less often given to women. These facts are particularly worrisome, because these therapies can reduce mortality and disability if performed in a timely manner.

Although these facts may partially explain the gender disparity, women also seem to be less aggressively treated than men for CVD from the outset. Women are told less often that they have CHD compared with men, leading to fewer steps taken to manage their associated risk factors. In a study of ambulatory treatment of hypertension,

Table 1				
Gender disparity in cardiovascular disease				
	Death Within 1 Year of a First Heart Attack[12]	**Death After Bypass Surgery**	**Heart Attack Within 6 Years of Prior Myocardial Infarction**	**Disabled Because of Heart Failure Within 6 Years**
Women	38%	Twice as likely as men	0	46%
Men	25%	N/A	18%	22%

Abbreviation: N/A, not applicable. Women Heart.
Data from WomenHeart: The National Coalition for Women with Heart Disease. Women & Heart Disease Fact Sheet. Available at: http://www.womenheart.org/resources/cvdfactsheet.cfm. Accessed December 4, 2008.

Table 2
Risks of events within 6 years of a myocardial infarction in men and women

	Second Myocardial Infarction (MI) After First MI	Sudden Death	Disabled With Heart Failure	Stroke
Men	18%	7%	22%	8%
Women	35%	6%	46%	11%

Data from Mosca L, Manson JE, Sutherland SE, et al. Cardiovascular disease in women. A statement for healthcare professionals from the American Heart Association. Circulation 1997;96:2468–82.

women were less likely than men to meet blood pressure control targets (54.0% vs. 58.7%) and elderly women were even less likely (53.4% vs. 63.2%) to do so. There was no significant difference in the use of specific antihypertensive medications or in initiating a new therapy among patients with uncontrolled hypertension. Women less commonly used angiotensin-converting enzyme inhibitors than men and more commonly received diuretics.[19]

Care of women who have established CVD also shows considerable gender bias. Cardiac rehabilitation is underused in myocardial infarction in women, because women were 55% less likely than men to participate.[20] One study of ambulatory post-myocardial infarction care showed that women were less likely to receive an aspirin (20.7% vs. 35.5%), a beta-blocker (31.9% vs. 44.5%), or a statin (28.5% vs. 35.3%), even after having had a heart attack.[19] These results are even more startling when you consider that this study was conducted in a primary care setting in which women saw their primary care providers more often than men.[19]

These health disparities exist not just in the United States but in other countries as well. European women show similar CVD mortality rates as US women. Research across Europe similarly demonstrates that women are less likely than men to undergo revascularization procedures.[21] One can conclude that medical professionals worldwide fail to identify pertinent cardiovascular risk factors and underdiagnose and undertreat women with such risks.[22]

PRESENTATION OF CARDIOVASCULAR DISEASE IN WOMEN

Heart disease presents differently in women than in men, which may explain the differences in treatment patterns. The term *Yentl syndrome* has been coined to describe how a woman with CAD must present like a man to receive the same medical treatment that a man would receive. It was coined after the heroine in Issac Bashevis Singer's short story of a young Jewish girl who disguised herself as a man to study the Talmud at an all-male school in nineteenth century Poland.[23] Chest pain is the most common symptom associated with CVD. Angina symptoms are actually higher among women than men when adjusted for age, but only 20% of myocardial infarctions are preceded by long-standing anginal symptoms. Although women may experience "classic" symptoms, including chest pain, diaphoresis, and shortness of breath, they may also experience more subtle symptoms, such as indigestion, back pain, dizziness, fatigue, and numbness (**Fig. 4**; **Table 3**).[24]

These differences in presentation may help to explain some of the disparities in CVD outcomes. Physicians may be less likely to consider CVD as part of the differential diagnosis in women with these symptoms, and are therefore less likely to pursue the proper investigation and offer appropriate treatments. Physicians need to have a higher vigilance for CVD when women present with these symptoms.

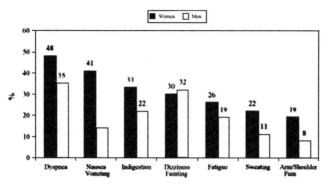

Fig. 4. Differences in symptom presentation among patients without chest pain. (*From* Milner KA, Funk M, Richards S, et al. Gender differences in symptom presentation associated with coronary heart disease. Am J Cardiol 1999;84:398; with permission.)

ASSESSING CARDIOVASCULAR DISEASE RISK

There are several well-recognized risk factors for CVD in women. Although age and hereditary are not modifiable and untreatable, there is considerable interplay among the other risk factors. For example, women who are more sedentary are more likely to gain weight, leading to an increased risk for developing additional comorbidities, including diabetes, hypertension, and hyperlipidemia. Current guidelines recommend a comprehensive assessment of cardiovascular risk factors. This evaluation should include a complete medical history to identify symptoms of undetected heart disease

Table 3
Gender differences in chest pain and non-chest pain symptoms

Symptoms	Women (n = 90)	Men (n = 127)	Odds Ratio	95% Confidence Interval	P Value
No chest pain	27 (30%)	37 (29%)	1.04	0.58–1.88	0.890
Chest pain symptoms					
Pain in center or left chest	36 (57%)	63 (70%)	0.58	0.30–1.12	0.101
Chest heaviness, pressure, or tightness/squeezing	27 (43%)	27 (30%)			
Non-chest pain symptoms					
Midback pain	12 (13%)	2 (2%)	9.61	2.10–44.11	0.001
Nausea or vomiting	27 (30%)	20 (16%)	2.29	1.19–4.42	0.012
Dyspnea	45 (50%)	45 (35%)	1.82	1.05–3.16	0.032
Palpitations	9 (10%)	4 (3%)	3.42	1.02–11.47	0.036
Indigestion	20 (22%)	15 (12%)	2.13	1.03–4.44	0.040
Fatigue	16 (18%)	12 (9%)	2.07	0.93–4.63	0.071
Arm/shoulder pain	34 (38%)	34 (27%)	1.66	0.93–2.96	0.085
Sweating	27 (30%)	29 (23%)	1.45	0.78–2.67	0.235
Jaw pain	4 (4%)	9 (7%)	0.61	0.18–2.04	0.419
Dizziness/fainting	19 (21%)	23 (18%)	1.21	0.61–2.38	0.581
Neck or throat pain	9 (10%)	11 (8%)	1.17	0.46–2.96	0.737

From Milner K. Gender differences in symptom presentation associated with coronary heart disease. Am J Cardiol 1999;84:398; with permission.

and screening for hypertension, hyperlipidemia, diabetes, and obesity. A family history should identify first-degree relatives with early-onset CVD (younger than the age of 55 years in men and younger than the age of 65 years in women). In women with known hyperlipidemia, a thyroid-stimulating hormone level should be drawn to rule out secondary causes.[25]

Several different models exist to help physicians assess a woman's risk for the development of CVD. One of the more common models, the Framingham Risk Assessment calculator (**Fig. 5**), is based on more than 40 years of data. This model is based on an in-office assessment along with a basic laboratory evaluation comprising a fasting serum lipid panel.

Age	Points
20-34	-7
35-39	-3
40-44	0
45-49	3
50-54	6
55-59	8
60-64	10
65-69	12
70-74	14
75-79	16

Total Cholesterol	Points				
	Age 20-39	Age 40-49	Age 50-59	Age 60-69	Age 70-79
<160	0	0	0	0	0
160-199	4	3	2	1	1
200-239	8	6	4	2	1
240-279	11	8	5	3	2
≥280	13	10	7	4	2

	Points				
	Age 20-39	Age 40-49	Age 50-59	Age 60-69	Age 70-79
Nonsmoker	0	0	0	0	0
Smoker	9	7	4	2	1

HDL (mg/dL)	Points
≥60	-1
50-59	0
40-49	1
<40	2

Systolic BP (mmHg)	If Untreated	If Treated
<120	0	0
120-129	1	3
130-139	2	4
140-159	3	5
≥160	4	6

Point Total	10-Year Risk %
<9	<1
9	1
10	1
11	1
12	1
13	2
14	2
15	3
16	4
17	5
18	6
19	8
20	11
21	14
22	17
23	22
24	27
≥25	≥30

10-Year risk _____%

Fig. 5. Framingham Risk Assessment. BP, blood pressure. (National Institutes of Health. ATP III guidelines at-a-glance quick desk reference. Available at: http://www.nhlbi.nih.gov/guidelines/cholesterol/atglance.pdf. Accessed December 4, 2008.)

Only 20% of women fall into a category of low risk, as defined by systolic blood pressure, serum cholesterol level, body mass index (BMI), presence of diabetes mellitus, and smoking status.[26]

There are some valid concerns regarding the use of the Framingham Risk Assessment calculator, although it remains one of most commonly used risk assessment tools in modern medicine. Up to 20% of heart attacks occur in women without any of the major risk factors studied by the Framingham model, possibly because that model does not inquire about markers of inflammation or heredity, both of which are important in risk-stratifying women for development of CVD.[27] Studies have shown that the Framingham model may overpredict CVD in higher risk groups.[28] Other models, such as the general practice model, based solely on age, systolic blood pressure, smoking status, and self-rated quality of health, may be easier to use and provide similar results.[28]

One large study of women to assess and track CVD risk was the Nurses Health Study (which examined more than 84,000 women free of CVD, cancer, and diabetes over 14 years). Women in this study who were defined as being at low risk had the following characteristics:

Not currently smoking
Had a BMI less than 25
Consumed an average of one-half drink of alcohol per day
Engaged in moderate to vigorous physical activity (including brisk walking) for at least 30 minutes a day
Scored highest in the cohort for consumption of cereal fiber, omega-3 fatty acids, and folate, with a high ratio of intake of polyunsaturated versus saturated fat.[29]

Only 3% of women were in the low-risk category, and they had a relative risk for CVD of 0.17 as compared with other women. Eighty-two percent of the coronary events could be attributed to a lack of adherence to lifestyle guidelines involving diet, exercise, and smoking. The most important risk factor was smoking three quarters of a pack of cigarettes per day or more, with a relative risk of 5.48 as compared with nonsmokers. Smoking 1 to 14 cigarettes per day tripled a woman's risk for having an acute coronary event. In this study, 41% of events were attributable to current smoking. Former smokers had a 1.53 relative risk compared with those women who had never smoked.

Other studies have found similar risk factors in women. The INTERHEART study tracked 15,000 patients, 25% of them being women, with acute myocardial infarctions across 52 countries. Nine factors accounted for 90% of patients' risks, including smoking, dyslipidemia, hypertension, diabetes, abdominal obesity, lack of physical activity, low daily fruit and vegetable consumption, alcohol overconsumption, and a psychosocial index.[30] A meta-analysis of three large trials involving more than 380,000 patients similarly showed that 90% of patients with known CAD have a prior exposure to at least one major risk factor, including hypertension, dyslipidemia, smoking, or diabetes.[31]

PRIMARY AND SECONDARY PREVENTION OF CARDIOVASCULAR DISEASE

The goal of primary prevention is to prevent diseases before they develop. In the case of CVD, primary prevention includes promoting proper dietary habits to lower cholesterol intake, increasing physical activity, and prevention of tobacco use and exposure.[32] Primary prevention also includes optimizing the treatment of hypertension, dyslipidemia, and diabetes. The AHA guidelines emphasize the need for women to participate in at least 30 minutes of moderate intense activity 5 days a week.[33] Aspirin is recommended for women at highest risk, in addition to statins if needed for cholesterol. Lifestyle changes are encouraged to help deal with obesity, including dietary control and exercise.

The AHA defines secondary prevention as "identifying and treating persons with established disease and those at very high risk for developing disease, and treating and rehabilitating patients who have had a heart attack to prevent a second cardiovascular event."[34] In the case of patients who have established or new CVD, aspirin and beta-blockers work equivalently in women as in men for secondary prevention. Beta-blockers reduce mortality by 21%, decrease sudden death by 30%, and lower reinfarction rates by 25%. Aspirin reduces the risk for reinfarction by 25%. Omega-3 fatty acids or supplements are suggested twice a week for women with CAD or three times a week for women with high triglycerides.[34]

HYPERTENSION

High blood pressure is one of the most common and most treatable risk factors for all forms of CVD. There is an age-related increase in the prevalence of hypertension in women and in men. After adolescence, men have a greater prevalence of hypertension than women until 50 to 60 years of age, when the prevalence becomes almost equal.[35] This prevalence differs with ethnicity, because African-American women have the highest prevalence, affecting up to 80% of women older than the age of 60 years (**Figs. 6** and **7**). High blood pressure is more common in women taking oral contraceptives, especially in obese women.

Pharmacologic treatment of hypertension has been shown to decrease the incidence of CVD (**Fig. 8**). Unfortunately, women are less likely to meet their blood pressure targets than men. The reasons for this discrepancy may be similar to why women are less likely to be aggressively treated for CVD in general.[36]

SMOKING

Cigarette smoking remains one the key preventable risk factors for CVD in women. It has been estimated that 50% of myocardial infarctions in middle-aged women are

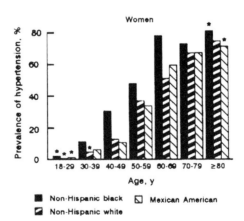

Fig. 6. Prevalence of high blood pressure by age and race/ethnicity for US women. (*From* Burt VL, Whelton P, Roccella EJ, et al. Prevalence of hypertension in the US adult population: results from the Third National Health and Nutrition Examination Survey, 1988–1991. Hypertension 1995;25:305; with permission.)

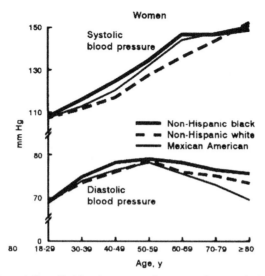

Fig. 7. Mean systolic and diastolic blood pressures by age and race/ethnicity for US women. (*From* Burt VL, Whelton P, Roccella EJ, et al. Prevalence of hypertension in the US adult population: results from the Third National Health and Nutrition Examination Survey, 1988–1991. Hypertension 1995;25:306; with permission.)

attributable to smoking and that women who continue to smoke after a myocardial infarction have a 50% higher risk for recurrent events compared with nonsmokers.[37] Women who smoke tend to develop CAD earlier than nonsmokers, up to 19 years earlier according to some studies.[38] Smoking may also increase a woman's risk for the development of another risk factor for CVD, specifically hypertension.[39] Secondhand smoke is also a risk for CVD. When compared with women who do not smoke and are not exposed to smoke, secondhand smoke increases a woman's risk by 25% to 60%.[40] There is no risk-free level of exposure to secondhand smoke, and even minor regular amounts should be avoided.[41]

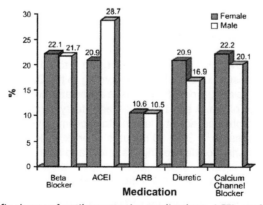

Fig. 8. Use of specific classes of antihypertensive medications. ACEI, angiotensin-converting enzyme inhibitor; ARB, angiotensin II receptor blocker. (*From* Keyhani S, Scobie JV, Hebert PL, et al. Gender disparities in blood pressure control and cardiovascular care in a national sample of ambulatory care visits. Hypertension 2008;51:e48; with permission.)

Smoking is twice as common in adults younger than the age of 35 years as compared with adults older than the age of 60 years. The prevalence of smoking has declined in both genders in the past 20 years.[42] Unfortunately, this decline has been slower among women than among men, because men had a decrease from 51% to 31% and women had a decrease from 41% to 29%.[43] That discrepancy emphasizes the need for physicians to continue aggressive screening and interventions.

The number of cigarettes smoked per day increases cardiovascular risks in a dose-dependent manner. Smoking 1 to 4 or 5 to 14 cigarettes per day was associated with a two- to threefold increase in the risk for fatal coronary heart disease or nonfatal infarction. Smoking more than 25 cigarettes per day increases the relative risk for fatal coronary heart disease to 5.5, nonfatal myocardial infarction to 5.8, and angina pectoris to 2.6. For women smoking more than 45 cigarettes per day, the relative risks for fatal heart disease and nonfatal myocardial infarction were 11 times greater than for women who had never smoked.[42] Overall, cigarette smoking was related to approximately one half of all of types of CVD, with the attributable risk for coronary heart disease caused by current smoking being highest among women who were older and had a parental history of myocardial infarction, a higher relative weight, hypertension, hypercholesterolemia, or diabetes.

Quitting smoking can substantially lower a woman's cardiovascular risk status.[44] That risk starts to decrease within a few months of quitting, with substantial risk reductions after 2 to 3 years.[45] Fifteen years after quitting, a woman's risk returns to that of a nonsmoker.[46] At the same time, the earlier a woman stops smoking, the greater is the minimization of CVD risk. Quitting smoking at the age of 50 years halves the risk for a tobacco-related death, and cessation at the age of 30 years avoids almost all risk.[47] Women who quit at the age of 35 years live up to 7.7 years longer compared with women who continue to smoke.[48] Structured intensive treatment programs have been shown to improve the odds of quitting significantly after a heart attack.[37]

PHYSICAL INACTIVITY

A lack of adequate exercise and a sedentary lifestyle also increase a woman's risk for CVD. This risk is independent of the contribution that being sedentary has on the risk for developing hypertension, high cholesterol, diabetes, and obesity. In the United States, only 28.9% of women get any leisure time physical activity, with minority women disproportionately affected by this problem. Although 39% of white women are sedentary and get no leisure time physical activity, 57% of African-American women, 57% of Hispanic women, and 49% of Asian/Pacific Islander women are similarly affected.[11]

The relative risk for CVD with physical inactivity is 1.5 to 2.4, which is comparable to dyslipidemia, hypertension, or smoking.[49] According to the Centers for Disease Control and Prevention, the annual cost for diseases associated with a lack of physical activity in 2000 was $76 billion. A short-term 8-week lifestyle modification program can successfully increase physical activity, leading to such improvements as a 10–mm Hg decrease in blood pressure.[50] Even 30 minutes of brisk walking can enhance insulin sensitivity, reduce the risk for developing diabetes, and improve dyslipidemia.[51]

OBESITY, ABDOMINAL OBESITY, AND WAIST CIRCUMFERENCE

Obesity is an independent risk factor for CVD in women[52] and represents the second most preventable cause of cardiovascular death after smoking. Obesity is especially important, given its epidemic status in the United States. Since 1991, the prevalence of obesity has increased by 75%; more than two thirds of US adults are now overweight, and more than one half are obese. The percentage of people with a BMI of 25 or greater has increased from 55.9% to 65.1%; the percentage of those with a BMI of 30 or higher has increased from 22.9% to 30.4%; and the percentage of those with a BMI greater than 40, consistent with morbid obesity, has increased from 2.9% to 4.9% (**Table 4**).[53] This increase in prevalence disproportionately affects minority women; whereas 23% of white women are obese, 38% of African-American women and 36% of Mexican-American women are obese.

Accompanying the increase in obesity over the past 15 years is a similar increase in abdominal obesity, a problem that now affects more than one half of US adults. Abdominal obesity can easily be measured by waist circumference or the waist-to-hip ratio. Increases in this measurement have been related to increased insulin resistance, elevated serum cholesterol levels, and an increase in systemic inflammation, all of which may increase the risk for CVD. Studies have also shown that waist circumference by itself is an independent risk factor for CVD independent of BMI and whether or not a woman is overweight or obese.[54]

HYPERCHOLESTEROLEMIA

Dyslipidemia is defined as elevated levels of total cholesterol, low-density lipoprotein cholesterol (LDL-C), or triglycerides, but it can also refer to decreased levels of high-density lipoprotein cholesterol (HDL-C). The association between LDL-C and CVD is well established, and evidence exists that lowering LDL-C can reduce the risk.[55] Given the significance of the issue, it is important to explore the various types of cholesterol in addition to treatment options. The current National Cholesterol Education Program (NCEP) guidelines are listed in **Box 1** and **Tables 5–7**.

One way to remember the statistics about women and cholesterol is to think of it as a rule of "halves." One half of US adult women have elevated cholesterol (50.9% or 57 million). Only one half of women with established CVD are currently taking lipid-lowering medications, indicating that women are undertreated for this condition.[11] In the Heart and Estrogen/Progestin Replacement Study (HERS), a trial of 2763 postmenopausal women investigating the effect of hormone replacement therapy (HRT) on heart disease, one half of women with established CVD were not receiving lipid-modifying medications.[56] Of the women who were prescribed lipid-lowering medications, one half stopped taking their medication after half a year.[57]

The Framingham Heart Study confirmed that low levels of HDL-C are an important predictor of cardiovascular death in women. For every 1-mg/dL increase in HDL-C,

Table 4
Annual cardiovascular disease incidence[a] according to body mass index in Framingham Heart Study adults aged 56 to 75 years: 44-year follow-up

End Point	Age in Years	Men, Body Mass Index (kg/m²)			Women, Body Mass Index (kg/m²)		
		<25	25–29.9	≥30	<25	25–29.9	≥30
CHD	56–65	3.2	4.8	4.4	1.8	2.2	3.4
	66–74	4.6	4.6	6.1	2.1	2.9	3.0
Stroke	56–65	1.5	2.5	2.2	1.0	1.6	2.3
	66–74	2.0	1.9	2.4	1.1	1.9	1.7
CVD	56–65	5.2	6.3	6.5	3.0	3.3	5.0
	66–74	7.9	7.9	9.9	4.5	5.3	6.0

[a] Rates per 1000 per year.
Data from Wilson PWF, Kannel WB. Obesity, diabetes, and risk of cardiovascular disease in the elderly. Am J Geriatr Cardiol 2002;11(2):121.

Box 1
Major risk factors that modify low-density lipoprotein goals

- Cigarette smoking
- Hypertension (blood pressure ≥ 140/90 mm Hg or on antihypertensive medication)
- Low HDL-C (<40 mg/dL)[a]
- Family history of premature CHD (CHD in male first-degree relative <55 years; CHD in female first-degree relative <65 years)
- Age (men ≥45 years; women ≥55 years)

Diabetes is regarded as a CHD risk equivalent.
[a] HDL cholesterol 60 mg/dL or greater counts as a "negative" risk factor; its presence removes one risk factor from the total count.
From National Institutes of Health. ATP III guidelines at-a-glance quick desk reference. Available at: http://www.nhlbi.nih.gov/guidelines/cholesterol/atglance.pdf. Accessed December 4, 2008.

---

there is a 3% decrease in cardiovascular risk. Additional studies have shown that low HDL-C and high triglycerides were better predictors of coronary risk and cardiovascular mortality in women than total cholesterol or LDL-C values.[58] Unfortunately, high levels of HDL-C may not predict CVD in women and do not protect women from it; one retrospective study of women with high HDL showed that they still develop CVD.[59] For that reason, when a women's HDL-C is elevated, physicians may underestimate her cardiovascular risk and symptoms, leading to underdiagnosis and undertreatment.

Two other risk factors for CVD include lipoprotein(a) and homocysteine. It seems that lipoprotein(a) may also be an independent risk factor for CVD. It is unaffected by diet, exercise, and most cholesterol-lowering medications, except niacin.[55] It is still controversial as to whether or not women should be screened for lipoprotein(a) and whether or not such screening adds to accurate risk stratification.

Table 5
Adult Treatment Panel III classification of low-density lipoprotein cholesterol, total cholesterol, and high-density lipoprotein cholesterol

LDL cholesterol	
<100	Optimal
100–129	Near or above optimal
130–159	Borderline high
160–189	High
≥190	Very high
Total cholesterol	
<200	Desirable
200–239	Borderline high
≥240	High
HDL cholesterol	
<40	Low
≥60	High

From National Institutes of Health. ATP III guidelines at-a-glance quick desk reference. Available at: http://www.nhlbi.nih.gov/guidelines/cholesterol/atglance.pdf. Accessed December 4, 2008.

Table 6	
Three categories of risk that modify low-density lipoprotein cholesterol goals	
Risk Category	**Low-Density Lipoprotein Goal (mg/dL)**
CHD and CHD risk equivalents	<100
Multiple (2+) risk factors[a]	<130
0–1 risk factor	<160

[a] Risk factors that modify the LDL are listed in Table 3.
From National Institutes of Health. ATP III guidelines at-a-glance quick desk reference. Available at: http://www.nhlbi.nih.gov/guidelines/cholesterol/atglance.pdf. Accessed December 4, 2008.

Additional controversies surround homocysteine as a modifiable risk factor for CVD (**Fig. 9**). Higher levels of the substance seem to correlate with higher degrees of CVD. Some studies have hypothesized that it may increase oxidative stress, increase endothelial cell dysfunction, and promote thrombogenesis.[60] Although folate has been successfully shown to reduce homocysteine levels,[61] to date, no large trial has successfully proved that supplementation with folate for primary or secondary prevention of CVD has been successful.[62] For that reason, it is still debatable as to whether or not homocysteine is a cause of CVD or simply an indication of its presence.

When faced with patients who have dyslipidemia, most physicians offer a trial of lifestyle modifications, including proper diet and exercise, to address the problem. In this regard, it becomes important for physicians to keep patients educated on the types of fats found in most diets. Saturated fats are found in animal products, such as meat, milk, cheese, and butter. Transfatty acids are created through hydrogenation and are thought to increase LDL-C substantially. Unsaturated fats include monounsaturated and polyunsaturated forms. When eaten in moderation, unsaturated fats can help to lower cholesterol types known to contribute to heart disease and heart attacks. Patients should reduce their intake of saturated fats (less than 7% of total daily calories) and limit total daily intake of cholesterol to less than 200 mg/d. Omega-3–rich foods can reduce triglycerides and increase HDL-C. They have also been shown to reduce sudden death, platelet adhesiveness, and the risk for arrhythmias.[63]

Until recently, women have been largely excluded from primary and secondary prevention trials of dyslipidemia for CVD. Women represented only 23% of all statin trials and 10% of primary prevention statin trials.[64] Women represent just 38% of subjects in cardiovascular studies funded by the National Institutes of Health (excluding single-gender trials).[65] Recent trials have attempted to correct that deficit. One recent study of pravastatin plus diet focused solely on women and followed almost 5400 women over 5 years to study statins as a means of primary prevention. It found that the occurrence of cardiovascular events was lower by 26% to 37% in the pravastatin plus diet group as compared with the diet group alone.[66]

Statins should be considered first-line therapy in helping women to achieve their cholesterol target goals. A meta-analysis of five primary and secondary prevention trials that included 4000 women found an overall risk reduction of 29%.[67] It is important to note that this value varies across individual studies. In the Cholesterol And Recurrent Event (CARE) trial, there was a 46% reduction in coronary events in women treated with pravastatin.[68] The Heart Protection Study (HPS) found an overall protection of major vascular events of 20% in women.[69]

The number needed to treat (NNT) was similar to that in men and women in the secondary prevention trials. The NNT was 176 for coronary heart disease in women older than 55 years of age and 106 for women older than 60 years of age. The NNT for the combined end points of coronary heart disease plus stroke was 109 for women older

Table 7
Summary of coronary events in women in secondary prevention trials with statins

	No. Participants	No. Major Coronary Events		Major Coronary Events by Gender	
		Placebo	Statin	Favors Treatment	Favors Control
Women					
4S	827	91	60		
CARE	576	39	23		
AFCAPS/TexCaps	997	13	7		
LIPID	1516	104	90		
Overall	3916	247	180		
HPS	5082	450	367		
Men					
4S	3617	531	371		
WOSCOPS	6595	248	174		
CARE	3583	235	189		
AFCAPS/TexCaps	5608	170	109		
LIPID	7498	611	467		
Overall	26,901	1795	1310		
HPS	15,454	2135	1666		

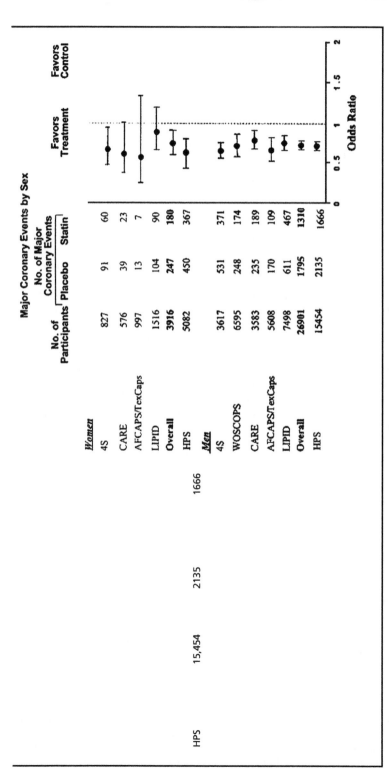

Major Coronary Events by Sex

	No. of Participants	No. of Major Coronary Events	
		Placebo	Statin
Women			
4S	827	91	60
CARE	576	39	23
AFCAPS/TexCaps	997	13	7
LIPID	1516	104	90
Overall	**3916**	**247**	**180**
HPS	5082	450	367
Men			
4S	3617	531	371
WOSCOPS	6595	248	174
CARE	3583	235	189
AFCAPS/TexCaps	5608	170	109
LIPID	7498	611	467
Overall	**26901**	**1795**	**1310**
HPS	15454	2135	1666

Favors Treatment — Favors Control

Odds Ratio: 0, 0.5, 1, 1.5, 2

Abbreviations: AFCAPS/TexCaps, Air Force/Texas Coronary Atherosclerosis Prevention Study; HPS, Heart Protection Study; LIPID, Long-Term Intervention with Pravastatin in Ischemic Disease; 4S, Scandinavian Simvastatin Survivaly Study; WOSCOPS, West Of Scotland COronary Prevention Study.

Adapted from LaRosa JC, He J, Vupputuri S. Effect of statins on risk of coronary disease: a meta-analysis of randomized controlled trials. JAMA 1999;282:2340–2346. Copyright © 1999 American Medical Association.

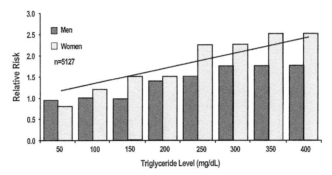

Fig. 9. Risk for CHD by triglyceride level in men and women.

than the age of 55 years and 61 for women older than the age of 60 years.[70] Statins are generally well tolerated, and the US Food and Drug Administration has been asked by manufacturers to allow over-the-counter sales.[71] Although their most common side effects include myopathy and hepatotoxicity, the incidence is low.[72]

Niacin has been shown to lower triglycerides modestly; to increase HDL-C; and, in some patients, to lower LDL-C minimally (**Table 8**). It is recommended for women with low HDL-C and high triglyceride values after an appropriate LDL-C goal has been reached.[25] Facial and truncal flushing are common side effects and are prostaglandin mediated. Avoiding substances that increase prostaglandins, such as caffeine-containing beverages and alcohol, can decrease this side effect. Aspirin taken 30 minutes before taking niacin can minimize these side effects,[73] yet it may also cause gastrointestinal symptoms, hyperuricemia, gout, and hyperglycemia. Niacin combined with a statin may induce myopathy, and these should used together with caution and frequent monitoring.

The fibrates are primarily used to lower triglycerides but can also increase HDL-C and have a modest effect on lowering LDL-C. Studies have proved that they reduce cardiovascular events, but these trials were primarily composed of men.[74] The fibrates are generally well tolerated, yet they carry a minimal risk for gastrointestinal side effects and an increased risk for gallstones. They may interfere with the metabolism of other medications, such as warfarin, because they are mostly protein bound.[75]

It is important that physicians understand the role that nutritional supplements may have in patients treated for high cholesterol. In the United States, up to 21% of adults taking prescription medications are also taking supplements for chronic conditions, including hyperlipidemia.[76] Two of the more common supplements used for this purpose are red yeast rice and garlic. Red yeast rice is the product of yeast grown on rice, and it is served as a dietary staple in some Asian countries. To date, there are no randomized controlled trials of red yeast rice in formulations without lovastatin proving that it lowers cholesterol or prevents CVD.[77] Garlic has also been promoted as a cholesterol-lowering agent; yet, studies have generally failed to confirm its efficacy at lowering LDL-C or improving the risk for CVD.[78]

DIABETES

Diabetes is a significant risk factor for CVD, and its prevalence is increasing in the United States. An estimated 11.5 million women, or 10.2% of all women aged 20 years or older, have diabetes, but 25% of them are unaware that they have it.[79] The risk for CVD is so significant in diabetics that diabetes is considered to be a CVD equivalent.

Table 8
Drugs used for treating dyslipidemia

Drug Class	Agents and Daily Doses	Lipid/Lipoprotein Effects		Side Effects	Contraindications
HMG CoA reductase inhibitors (statins)	Lovastatin (20–80 mg) Pravastatin (20–40 mg) Simvastatin (20–80 mg) Fluvastatin (20–80 mg) Atorvastatin (10–80 mg) Cerivastatin (0.4–0.8 mg)	LDL HDL TG	↓18%–55% ↑5%–15% ↓7%–30%	Myopathy Increased liver Enzymes	Absolute: active or chronic liver disease Relative: concomitant use of certain drugs
Bile acid sequestrants	Cholestyramine (4.16 g) Colestipol (5.20 g) Colesevelam (2.6–3.8 g)	LDL HDL TG	↓15%–30% ↑3%–5% No change or increase	Gastrointestinal distress Constipation Decreased absorption of other drugs	Absolute: dysbeta-lipoproteinemia, TG >400 mg/dL Relative: TG >200 mg/dL
Nicotinic acid	Immediate release (crystalline) nicotinic acid (1.5–3 gm), extended release nicotinic acid (Niaspan; 1.2 g), sustained release nicotinic acid (1–2 g)	LDL HDL TG	↓5%–25% ↑15%–35% ↓20%–50%	Flushing Hyperglycemia Hyperuricemia (or gout) Upper gastrointestinal distress Hepatotoxicity	Absolute: chronic liver disease, severe gout Relative: diabetes, hyperuricemia, peptic ulcer disease
Fibric acids	Gemfibrozil (600 mg BID) Fenofibrate (200 mg) Clofibrate (1000 mg BID)	LDL HDL TG	↓5%–20% ↑10%–20% ↓20%–50%	Dyspepsia Gallstones Myopathy	Absolute: severe renal disease, severe hepatic disease

Abbreviations: CoA, coenzyme A; BID, twice daily; TG, triglycerides.
From National Institutes of Health. ATP III guidelines at-a-glance quick desk Reference. Available at: http://www.nhlbi.nih.gov/guidelines/cholesterol/atglance.pdf. Accessed December 4, 2008.

CVD affects diabetics twice as often as those without diabetes.[80] Two of three diabetics die from heart disease or stroke. Diabetics are two to four times more likely to have a stroke and are two to four times more likely to have a recurrent stroke after their first one compared with nondiabetics. Death from heart disease in women with diabetes has increased 23% over the past 30 years compared with a 27% decrease in women without diabetes.

Women with diabetes are at a greater risk for CVD than men with the same condition,[81] with a risk ratio of 2.4 to 3.5 (**Figs. 10** and **11**). This same gender disparity also relates to survival after a myocardial infarction, in which women with diabetes are less likely to survive than men with the same condition.[12]

Epidemiologic studies have shown a relation between high glycosylated hemoglobin levels and cardiovascular events. The increased risk for CVD is directly related to the degree of hyperglycemia. After adjustment for other risk factors, an increase of 1% in the glycosylated hemoglobin level is associated with an increase of 18% in the risk for cardiovascular events.[82]

One of the most important concerns in women with diabetes is whether or not intensive glycemic control reduces overall CVD risk. The Action in Diabetes and Vascular Disease (ADVANCE) trial assigned 11,140 patients from 20 countries across Asia, Australia, Europe, and North America with type 2 diabetes to undergo standard glucose control or intensive glucose therapy to achieve a glycosylated hemoglobin value of 6.5% or less. Forty-two percent of the trial participants were women. There was no significant improvement in cardiovascular risk with the intensive therapy group.[83] The Action to Control Cardiovascular Risk in Diabetes (ACCORD) trial followed 10,000 patients from North America, randomized to receive intensive therapy (glycosylated hemoglobin less than 6.0%) or standard therapy (glycosylated hemoglobin from 7.0% to 7.9%) (**Fig. 12**). Thirty-eight percent of trial participants were women. The finding of higher mortality in the intensive therapy group led to early termination of the study.[84] The conclusion of both studies is that the goal for glycosylated hemoglobin should stay at 7% for patients who have diabetes.[85]

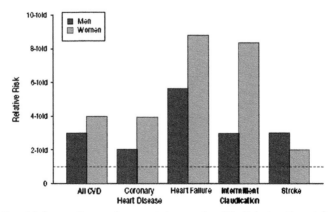

Fig. 10. Relative risk for cardiovascular events in people with diabetes. Except for stroke, the relative risk for CVD associated with diabetes is greater for women than for men. The dashed line represents a relative risk of 1 (ie, relative risk expected of a control group). (*Adapted from* Barrett-Connor E, Giardina EV, Gitt AK, et al. Women and heart disease: the role of diabetes and hyperglycemia. Arch Intern Med 2004;164:935; with permission.)

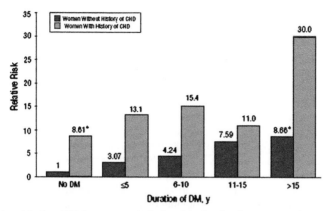

Fig. 11. Relative risks for CHD in women. Relative risks for fatal CHD according to duration of diabetes mellitus (DM) and stratified by a history of CHD. The asterisk indicates that women without a history of CHD who have diabetes for more than 15 years share the relative risk of those with a history of CHD. (*Adapted from* Barrett-Connor E, Giardina EV, Gitt AK, et al. Women and heart disease: the role of diabetes and hyperglycemia. Arch Intern Med 2004;164:936; with permission.)

DIET

A woman's diet can play a key role in the development of many CVD risks, including dyslipidemia, obesity, and hypertension. The American diet tends to be high in fats and carbohydrates, and the average adult now consumes 300 more calories per day than in 1985, adding to weight gain and the risk for obesity and its related CVD risks. It is important that physicians explore aspects of a women's diet to determine the number of servings each day of meat, grains, dairy products, and various fruits and vegetables. Several studies have attempted to investigate diet as a means of lowering CVD risk.

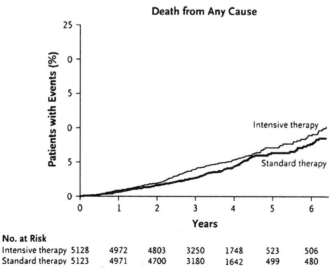

Fig. 12. The Action to Control Cardiovascular Risk in Diabetes (ACCORD) trial. (*From* The Action to Control Cardiovascular Risk in Diabetes Study Group. Effects of intensive glucose lowering in type 2 diabetes. N Engl J Med 2008;358:2554; with permission.)

The Woman's Health Initiative (WHI) had a dietary intervention arm designed to test the effects of a diet low in fat and high in vegetables, fruits, and grains on CHD risk. The trial is the largest long-term randomized trial of dietary intervention. Over an 8.1-year period, the dietary intervention group showed small but significant reductions in weight, waist circumference, diastolic blood pressure, and LDL-C levels. There was a nonsignificant trend toward lower CHD rates in the dietary intervention arm in the later years, which was more pronounced in women without baseline CHD. These results developed even though the study failed in its goal to lower total fat intake by 8.2% (the goal was 20%).[86] Another study followed 3588 men and women older than 65 years of age over an 8.6-year follow-up period to assess CVD risk compared with dietary fiber intake. The study adjusted for age, gender, education, diabetes, tobacco use, physical activity, alcohol intake, and fruit and vegetable fiber consumption. Cereal fiber consumption was found to be inversely associated with incident CVD, with a 21% lower risk in the highest quintile of intake compared with the lowest quintile. Cereal fiber was also found to lower the risk for all strokes, ischemic stroke in particular. Fruit and vegetable fiber intake did not, however, lower risks in this study.[87]

ANTIPLATELET THERAPY

Antiplatelet therapy is essential for the treatment of CVD and usually consists of aspirin as first-line therapy but may also include Plavix or Aggrenox (a fixed-dose combination of aspirin and dipyridamole). Aspirin is quite effective and economic. When discussing aspirin with patients, it is important to distinguish if it is being used for primary or secondary prevention. Until recently, most of the primary prevention studies had been done on men and demonstrated an approximated 32% reduction in the risk for myocardial infarction.[88]

One large primary prevention study of aspirin for CVD was The Women's Health Study (**Fig. 13**). It evaluated the effect of low-dose aspirin (100 mg every other day) versus placebo on nearly 40,000 women who were at least 45 years old. The study monitored these women for 10 years for major cardiovascular events, including

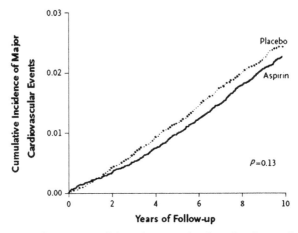

Fig. 13. Cumulative incidence rates of the primary end point of major cardiovascular events (defined as a nonfatal myocardial infarction, a nonfatal stroke, or death from cardiovascular causes). (*From* Ridker PM, Cook NR, Lee IM, et al. A randomized trial of low-dose aspirin in the primary prevention of cardiovascular disease in women. N Engl J Med 2005;352(13):1298; with permission.)

nonfatal myocardial infarction, nonfatal stroke, or death from cardiovascular causes. Overall, aspirin had a 17% risk reduction for first strokes without any significant effect on the risk for fatal or nonfatal myocardial infarction or death from cardiovascular causes. A subgroup analysis of women older than 65 years of age, however, did show a significantly reduced risk for major cardiovascular events (26% risk reduction), ischemic stroke (30% risk reduction), and myocardial infarction (34% risk reduction).[89] Gastrointestinal bleeding was more common in the group that received aspirin. This study confirmed the cost-effectiveness of aspirin in high-risk women, although the data on moderate-risk women remain controversial.[90]

Using aspirin for secondary prevention of heart disease has more established data. A meta-analysis of multiple studies on men and women found that aspirin used for secondary prevention reduced the combined outcome of serious vascular events by approximately one quarter, nonfatal myocardial infarctions by one third, nonfatal strokes by one quarter, and vascular mortality rate by one sixth.[91] Unfortunately, women are less likely than men to be discharged from the hospital on aspirin after an acute myocardial infarction, and less than one half of postmenopausal women with CVD are using aspirin.[92]

The use of clopidogrel as a means of preventing heart disease should also be considered. The Clopidogrel for High Atherothrombotic Risk and Ischemic Stabilization, Management, and Avoidance (CHARISMA) trial examined whether combination therapy of clopidogrel with aspirin provided any therapeutic benefit over aspirin alone in patients at high risk for CVD. Although the combination therapy had a suggestion of benefit in patients who had CAD, it was not found to be significantly more effective than aspirin alone in reducing the rate of myocardial infarction, stroke, or death from cardiovascular causes in patients who did not have CAD. The CHARISMA investigators conclude that dual antiplatelet therapy should not be used in patients without a history of established vascular disease.[93]

HORMONE REPLACEMENT THERAPY

There has been a lot of excitement in the recent past about the potential for HRT as a means to reduce CVD in women. This excitement stemmed from the observation that the incidence of CVD and many of its risk factors increases precipitously after menopause, at a time when estrogen levels decrease significantly. Moreover, HRT has been shown to increase levels of HDL-C and lower levels of LDL-C.[94] Several observational studies in the past seemed to confirm these theories and showed some reduced risk for CHD with the use of HRT.[95]

The WHI and HERS examined the role of HRT to help protect women from CHD. The WHI trial had several treatment arms, including a combined estrogen-progesterone group and an estrogen-only group. The combination arm was stopped early, however, because a midtrial analysis showed a 26% increase in the incidence of breast cancer and a 29% increase in CHD, which were predominantly nonfatal myocardial infarctions, with most occurring during the first year of therapy. The estrogen-only arm of the WHI trial (women with a prior hysterectomy) was terminated because of lack of CVD protection and an increased risk for stroke. The HERS showed a similar increase in CHD events. Both of these trials showed a trend toward a decrease in the relative risk for CHD after several years on hormonal therapy.[86] Based on these results, HRT is not recommended for CVD prevention and may increase the risk for CVD and for ovarian and breast cancer.

TESTING WOMEN FOR CARDIOVASCULAR DISEASE

Testing options for women with suspected CVD are identical to those of men but are not without controversy. These options include exercise stress tests, stress nuclear imaging, stress echocardiography, computed tomographic angiography/electron beam CT, and MRI. Each of these tests has a different sensitivity and specificity for detecting CVD (**Table 9**). Researchers have shown that some of these tests may have poorer diagnostic accuracy in women than in men. Several studies have shown that women with existing heart disease are more likely than men to have a normal electrocardiogram. At the same time, the specificity of exercise stress electrocardiography for CAD is lower in women than in men (64% vs. 74%),[96] while also having a higher false-positive rate.[97] The problem may lie in the fact that women are more likely to have single-vessel disease and are less likely than age-matched men to have triple-vessel disease or atherosclerosis of the left main coronary artery.[98]

According to the AHA, an exercise stress test is not particularly sensitive or specific at detecting single-vessel coronary disease, which is more common in women than in men. At the same time, studies have shown that the Duke Treadmill Score (DTS), the most common scoring system in use in the United States, may, in fact, have diagnostic and prognostic equivalence in both genders.[99] Another study confirmed that the DTS can accurately risk-stratify women for the presence of CVD, especially in younger women with a lower pretest probability of disease. It seems that the test is most useful for excluding CAD (eg, a high negative predictive value) in low-risk women.[99] Currently, exercise stress electrocardiography is recommended for all women who report anginal symptoms and have a normal resting electrocardiogram. When the resting study is abnormal and the history suggests probable or atypical angina, thallium or other perfusion testing is recommended.[100]

CEREBROVASCULAR DISEASE

Stroke is the third leading cause of death in the United States and is the leading cause of disability. On average, someone in the United States has a stroke every 45 seconds, with approximately 30% being new strokes and 70% being recurrent strokes. Of those strokes, 88% are ischemic, 9% are intracerebral hemorrhages, and 3% are subarachnoid hemorrhages. Women have more strokes than men and have higher mortality. The lifetime risk for dying from a stroke is 16% in women compared with 8% in men, and this is possibly related to women's older age and higher comorbidities. Overall, women account for 61.5% of stroke deaths. The ratio of strokes in men to women is related to age and is 1.59 for the age of 65 to 69 years, 1.35 for the age of 70 to 74 years, and 0.74 for the age of 75 years and older. African-American women have twice the stoke risk of white women.[101]

The risks for stroke are similar to those of CVD and include smoking, diabetes, hypertension, and inactivity. Heavy smokers (more than two packs per day) have twice the rate

| Table 9 | | |
| Sensitivity and specificity of stress tests in women | | |
	Sensitivity (%)	Specificity (%)
Stress electrocardiography	61	70
Stress echocardiography	86	90
Nuclear (gated SPECT)	84	90

Abbreviation: SPECT, single photon emission computed tomography.

Data from Mieres JH. Does the Treadmill Test Work in Women? Available at: http://www.cardiosource.com/ExpertOpinions/Programhlts/interviewDetail.asp?interviewID=360. Accessed December 4, 2008.

as compared with light smokers (half a pack per day). After quitting, stroke risk decreases to the level of nonsmokers after 5 years. Diabetics have twice the risk for ischemic strokes compared with nondiabetics. Uncontrolled hypertension increases stroke risk, with a 46% increase in stroke risk for every 7.5–mm Hg increase in diastolic blood pressure.[102] Stroke risk decreases with increasing physical activity. According to the Nurses Health Study, women in the highest quartile of physical activity had a 0.66 relative risk.[103]

The prevalence for transient ischemic attacks increases with age and is 1.6% for the age of 65 to 60 years and 4.1% for the age of 75 to 79 years. Approximately 10% of patients who have a TIA develop a stroke within 90 days. The risk for stroke is 13 to 14 times higher in the first year after a TIA and 7 times higher during the first 5 years. Strokes occurring after a TIA are more common in women older than the age of 60 years, diabetics, women who have focal symptoms of weakness of speech impairment, and women in whom the symptoms last for longer than 10 minutes.[104]

SUMMARY

CVD remains the most important health issue facing women and continues to be their number one cause of morbidity and mortality. Women are disproportionately affected by CVD compared with men. It is diagnosed less often and treated less aggressively in the inpatient and outpatient settings; as a result, women have poorer outcomes. It is therefore imperative that physicians take steps to screen women for the risks associated with CVD and actively education them on primary and secondary prevention.

REFERENCES

1. American Heart Association. Heart disease and stroke statistics—2003, update. Available at: http://www.americanheart.org/downloadable/heart. Accessed December 1, 2008.
2. Rogers CC. Changes in the social and economic status of women by metro-nonmetro residence. Available at: http://www.ers.usda.gov/publications/aib732/AIB732a.PDF. Accessed December 1, 2008.
3. Wenger NK, Speroff L, Packard B. Cardiovascular health and disease in women. N Engl J Med 1993;329:247–56.
4. CDC. Preventing heart disease and strokes. Available at: http://www.cdc.gov/nccdphp/publications/factsheets/Prevention/dhdsp.htm. Accessed December 1, 2008.
5. Mosca L, Jones WK, King KB, et al. Awareness, perception, and knowledge of heart disease risk and prevention among women in the United States. Arch Fam Med 2000;9:506–15.
6. Mosca L, Ferris A, Fabunmi R. Tracking women's awareness of heart disease. Circulation 2004;109:573–9.
7. Jackson SA, Burke GL. Heart disease prevention in US women: there is more work to be done. Arch Fam Med 2000;9(6):516–7.
8. Kaplan GA, Salonen JT, Cohen RD, et al. Social connections and mortality from all causes and from cardiovascular disease: prospective evidence from eastern Finland. Am J Epidemiol 1988;128(2):370–80.
9. Bello N, Mosca L. Epidemiology of coronary heart disease in women. Prog Cardiovasc Dis 2004;46:287–95.
10. American Heart Association. Heart and stroke statistical update. Dallas (TX): American Heart Association; 1999.
11. American Heart Association. Heart disease and stroke statistics—2006 update. Available at: http://www.americanheart.org/downloadable/heart/1105390918119HDSStats2005Update.pdf. Accessed December 1, 2008.

12. Sowers. Diabetes mellitus and cardiovascular disease in women. Arch Intern Med 1998;158:617–21.
13. Vaccarino V, Parsons L, Every NR, et al. Sex-based differences in early mortality after myocardial infarction. N Engl J Med 1999;341:217–25.
14. Lerman G, Sopko G. Women and cardiovascular heart disease: clinical implications from the Women's Ischemia Syndrome Evaluation (WISE) study: are we smarter? J Am Coll Cardiol 2006;47(Suppl 3):S59–62.
15. Mosca L, Manson JE, Sutherland SE, et al. Cardiovascular disease in women. A statement for healthcare professionals from the American Heart Association. Circulation 1997;96:2468–82.
16. Jani SM, Montoye C, Mehta R, et al. Sex differences in the application of evidence-based therapies for the treatment of acute myocardial infarction. Arch Intern Med 2006;166:1164–70.
17. Greenland P, Gulati M. Improving outcomes for women with myocardial infarction. Arch Intern Med 2006;166:1162–3.
18. American Heart Association Scientific Statement. Percutaneous coronary intervention and adjunctive pharmacotherapy in women. Circulation: journal of the American Heart Association 2005;111:940–53.
19. Keyhani, Scobie JV, Hebert PL, et al. Gender disparities in blood pressure control and cardiovascular care in a national sample of ambulatory care visits. Hypertension 2008;51:1149–55.
20. Witt BJ, Jacobsen SJ, Weston SA, et al. Cardiac rehabilitation after myocardial infarction in the community. J Am Coll Cardiol 2004;44:988–96.
21. Daly C, Clemens F, Lopez Sendon JL. Cardiovascular disease in women: gender differences in the management and clinical outcome of stable angina. Circulation 2006;113:490–8.
22. Weisz D, Gusmano MK, Rodwin VG. Gender and the treatment of heart disease in older persons in the United States, France, and England: a comparative, population-based view of a clinical phenomenon. Gend Med 2004;1:29–40.
23. Healy B. The Yentl syndrome. N Engl J Med 1991;325:274–6.
24. Milner KA, Funk M, Richards S, et al. Gender differences in symptom presentation associated with coronary heart disease. Am J Cardiol; 84(4);396–9.
25. Mosca L, Appel LJ, Benjamin EJ, et al. Evidence based guidelines for cardiovascular disease prevention in women. Circulation 2004;109:672–93.
26. Daviglus ML, Stamler J, Pirzada A, et al. Favorable cardiovascular risk profile in young women and long-term risk of cardiovascular and all-cause mortality. JAMA 2004;292:1588–92.
27. The Harvard Medical School Family Health Guide. A better way to predict cardiovascular risk. Available at: http://www.health.harvard.edu/fhg/updates/a-better-way-to-predict-cardiovascular-risk.shtml. Accessed December 2, 2008.
28. May M, Lawlor DA, Brindle P, et al. Cardiovascular disease risk assessment in older women: can we improve on Framingham? British Women's Heart and Health Prospective Cohort Study. Heart 2006;92:1396–401.
29. Stampfer MJ, Hu FB, Mansonx JE, et al. Primary prevention of coronary heart disease in women through diet and exercise. N Engl J Med 2000;343:16–22.
30. Yusuf S, Hawken S, Ounpuu S, et al. Effect of potentially modifiable risk factors associated with myocardial infarction in 52 countries (the INTERHEART study): case-control study. Lancet 2004;364(9438):937–52.
31. Greenland P, Knoll MD, Stamler J, et al. Major risk factors as antecedents of fatal and nonfatal coronary heart disease events. JAMA 2003;290:891–7.

32. U.S. Department of Health and Human Services. Healthy people 2000: national health promotion and disease prevention objectives. DHHS Pub. No. (PHS) 91-50212. Washington, DC: U.S. Government Printing Office; 1991. Sclar ED. Community economic structure and individual well-being: a look behind the statistics. International Journal of Health Services 1980;10:563–79.

33. Haskell WL, Lee IM, Pate RR, et al. Physical activity and public health—updated recommendation for adults from the American College of Sports Medicine and the American Heart Association. Circulation 2007;116:1081–93.

34. American Heart Association. 1998 heart and stroke statistical update. Dallas (TX): American Heart Association; 1997.

35. Anastos K, Charney P, Charon RA. Hypertension in women: what is really known? The Woman's Caucus, Working Group on Women's Health of the Society of General Internal Medicine. Ann Intern Med 1991;115:287–93.

36. Keyhani S, Scobie JV, Hebert PL, et al. Gender disparities in blood pressure control and cardiovascular care in a national sample of ambulatory care visits. Hypertension 2008;51:1149–55.

37. Mohiuddin SM, Mooss AN, Hunter CB, et al. Intensive smoking cessation intervention reduced mortality in high risk smokers with cardiovascular disease. Chest 2007;131:446–52.

38. Al-Delaimy WK, Manson JE, Solomon CG, et al. Smoking and risk of coronary heart disease among women with type 2 diabetes mellitus. Arch Intern Med 2002;162:273–9.

39. Bowman TS, Gaziano JM, Buring JE, et al. A prospective study of cigarette smoking and risk of incident hypertension in women. J Am Coll Cardiol 2007; 50:2085–92.

40. Centers for Disease Control and Prevention. The health consequences of involuntary exposure to tobacco smoke: a report of the Surgeon General. Atlanta (GA): U.S. Department of Health and Human Services, Coordinating Center for Health Promotion, National Center for Chronic Disease Prevention and Health Promotion, Office on Smoking and Health; 2006.

41. Whincup PH, Gilg JA, Emberson JR, et al. Passive smoking and risk of coronary heart disease and stroke: prospective study with cotinine measurement. BMJ 2004;329(7459):200–5.

42. Fielding JE. Smoking and women. Tragedy of the majority. N Engl J Med 1987; 317:1343–5.

43. Tobacco use: United States, 1900–1999, from morbidity and mortality weekly report. Available at: http://www.cancernetwork.com/display/article/10165/81348. Accessed December 3, 2008.

44. Willett WC, Green A, Stampfer MJ, et al. Relative and absolute excess risks of coronary heart disease among women who smoke cigarettes. N Engl J Med 1987;317:1303–9.

45. Centers for Disease Control and Prevention. Women and smoking: a report of the Surgeon General. Atlanta (GA): U.S. Department of Health and Human Services, CDC, National Center for Chronic Disease Prevention and Health Promotion, Office on Smoking and Health; 2001.

46. Centers for Disease Control and Prevention. The health consequences of smoking: a report of the Surgeon General. Atlanta (GA): Department of Health and Human Services, Centers for Disease Control and Prevention, National Center for Chronic Disease Prevention and Health Promotion, Office on Smoking and Health; 2004.

47. Doll R, Peto R, Boreham J, et al. Mortality in relation to smoking: 50 years' observations on male British doctors. Available at: http://www.bmj.com/cgi/reprint/328/7455/1519. Accessed December 3, 2008.
48. Taylor DH Jr, Hasselblad V, Henley SJ, et al. Benefits of smoking cessation for longevity. Am J Public Health 2002;92(6):990–6.
49. Pate RR, Pratt M, Blair SN, et al. Physical activity and public health. A recommendation from the Centers for Disease Control and Prevention and the American College of Sports Medicine. JAMA 1995;273:402–7.
50. Pazoki P, Nabipour I, Seyednezami N, et al. Effects of a community-based healthy heart program on increasing women's physical activity: a controlled trial guided by community-based participatory research (CBPR). BMC Public Health 2007;7:216.
51. Gaillard. Importance of aerobic fitness in cardiovascular risks in sedentary overweight and obese African-American women. Nurse Res Prev Cardiol 2007.
52. Lerner DJ, Kannel WB. Patterns of coronary heart disease morbidity and mortality in the sexes: a 26 year follow-up of the Framingham population. Am Heart J 1986;111:383–90.
53. Hedley AA, Ogden CL, Johnson CL, et al. Prevalence of overweight and obesity among US children, adolescents, and adults, 1999–2002. JAMA 2004;291:2847–50.
54. Zhang C, Rexrode KM, van Dam RM, et al. Abdominal obesity and risk of all-cause cardiovascular, and cancer mortality. Circulation 2008;117:1658–67.
55. Grundy SM, Becker D, Clark LT, et al. Expert Panel on Detection, Evaluation and Treatment of High Blood Cholesterol. Circulation 2002;106:3143–421.
56. Schrott HG, Bittner V, Herrington DM, et al. Adherence to National Cholesterol Education Program treatment goals in postmenopausal women with heart disease. The Heart and Estrogen/Progestin Replacement Study (HERS). The HERS Research Group. JAMA 1997;277(16):1281–6.
57. Safeer RS, Lacivita CL. Choosing drug therapy for patients with hyperlipidemia. Am Fam Physician 2000;61(11):3371–82.
58. Bass KM, Newschaffer CJ, Klag MJ, et al. Plasma lipoprotein levels as predictors of cardiovascular death in women. Arch Intern Med 1993;153(19):2209–16.
59. Baron AA, Baron SB. High levels of HDL cholesterol do not predict cardiovascular disease in women. Prev Cardiol 2007;10(3):125–7.
60. Moat. Plasma total homocysteine: instigator or indicator of cardiovascular disease? Ann Clin Biochem 2008;45:345–8.
61. Ward M, McNulty H, McPartlin J, et al. Plasma homocysteine, a risk factor for cardiovascular disease, is lowered by physiological doses of folic acid. QJM 1997;90:519–24.
62. Bazzano LA, Reynolds K, Holder KN, et al. Effect of folic acid supplementation on risk of cardiovascular diseases: a meta-analysis of randomized controlled trials. JAMA 2006;296:2720–6.
63. Wijendran V, Hayes KC. Dietary n-6 and n-3 fatty acid balance and cardiovascular health. Annu Rev Nutr 2004;24:597–615.
64. Bandyopadhyay S, Bayer A, O Mahony M. Age and gender bias in statin trials. QJM 2001;94:127–32.
65. Harris DJ, Douglas PS. Enrollment of women in cardiovascular clinical trials funded by the National Heart, Lung, and Blood Institute. N Engl J Med 2000;343:475–80.
66. Mizuno K, Nakaya N, Ohashi Y, et al. Usefulness of pravastatin in primary prevention of cardiovascular events in women: analysis of the management of elevated cholesterol in the primary prevention group of adult Japanese (MEGA Study). Circulation 117:494–502.

67. LaRosa. Effects of statins on risk of coronary disease: a meta analysis of randomized trials. JAMA 1999;282:2340–6.
68. Lewis SJ, Sacks FM, Mitchell JS, et al. Effect of pravastatin on cardiovascular events in women after myocardial infarction: the cholesterol and recurrent events (CARE) trial. J Am Coll Cardiol 1998;32:140–6.
69. Heart Protection Collaborative Group MRC/BHF Heart Protection Study of cholesterol lowering with simvastatin in 20,536 high-risk individuals: a randomised placebo-controlled trial. Lancet 2002;360:7–22.
70. Walsh JM, Pignone M. Drug treatment of hyperlipidemia in women. JAMA 2004; 219:2243–52.
71. Strom BL. Statins and over-the-counter availability. N Engl J Med 2005;352: 1403–5.
72. Pasternak RC, Smith SC Jr., Bairey-Merz CN, et al. ACC/AHA/NHLBI clinical advisory on the use and safety of statins. J Am Coll Cardiol 2002;40:567–72.
73. Whelan AM, Price SO, Fowler SF, et al. The effect of aspirin on niacin-induced cutaneous reactions. J Fam Pract 1992;34:165–8.
74. Frick MH, Elo O, Haapa K, et al. Helsinki heart study primary-prevention trial with gemfibrozil in middle-aged men with dyslipidemia. N Engl J Med 1987;317: 1237–45.
75. Meagher EA. Addressing cardiovascular disease in women: focus on dyslipidemia. The Journal of the American Board of Family Practice 2004;17:424–37.
76. Gardiner P, Graham RE, Legedza AT, et al. Factors associated with dietary supplement use among prescription medication users. Arch Intern Med 2006;166: 1968–74.
77. U.S. Food and Drug Administration. Avoid red yeast rice promoted for high cholesterol. Available at: http://www.fda.gov/consumer/updates/redyeastrice081007. html. Accessed December 4, 2008.
78. Gardner CD, Lawson LD, Block E, et al. Effect of raw garlic vs commercial garlic supplements on plasma lipid concentrations in adults with moderate hypercholesterolemia: a randomized clinical trial. Arch Intern Med 2007;167(4): 346–53.
79. American Diabetes Association. Available at:http://www.diabetes.org/diabetes-statistics/prevalence.jsp. Accessed December 5, 2008.
80. Barrett-Conner E, Cohn B, WingardSeyednezami DN, et al. Why is diabetes mellitus a stronger risk factor for fatal ischemic heart disease in women than in men? JAMA 1991;265:627–31.
81. American Diabetes Association. Available at: http://www.diabetes.org/diabetes-statistics/heart-disease.jsp. Accessed December 4, 2008.
82. Selvin E, Marinopoulos S, Berkenblit G, et al. Meta-analysis: glycosylated hemoglobin and cardiovascular disease in diabetes mellitus. Ann Intern Med 2004; 141:421–31.
83. The ADVANCE Collaborative Group. Intensive blood glucose control and vascular outcomes in patients with type 2 diabetes. N Engl J Med 2008;358(24): 2560–2572.
84. Gerstein HC, Miller ME. Effects of intensive glucose lowering in type 2 diabetes. N Engl J Med 2008;358(24):2545–59.
85. American Diabetes Association. Standards of medical care in diabetes—2008. Diabetes Care 2008;31(Suppl 1):S12–54.
86. Mohandas B, Mehta JL, et al. Lessons from the hormone replacement therapy trials for primary prevention of cardiovascular disease. Curr Opin Cardiol 2007;22:434–42.

87. Mozaffarian D, Kumanyika SK, Lemaitre RN, et al. Cereal, fruit, and vegetable fiber intake and the risk of cardiovascular disease in elderly individuals. JAMA 2003;289:1659–66.

88. Hayden M, Pignone M, Phillips C, et al. Aspirin for the primary prevention of cardiovascular events: a summary of the evidence for the US Preventive Services Task Force. Ann Intern Med 2002;136:161–72.

89. Ridker PM, Cook NR, Lee IM, et al. A randomized trial of low-dose aspirin in the primary prevention of cardiovascular disease in women. N Engl J Med 2005; 352(13):1293–1304.

90. Pignone M, Earnshaw S, Pletcher MJ, et al. Aspirin for primary prevention of cardiovascular disease in women. Arch Intern Med 2007;167(3):290–5.

91. Antithrombotic Trialists' Collaboration. Collaborative meta-analysis of randomised trials of antiplatelet therapy for prevention of death, myocardial infarction, and stroke in high risk patients. BMJ 2002;324:71–86.

92. Lawlor DA, Bedford C, Taylor M, et al. Aspirin use for the prevention of cardiovascular disease: the British Women's Heart and Health Study. Br J Gen Pract 2001;51(470):743–5.

93. Bhatt DL, Fox KA, Werner Hacke CB, et al. Clopidogrel and aspirin versus aspirin alone for the prevention of atherothrombotic events. NEJM 2006;354(16): 1706–17.

94. Walsh BW, Schiff I, Rosner B, et al. Effects of postmenopausal estrogen replacement on the concentrations and metabolism of plasma lipoproteins. N Engl J Med 1991;325(17):1196–204.

95. Petitti DB, Sidney S, Quesenberry CP, et al. Hormone replacement therapy and heart disease prevention: experimentation trumps observation. JAMA 1998; 280(7):650–2.

96. Gibbons RF. Electrocardiography testing with and without radionuclide studies. In: Wenger NK, Speroff L, Packard B, editors, Cardiovascular health and disease in women, 73. Greenwich (CT): Lejaq Comms; 1993.

97. Travin MI, Johnson LL. Assessment of coronary artery disease in women. Curr Opin Cardiol 1997;12:587–94.

98. Mieres JH, Shaw LJ, Arai A, et al. Role of noninvasive testing in the clinical evaluation of women with suspected coronary artery disease. Circulation 2005;111: 682–96.

99. Alexander KP, Shaw LJ, DeLong ER, et al. Value of exercise treadmill testing in women. J Am Coll Card 1998;32:1657–64.

100. DeCara JM. Noninvasive cardiac testing in women. J Am Med Womens Assoc 2003;58(4):254–63.

101. Rosamond W, Flegal K, Furie K, et al. Heart disease and stroke statistics—2008 update. American Heart Association. Available at: http://circ.ahajournals.org/cgi/content/full/117/4/e25. Accessed December 4, 2008.

102. MacMahon S, Peto R, Cutler J, et al. Blood pressure, stroke, and coronary heart disease. Part 1. Prolonged differences in blood pressure: prospective observational studies corrected for the regression, dilution bias. Lancet 1990;335: 765–74.

103. Hu FB, Stampfer MJ. Physical activity—nurses health study. JAMA 2000;283: 2961–7.

104. Johnston SC, Gress DR. Short-term prognosis after emergency department diagnosis of TIA. JAMA 2000;284(22):2901–6.

Common Breast Concerns

Ann M. Rodden, DO, MS

KEYWORDS

- Breast pain • Mastalgia • Nipple discharge
- Galactorrhea • Breast mass • Breasty cyst

Breast concerns commonly occur in the outpatient setting and predominantly consist of breast pain, nipple discharge, and breast masses.[1] Many of these concerns can be treated with reassurance and reevaluation, but not if the patient has risk factors for an underlying pathology. This article reviews the diagnosis and treatment of the three most common breast concerns encountered in primary care practices.

BREAST PAIN (MASTALGIA)

Breast pain, or mastalgia, can be categorized into one of three types: cyclic, noncyclic, or nonbreast (musculoskeletal). A thorough history consisting of a description of the pain, location, radiation, relation to menstrual cycle or physical activity, interference with activities of daily living, and family history of breast cancer directs the diagnosis. Differentiating between breast and musculoskeletal pain can be difficult; the best way to determine true origin of pain is to have the woman explain and show where she perceives the pain to be originating. In addition to a history of pain, a history of medications, medical conditions, caffeine intake, stress, and smoking status should be collected. Many medications, including antipsychotics and antimicrobials, are believed to cause mastalgia.[2,3] The predominant pharmacologic agents are usually hormones, such as estrogens, progesterones, oral contraceptives, or clomiphene.[4] If a medication change has occurred or an association is being considered, a trial off of the medication (if possible) may be warranted. After the history is obtained, physical examination of the breasts, regional lymph nodes, chest wall, cervical and thoracic spine, and upper extremities should be performed. The patient should be examined in the supine and seated positions to differentiate chest wall versus breast pain.[5] If a breast mass is palpable on examination, an appropriate radiographic work-up should follow.

Most cases of breast pain are attributable to cyclic mastalgia.[6] It is characterized as a diffuse, bilateral tenderness that occurs during the luteal phase of the menstrual cycle predominantly in women during their 30s and 40s and is uncommon in postmenopausal women. The pain is sometimes described as heaviness, soreness, or an

Department of Family Medicine, Medical University of South Carolina, PO Box 250192, 295 Calhoun Street, Charleston, SC 29425, USA
E-mail address: rodden@musc.edu

Prim Care Clin Office Pract 36 (2009) 103–113
doi:10.1016/j.pop.2008.10.006
0095-4543/08/$ – see front matter
primarycare.theclinics.com

aching sensation occurring just before menses that improves as the cycle continues. On occasion, the pain is worse in one breast. Noncyclic mastalgia tends to be a sharp, burning, localized, and unilateral pain. This condition tends to affect an older population of women in their 40s and 50s and can occur in the postmenopausal state, unlike cyclic mastalgia. The cause of noncyclic mastalgia is unknown.

Diagnosis

The diagnosis of mastalgia can be made by history and physical examination alone in most cases. If the clinician is unable to differentiate between mastalgia of a cyclic versus a noncyclic nature, a breast pain diary may assist in making the accurate diagnosis. Patients are asked to document time that pain occurs, relationship to activity, and relationship to menstrual cycles. In addition to determining a pain rating and overall interference in daily life, this tool can often identify treatment effects. The only laboratory study that should be performed is a urine pregnancy test. Serum hormone assays are not useful in making the diagnosis of mastalgia or in managing the condition.[2] Radiographic imaging studies are at the discretion of the clinician. If the patient is 30 years of age or older and has notable mastalgia, she should undergo a mammogram if one has not been performed in the previous 12 months.[7,8] If a woman has a family history of early breast cancer or localized pain, a mammogram or ultrasound evaluation should be considered. The prevalence of breast cancer in patients who have mastalgia is estimated to be 0 to 3.2%.[9–11]

Treatment

The initial treatment of cyclic and noncyclic mastalgia is to offer the patient reassurance; 70% to 85% of these cases are self-limited.[12] The use of well-fitted brassieres and sports bras may limit breast movement and improve mastalgia. If the pain interferes with sleep, a well-fitted sports bra worn while sleeping may also alleviate symptoms. Lifestyle changes, such as smoking cessation and caffeine avoidance, have been recommended as a treatment of mastalgia, despite a lack of evidence demonstrating a benefit to caffeine or nicotine reduction with respect to long-term outcomes.[2] Decreasing saturated fat intake and sodium are also recommended, but no studies have found these to be beneficial measures.[5,13] Relaxation therapy was found to reduce mastalgia symptoms compared with a control group,[14] and massage with ice or heat may also reduce pain symptoms.[2,5] A trial off of any potentially offending medications may alleviate mastalgia symptoms also.

If conservative treatment does not improve the symptoms, and no underlying pathology is identified with imaging, further treatment consists of several medication options. Individuals who have noncyclic mastalgia may not respond to medications as well as those who have cyclic mastalgia, but the same medications can be used.[15] Evening primrose up to 3 g a day in divided doses (equivalent to 240 mg gamma-linolenic acid) has been shown to be safe with only minimal side effects.[15] Different doses have been studied, and the results are conflicting even at the 3-g dose.[2,15–17] This treatment may take up to 4 months to see improvement of symptoms, and should be stopped after 6 months of treatment. If conservative measures do not improve mastalgia, evening primrose should be a second-line option because of the minimal side effect profile compared with other treatments.[5,15]

Danazol, a synthetic androgen, is the only current medication approved for the treatment of mastalgia by the US Food and Drug Administration (FDA). The typical starting dose is 200 mg per day beginning the second day of the menstrual cycle, but a range of 100 to 400 mg per day can be used for cases of moderate to severe mastalgia. If a response is seen after 2 months, the dose should be decreased to 100 mg per day. If after

2 or more months a further response is seen with this dose, the dose can be further decreased to 100 mg every other day or 100 mg on the last 2 weeks of each menstrual cycle.[15] Another study determined that 200 mg daily given only during the luteal phase (days 14 to 28) of the menstrual cycle improved cyclic mastalgia compared with a placebo.[18] Common reported side effects include menstrual irregularities, a decrease in breast size, acne, weight gain, bloating, voice changes, hair loss or hirsutism, depression, and irritability. Danazol is teratogenic, so when it is used for treatment of mastalgia, a barrier method of birth control should be encouraged.

Another treatment option is bromocriptine, a dopamine agonist, with a therapeutic goal of 2.5 mg twice daily. By starting out at 1.25 mg at night and increasing by 1.25 mg daily every few days over 2 weeks or more, the side effects can be minimized.[15,19] Dizziness and nausea are major side effects with bromocriptine treatment. In a study comparing evening primrose, danazol, and bromocriptine, approximately one third of women taking danazol or bromocriptine stop taking the medication secondary to side effects.[15] Danazol has been found to be most effective of these three medications, whereas evening primrose offers the best side-effect profile.[15]

Tamoxifen also is not FDA approved for the treatment of mastalgia but has been found to be an effective treatment option.[2,20] This selective estrogen receptor modulator (SERM) improves pain at doses of 10 mg or 20 mg daily, but the 10-mg dose has been shown to have equal efficacy in symptomatic control compared with the 20 mg dose, with fewer side effects.[21] Tamoxifen should be reserved for severe mastalgia because the side-effect profile includes deep venous thrombosis, pulmonary emboli, endometrial cancer, hot flashes, weight gain, menstrual irregularities, vaginal dryness, and nausea. Afimoxifene, a metabolite of tamoxifen, applied as gel dosed 2 to 4 mg daily improves symptoms with minimal side effects compared with a placebo gel.[22] This study investigated pain scores over a 4-month period and long-term pain control needs to be studied further. Another SERM, toremifene, in doses of 20 to 30 mg daily over three menstrual cycles, improves moderate to severe cyclic mastalgia compared with placebo.[23,24]

Lisuride is another medication with some data in its favor. This dopamine agonist has been studied in a double-blinded, placebo-controlled trial and found to be superior to placebo in pain control after 2 months at 0.2 mg per day.[25] Longer studies need to be performed as with many of the medications currently being used to determine long-term pain control.

For mastalgia that has been refractory to other treatments or is recurrent, goserelin (Zoladex), a luteinizing hormone–releasing hormone, at a dose of 3.6 mg by injection each month may improve symptoms rapidly so that an alternative therapy may be initiated.[26,27] In one study, participants received a monthly injection of goserelin or sham injection for 6 months. After the treatment, those receiving goserelin reported lower pain scores, but 6 months later no significant statistical difference in pain scores was noted between the two groups.[26] Side effects of this medication consist of vaginal dryness, decreased libido, hot flashes, skin changes, and decreased breast size. With a favorable side-effect profile and a quick initial response, goserelin works as a short-term bridging treatment to other modalities when other medications have not been effective alone.

Other medications may be useful as sole or adjunctive therapy. Oral or topical NSAIDs can be considered for pain control. Topical NSAIDS have been studied in randomized and nonrandomized studies, demonstrating that topical NSAIDs, including diclofenac diethylammonium and piroxicam gel are effective treatments of mastalgia, and have similar therapeutic responses compared with evening primrose oil.[28–30] Oral NSAIDs may not be feasible for some patients because of gastrointestinal side effects.

If a medication initially improves the symptoms of mastalgia but they return after the medication is stopped, then another trial of the medication may be attempted before changing medications. Patients who have refractory mastalgia that does not respond to conservative treatment and medications may be candidates for surgery. A few cases have improved with bilateral mastectomy and breast reconstruction but surgical management should remain a last resort option for severe, refractory mastalgia.[31]

NIPPLE DISCHARGE (GALACTORRHEA)

Nipple discharge can be either physiologic or pathologic in nature. The first step in determining the cause of galactorrhea is to obtain a careful history consisting of timing, need of compression/stimulation to occur, unilateral or bilateral leakage, relation to a mass, number of ducts that expel discharge, and a description of the discharge (eg, clear, milky, bloody, purulent) (**Box 1**). Other pertinent information includes the relationship of the nipple discharge to menses, pregnancy, trauma, thyroid disease, exercise, and medications. A history of visual changes, headaches, fatigue, cold intolerance, constipation, weight gain, amenorrhea, and changes in libido may focus the evaluation toward an underlying cause of the nipple discharge.

The physical examination should provide additional information on the presence of a mass, number of ducts that expel discharge, type of discharge, and if the discharge is unilateral or bilateral. Discharge that is spontaneous, watery, serous, or sanguineous may be pathologic and requires further evaluation. Pathologic nipple discharge tends to be unilateral and from a single duct. Causes of pathologic nipple discharge are benign intraductal papillomas, duct ectasia, carcinoma, breast abscesses, and breast infections. The most worrisome of these causes is the infiltrating ductal carcinoma that makes up 8% to 15% of pathologic nipple discharges.[1] Physiologic discharge occurs with stimulation or compression of the nipple, is expressed from multiple ducts, and tends to be bilateral in nature. The discharge may be various colors, including green, yellow, gray, brown, black, or white, and may be of a sticky consistency. The underlying cause of physiologic nipple discharge may not be identified. Medications, hypothyroidism, pituitary adenoma, and pregnancy, along with chronic stimulation of the nipple and postthoracotomy syndrome may cause a physiologic nipple discharge.

In addition to a detailed breast and axillary examination, the physical examination should include an inspection of the thyroid gland for enlargement or nodules; eyebrows for thinning; eyes for visual field deficits, papilledema, or proptosis; hands for tremors; skin for dryness, acne, or hirsutism; and heart rate for bradycardia or tachycardia.

Diagnosis

Laboratory evaluation for nipple discharge is often left to the discretion of the physician. In cases of a milky to yellow discharge, laboratory tests, such as a urine pregnancy test, thyroid function studies, and serum prolactin levels, may determine whether the cause of the discharge is pregnancy, hypothyroidism, or a pituitary adenoma.[5] Medications that may cause a physiologic discharge include oral contraceptives, antihypertensive medications (eg, angiotensin-converting enzyme inhibitors), and some psychotropic medications (**Table 1**). Discharges that are green, gray, or milky may be due to ductal ectasia and fibrocystic change.

Cytologic evaluation of pathologic discharge is often used to rule out malignancy. A negative cytology report does not necessarily rule out malignancy and further evaluation should continue until a definitive cause can be determined. A positive cytology

| Box 1 |
| Important information to evaluate nipple discharge |

History

   Discharge description

      Timing of discharge

      Spontaneously/by stimulation

      Unilateral/bilateral

      Presence of a mass

      Color

   Reproduction

      Relationship to menses

      Pregnancy

      Amenorrhea

   Medical Conditions

      Medications

      Thyroid disease

   Stimulating events

      Trauma

      Exercise

   Review of symptoms

      Headaches

      Visual changes

      Fatigue

      Weight gain

      Constipation

      Changes in libido

Physical

   Breast examination

      Mass

      Number of ducts involved

      Type of discharge

      Unilateral/bilateral

   Further examination

      Thyroid

         Nodules/enlargement

      Eyes

         Visual fields

         Papilledema

         Proptosis

Eyebrows

   Thinning

Hands

   Tremor

Skin

   Dryness

   Acne

   Hirsutism

Heart rate

   Bradycardia

   Tachycardia

report cannot distinguish between the types of cancer so further evaluation is warranted.[7,8] If the nature of the discharge is difficult to determine, performing a guaiac test of the discharge can identify the presence of blood. A diagnostic mammogram or ultrasound should be performed in the evaluation of pathologic nipple discharge but this should not delay a prompt surgical evaluation. Any woman older than 30 years of age who has a new-onset nipple discharge should have imaging performed.[8]

Treatment

For women who have physiologic nipple discharge, reassurance is the primary treatment. Education about cessation of nipple stimulation is paramount to promoting

Table 1
Medications associated with nipple discharge

H2 Receptor Antagonists	Cimetidine
Hormones	Oral contraceptives Estrogen Thyrotropin-releasing hormone
Antiemetics	Domperidone Metoclopramide Sulpiride
Antihypertensives	Methyldopa Resperpine
Opiates	Methadone
Psychotropics	Phenothiazine Olanzapine Haloperidol Risperidone[a] Molindone Tricyclic antidepressants Selective serotonin reuptake inhibitors Monoamine oxidase inhibitors

Medication list obtained from MICROMEDEX search.
[a] Medication not noted on MICROMEDEX. MICROMEDEX.[42,45]

nipple discharge resolution. If a woman continually checks her nipples for discharge, this practice prolongs the discharge and subsequent anxiety of having the discharge. Physiologic nipple discharge tends to resolve spontaneously when the nipple is not stimulated. A well-fitted bra reduces stimulation to the nipples. Medication changes may be indicated if the patient is currently taking a medication known to cause a nipple discharge. If the discharge does not resolve or if the patient is anxious about the discharge, referral to a breast surgeon is appropriate. Excisional biopsy can offer diagnosis and treatment of benign cases of nipple discharge.[32,33] Women who have pathologic discharge should be referred to a breast surgeon for evaluation of possible duct excision. Ductography can be performed for more detailed evaluations, but its use is controversial.[34]

BREAST MASS

Breast masses range from benign causes, including fibroadenomas, macrocysts, prominent areas of fibrocystic change, normal nodularity, fat lobules, and inframammary lymph nodes, to infectious causes, such as an abscess, to malignant causes. Risk factors for breast cancer should be ascertained with a detailed history (**Box 2**). In premenopausal women, a history of changes in the mass with the menstrual cycle should be determined. A thorough physical examination of the breasts should determine size, mobility, demarcation, and texture of the mass. Benign masses tend to be smooth, well-defined, soft in consistency, and mobile. Malignant masses tend to be immobile and fixed to the surrounding tissues, poorly defined, and hard in nature. A patient may also present with a vague nodularity that feels like an irregularity or

---

Box 2
Risk factors for breast cancer

Unchangeable risk factors

> Age
>
> Age of menarche (<12 years of age)
>
> Age of menopause (>55 years of age)
>
> First-degree relatives who have breast cancer
>
> History of breast cancer
>
> Breast biopsy with atypical hyperplasia
>
> Race
>
> Previous chest radiation for another cancer treatment
>
> Diethylstilbestrol exposure

Lifestyle risk factors

> Nulliparity
>
> Age at first live birth (>30 years of age)
>
> Alcohol use
>
> Hormone therapy (oral contraception or hormone replacement therapy)
>
> Overweight or obese

Data from Refs.[41,43,44]

prominence but not a defined mass. Also, the mass that the patient felt on examination may occasionally not be confirmed with physical examination in the office setting. When a woman discovers a breast mass, it is common for her to have significant anxiety about breast cancer. If the patient remains anxious during the evaluation, it is appropriate at any stage to refer her to a breast surgeon or specialist.

Diagnosis and Treatment

Defined mass

In women younger than 30 years of age who have a suspicious breast mass, an ultrasound is the preferred first step in the diagnosis.[7,8] An ultrasound will likely differentiate between a solid and a cystic mass. If the suspicion for a cyst is high and the provider is comfortable performing the procedure, a fine needle aspiration can be attempted before imaging. The radiologist needs to be aware of the procedure, any complications, and the area where the mass has been identified on examination to improve diagnostic accuracy. If the mass is found to be solid and not cystic on fine needle aspiration, cytology should be sent; however, only fibroadenomas can be diagnosed in this manner without further work-up.[8] One study identified that fine needle aspiration of a breast mass has a false-positive rate of less than 1% and a false-negative rate of 9%, whereas another study using fine needle aspiration concluded that the adequacy of the sample may ultimately affect the cytology results.[35,36] If the breast mass is suspicious for cancer and the cytology is negative, the evaluation should continue. If the provider is not skilled in performing a fine needle aspiration, the patient will benefit more from additional imaging and an image-guided biopsy rather than an attempted fine needle aspiration.

If the mass is solid and suspicious or indeterminate, a mammogram should be considered along with histologic sampling by core needle biopsy or excision. If the result is highly suspicious of malignancy, an open excisional biopsy is preferred.[5] Mammography in women younger than 30 years of age has limited diagnostic sensitivity and specificity but may be helpful in these cases.[8] If the mass is not suspicious and is less than 2 cm in size, the patient can either be monitored every 6 to 12 months for 2 years for changes in physical examination and imaging or undergo a tissue biopsy by core needle or excision.[7]

In women 30 years of age or older, a mammogram should be the first step in diagnosis because the suspicion of malignancy is increased in women older than 30 years of age. The only exception to this guideline is in cases with a high suspicion of a cystic lesion because of past history of cysts, and then a fine needle aspiration may be attempted.[7] If mammography is to follow an attempt at aspiration, the procedure may interfere with the results of the imaging up to 2 weeks after the procedure because of trauma and inflammation to the area and formation of hematomas.[8]

If the results of the mammogram are suspicious (Breast Imaging Reporting and Data System [BI-RADS] category 4–5) then the patient should be referred to a breast surgeon immediately. If the mammogram results are normal to probably benign (BI-RADS category 1–3), an ultrasound is the next step to determine if the mass is cystic or solid in nature. Solid masses that are suspicious for cancer by ultrasound should be referred to a breast surgeon. If the mass is believed to be benign, the options consist of undergoing core needle biopsy or observation on a regular schedule every 6 to 12 months with physical examination and imaging for up to 2 years to determine stability. If the mass changes during any of these examinations or imaging, a biopsy and referral to a surgeon is necessary. When the mammogram and ultrasound are negative but a mass is palpable, the patient should be referred to a breast surgeon because some cancers are not identified by imaging.

The triple test, which consists of the breast examination with imaging and some form of tissue sampling, has been adapted to determine risk for cancer in a palpable breast mass.[37–40] Each part of the test has a score attached: 1 = benign, 2 = suspicious for malignancy, and 3 = malignant findings.[37] A score of 6 or more is 100% diagnostic for malignancy, whereas a score of 3 or 4 means the mass is benign and can be followed.[37,41] A score of 5, however, is not diagnostic or exclusive. The original combination consisted of fine needle aspiration as the tissue sampling modality. Fine needle aspirate cytology is not always conclusive and a core needle biopsy may have to be performed. The core needle biopsy has better accuracy than the fine needle aspirate and may improve the triple test results.[40] Guideline recommendations are moving away from fine needle aspiration toward image-guided core needle biopsy or excisional biopsy, because visualization of the mass with imaging while collecting the sample improves the diagnostic yield.

Cysts
In women who have a history of recurrent cystic lesions or in whom the provider identifies the mass as cystic, fine needle aspiration can be performed before imaging. If the cyst disappears with aspiration, further imaging is not necessary. If the fluid from the cyst is bloody and not due to trauma, or if the cyst does not resolve with aspiration of the fluid, the patient should be referred to a breast surgeon for further evaluation and treatment. If the fluid was not bloody and the cyst resolved, the patient should return to the clinic for reevaluation 4 to 6 weeks after the procedure. Performing a breast examination will determine if the mass has returned. If the mass is palpable, the patient should be referred to a breast surgeon. Routine cytology of breast cyst aspirate is not necessary unless the fluid is bloody.

Vague nodularity
Vague nodularity tends to have a lower suspicion for cancer, especially in premenopausal women. These nodularities can be followed as an outpatient over 1 to 2 months with a follow-up examination performed a week after menses. If the area remains abnormal, imaging studies with or without a fine needle aspiration of the mass should be performed.[13]

Vanishing mass
If a patient presents for a breast mass but nothing is palpable during the examination, the patient should be encouraged to return in a few weeks to re-examine the area.[13]

SUMMARY

The evaluation of common breast concerns differs according to the patient's risk factors, her current age, and her level of anxiety. For many common breast concerns, reassurance and conservative measures are the standard treatment. Being able to identify when to offer conservative measures versus further evaluation and treatment is paramount in the treatment of breast pain, nipple discharge, and breast masses.

REFERENCES

1. Hussain AN, Policarpio C, Vincent MT. Evaluating nipple discharge. Obstet Gynecol Surv 2006;61(4):278–83.
2. Smith RL, Pruthi S, Fitzpatrick LA. Evaluation and management of breast pain. Mayo Clin Proc 2004;79(3):353–72.
3. Bhatia SC, Bhatia SK, Bencomo L. Effective treatment of venlafaxine-induced noncyclical mastalgia with bromocriptine. J Clin Psychopharmacol 2000;20(5):590–1 [Case Report].

4. Crochetiere C. Breast pain diagnosis & treatment. AWHONN Lifelines 2005;9(4): 298–304.
5. Institute for Clinical Systems Improvement. Health care guideline: diagnosis of breast disease. 12th edition. Available at: http://www.icsi.org/breast_disease_diagnosis/ diagnosis_of_breast_disease_2.html. Accessed June 24, 2008.
6. Millett AV, Dirbas FM. Clinical management of breast pain: a review. Obstet Gynecol Surv 2002;57(7):451–61.
7. Comprehensive Cancer Network. NCCN clinical practice guidelines in oncology: breast cancer screening and diagnosis guidelines vol. 1,2008. Available at: http:// www.nccn.org/professionals/physician_gls/PDF/breast-screening.pdf. Accessed June 24, 2008.
8. University of Michigan Health System. Guidelines for clinical care: common breast problems. Available at: http://cme.med.umich.edu/pdf/guideline/breast. pdf. AccessedJune 24, 2008.
9. Tumyan L, Hoyt AC, Bassett LW. Negative predictive value of sonography and mammography in patients with focal breast pain. Breast J 2005;11(5):333–7.
10. Lumanchi F, Ermani M, Brandes AA, et al. Breast complaints and risk of breast cancer. Population-based study of 2,879 self-selected women and long-term follow-up. Biomed Pharmacother 2002;56(2):88–92.
11. Duijm LEM, Guit GL, Hendriks JHCL, et al. Value of breast imaging in women with painful breasts: observational follow up study. BMJ 1998;317(7171):1492–5.
12. Barros AC, Mottola J, Ruiz CA, et al. Reassurance in the treatment of mastalgia. Breast J 1999;5(3):162–5.
13. Cady B, Steele GD, Morrow M, et al. Evaluation of common breast problems: guidance for primary care providers. CA Cancer J Clin 1998;48(1):49–63.
14. Fox H, Walker LG, Heys SD, et al. Are patients with mastalgia anxious, and does relaxation therapy help? Breast 1997;6(3):138–42.
15. Gateley CA, Miers M, Mansel RE, et al. Drug treatments for mastalgia: 17 years experience in the Cardiff mastalgia clinic. J R Soc Med 1992;85(1):12–5.
16. Goyal A, Mansel RE. A randomized multicenter study of gamolenic acid (Efamast) with and without antioxidant vitamins and minerals in the management of mastalgia. Breast J 2005;11(1):41–7.
17. Blommers J, de Lange-de Klerk ESM, Kuik DJ, et al. Evening primrose oil and fish oil for severe chronic mastalgia: a randomized, double-blind, controlled trial. Am J Obstet Gynecol 2002;187(5):1389–94.
18. O'Brien PMS, Abukhalil IEH. Randomized controlled trial of the management of premenstrual syndrome and premenstrual mastalgia using luteal-only danazol. Am J Obstet Gynecol 1999;180(1):18–23.
19. Mansel RE, Dogliotti L. European multicentre trial of bromocriptine in cyclical mastalgia. Lancet 1990;335(8683):190–3.
20. Kontostolis E, Stefanidis K, Navrozoglou I, et al. Comparison of tamoxifen with danazol for treatment of cyclical mastalgia. Gynecol Endocrinol 1997;11(6):393–7.
21. GEMB Group (Grupo de Estudio de Mastopatias Benignas), Argentine. Tamoxifen therapy for cyclical mastalgia: dose randomized trial. Breast 1997;6(4):212–3
22. Mansel R, Goyal A, Nestour EL, et al. Afimoxifene (4-OHT) Breast Pain Research Group. A phase II trial of afimoxifene (4-hydroxytamoxifen gel) for cyclical mastalgia in premenopausal women. Breast Cancer Res Treat 2007;106(3):389–97.
23. Oksa S, Luukkaala T, Maenpaa J. Toremifene for premenstrual mastalgia: a randomized, placebo-controlled crossover study. BJOG 2006;113(6):713–8.
24. Gong C, Song E, Jia W, et al. A double-blind randomized controlled trial of toremifene therapy for mastalgia. Arch Surg 2006;141(1):43–7.

25. Kaleli S, Aydin Y, Erel CT, et al. Symptomatic treatment of premenstrual mastalgia in premenopausal women with lisuride maleate: a double-blind placebo-controlled randomized study. Fertil Steril 2001;75(4):718–23.
26. Mansel RE, Goyal A, Preece P, et al. European randomized, multicenter study of goserelin (Zoladex) in the management of mastalgia. Am J Obstet Gynecol 2004; 191(6):1942–9.
27. Hamed H, Caleffi M, Chaudary MA, et al. LHRH analogue for treatment of recurrent and refractory mastalgia. Ann R Coll Surg Engl 1990;72(4):221–4.
28. Colak T, Ipek T, Kanik A, et al. Efficacy of topical nonsteroidal antiinflammatory drugs in mastalgia treatment. J Am Coll Surg 2003;196(4):525–30.
29. Qureshi S, Sutlan N. Topical nonsteroidal anti-inflammatory drugs versus oil of evening primrose in the treatment of mastalgia. Surgeons 2005;3(1):7–10.
30. Irving AD, Morrison SL. Effectiveness of topical non-steroidal anti-inflammatory drugs in the management of breast pain. J R Coll Surg Edinb 1998;43(3):158–9.
31. Salgado CJ, Mardini S, Chen H. Mastodynia refractory to medical therapy: is there a role for mastectomy and breast reconstruction? Plast Reconstr Surg 2005;116(4):978–83.
32. Morrow M. The evaluation of common breast problems. AAFP 2000;61(8):2371–8.
33. King TA, Carter KM, Bolton JS, et al. A simple approach to nipple discharge. Am Surg 2000;66(10):960–5.
34. Dawes LG, Bowen C, Venta LA, et al. Ductography for nipple discharge: no replacement for ductal excision. Surgery 1998;124(4):685–91.
35. Ariga R, Bloom K, Reddy VB, et al. Fine-needle aspiration of clinically suspicious palpable breast masses with histopathologic correlation. Am J Surg 2002;184(5): 410–3.
36. Saxe A, Phillips E, Orfanou P, et al. Role of sample adequacy in fine needle aspiration biopsy of palpable breast lesions. Am J Surg 2002;182(4):369–71.
37. Morris KT, Vetto JT, Petty JK, et al. A new score for the evaluation of palpable breast masses in women under age 40. Am J Surg 2002;184(4):346–7.
38. Vetto J, Pommier R, Schmidt W, et al. Use of the "triple test" for palpable breast lesions yields high diagnostic accuracy and cost savings. Am J Surg 1995; 169(5):519–22.
39. Steinberg JL, Trudeau ME, Ryder DE, et al. Combined fine-needle aspiration, physical examination and mammography in the diagnosis of palpable breast masses: their relation to outcome for women with primary breast cancer. Can J Surg 1996;39(4):302–11.
40. Clarke D, Sudhakaran N, Gateley CA. Replace fine needle aspiration cytology with automated core biopsy in the triple assessment of breast cancer. Ann R Coll Surg Engl 2001;83(2):110–2.
41. Klein S. Evaluation of palpable breast masses. AAFP 2005;71(9):1731–8.
42. Bobes J, Garcia-Portilla MP, Rejas J, et al. Frequency of sexual dysfunction and other reproductive side-effects in patients with schizophrenia treated with risperidone, olanzapine, quetiapine, or haloperidol: the results of the EIRE study. J Sex Marital Ther 2003;29(2):125–47.
43. American Cancer Society. Overview: breast cancer. Available at: http://www.cancer.org/docroot/CRI/content/CRI_2_2_3X_How_is_breast_cancer_found_5.asp?sitearea=. Accessed June 24, 2008.
44. National Cancer Institute. Breast cancer risk assessment tool. Available at: http://www.cancer.gov/bcrisktool/. Accessed June 24, 2008.
45. MICROMEDEX. Available at: http://www.thomsonhc.com/hcs/librarian. Accessed June 24, 2008.

Gynecologic Cancers

Amy R. Blair, MD*, Cheyanne M. Casas, MD

KEYWORDS

- Vulvar cancer • Cervical cancer • Ovarian cancer
- Endometrial cancer

VULVAR CANCER
Epidemiology and Etiology

The rarest of gynecologic cancers, the American Cancer Society (ACS) estimates a total of 3460 cases of vulvar cancer and 2210 cases of vaginal and other genital cancers will be diagnosed in 2008.[1] Vulvar cancer is primarily a diagnosis of postmenopausal women, with the average age at diagnosis being 65 years old. Between 80% and 90% of vulvar cancers are squamous cell carcinomas. Premalignant precursor lesions to vulvar carcinoma, or vulvar intraepithelial neoplasia (VIN), have a younger peak incidence of 40 years. The mean age for women who have carcinoma in situ of the vulva is 10 years less than those who have invasive disease.

In recent years, the incidence of VIN among women 20 to 40 years of age has been increasing. This increase parallels the incidence of diagnosed dysplasia of the cervix, both correlating strongly with the rates of human papillomavirus (HPV) infection. Approximately 80% of vulvar intraepithelial neoplasias are positive for HPV. On the other hand, vulvar cancers in older women are multicentric, with less association with HPV and sexual risk factors. These are often nonneoplastic epithelial disorders, such as chronic inflammation or lichen sclerosis, that act as precursors in this second class of vulvar cancer. Other strong associations for vulvar cancer are immunosuppression, HPV infection, and advanced age.[2] Additional risk factors include current smoking, infection with HPV serotype 16, and infection with herpes simplex virus (HSV) type 2. Of these, HPV serotype 16 infection and smoking are considered to be the strongest risk factors for both in situ and invasive disease.[3]

Screening

There are no current specific screening recommendations or guidelines from the US Preventative Services Task Force (USPSTF) or American College of Obstetricians and Gynecologists (ACOG) with regard to vulvar or vaginal cancers. Expert opinion recommends that examination of the vulva should be routinely performed at the time of Papanicolaou (Pap) testing and pelvic examinations, thus mirroring the

Department of Family Medicine, Loyola University, Chicago Stritch School of Medicine, 2160 South 1st Avenue, Building 54, Maywood, IL 60153, USA
* Corresponding author.
E-mail address: ablair1@lumc.edu (A.R. Blair).

Prim Care Clin Office Pract 36 (2009) 115–130
doi:10.1016/j.pop.2008.10.001
0095-4543/08/$ – see front matter © 2009 Elsevier Inc. All rights reserved.
primarycare.theclinics.com

screening schedule of cervical cancer screening.[4] Screening for vaginal cancer is often performed inadvertently. Pap testing among women who do not have a cervix is essentially a screen for vaginal cancer; this results in cytologic screening for a cancer that is less common than cancer of the tongue or small intestine. Given the low incidence of these cancers, emphasis should focus on symptom recognition and early diagnosis of vulvar lesions, rather than general population screening guidelines.

Diagnosis

Although most vulvar cancers are diagnosed in the early stages of the disease, many women fail to report symptoms of vulvar cancer until the cancer has reached advanced stages, especially older patients.[5] Physicians also may contribute to delayed diagnosis because of prolonged treatment of one of the most common symptoms of vulvar cancer, pruritus. Other symptoms may include pain, bleeding, or ulceration.[6] Colposcopy and biopsy are the gold standard for diagnosis. On examination, preinvasive lesions may appear white and hyperkeratotic, or varying shades or pink or brown, and are often flat. The appearance of squamous cell carcinoma of the vulva may appear as a large exophytic lesion or small ulcer superimposed on an atypical base.

Any atypical vulvar lesions should be evaluated by punch biopsy or excision and histologic review. Squamous cell cancers are graded histologically from I (well differentiated) to III (poorly differentiated). The staging is surgical, using International Federation of Gynecology and Obstetrics (FIGO) staging classification (**Table 1**).

Management

The treatment of VIN and early vulvar carcinoma in situ is by surgical excision. VIN I lesions generally do not require treatment, whereas VIN II and III can be treated by laser ablation or excision. If multifocal disease is present, topical 5-fluorouracil may be used. Cure rates of preinvasive disease approach 100%.[7]

In cases of vulvar carcinoma, FIGO stage 0 (in situ) and stage IA (<2 cm) may be treated by superficial partial vulvectomy. Stages IIB (stromal invasion >1 cm) and stage II (>2 cm) may be treated with lymphadenectomy in addition to partial vulvectomy. Stage III (any size with adjacent spread) and stage IVA (spread to other organs)

Table 1
International Federation of Gynecology and Obstetrics staging for carcinoma of the vulva (surgical staging)

FIGO Stage	Criteria
0	Carcinoma in situ (vulvar intraepithelial neoplasia III, preinvasive)
IA	Confined to vulva/perineum, ≤2 cm greatest dimension, stromal invasion ≤1 mm
IB	Confined to vulva/perineum, ≤2 cm greatest dimension, stromal invasion >1 mm
II	Confined to vulva/perineum >2 cm greatest dimension
III	Tumor involves lower urethra, vagina, anus, and/or unilateral groin nodes
IVA	Tumor involves bladder or rectal mucosa, upper urethral mucosa, fixed to bone, and/or bilateral groin nodes
IVB	Any distant metastatic disease, including pelvic nodes

From Benedet JL, Bender H, Jones III H, et al. FIGO staging classifications and clinical practice guidelines in the management of gynecologic cancers. FIGO Committee on Gynecologic Oncology. Int J Gynaecol Obstet 2000;70(2):209–62; with permission.

should be treated with radical vulvectomy and lymphadenectomy. Stage III and IV cancers should be treated with preoperative pelvic irradiation, and therapies using chemotherapeutic agents (eg, cisplatin, 5-fluorouracil) have been combined with radiation for treatment of advanced-stage cancers.[8] Novel approaches using lymphatic mapping with sentinel node dissection seem promising for the future treatment of early vulvar cancers.[9]

Five-year survival rates for vulvar carcinoma are 55% to 77% if confined to the vulva and perineum (stages I–II). The status of inguinofemoral lymph nodes is the most important prognostic factor for survival. When inguinofemoral lymph nodes are positive or when the tumor extends to adjacent tissues, the survival rates decrease to 30% for stage III and 8% for stage IV cancers.[10]

CERVICAL CANCER
Epidemiology and Etiology

The incidence and mortality rates of cervical cancer in the United States have declined dramatically with the inception of cervical cancer screening programs. The ACS estimates that 11,070 cases of invasive cervical cancer will be diagnosed in 2008. Of those cases, 3870 deaths from cervical cancer are predicted. This mortality reflects that although the 5-year survival rate of localized disease approaches 92%, the deaths that continue to occur in the United States are a result of late presentation in the course of the disease.[1] On the other hand, the worldwide incidence and mortality rate from cervical cancer are alarming and reflect a serious burden of disease. Cervical cancer is the second leading cause of cancer deaths worldwide with almost 500,000 cases in 2002, with more than 80% of cervical cancer deaths occurring in developing countries.

A definitive causal relationship exists between HPV, cancer precursors, and cervical cancer.[11] Among the approximately 100 identified strains of HPV, the high-risk HPV serotypes 16 and 18 account for more than 70% of cervical cancers. The rate of HPV infection in the female population, estimated at 40% for ages 20 to 29 years, far exceeds the predicted number of cases of cervical cancer. The natural history of HPV infection demonstrates that spontaneous resolution occurs in 90% of immunocompetent women within the course of 2 years.[12] The development of invasive cancer from initial HPV acquisition to cancer precursors is a process that takes an average of 20 years. Characteristics that are predictive of progression of HPV infection to cervical intraepithelial neoplasia (CIN) and subsequent invasion include age, cigarette smoking, immunosuppression, and nutritional factors.[13]

Screening

The USPSTF recommends routine screening for cervical cancer with a Pap test for all women who are or have been sexually active and have a cervix.[14] The optimal age for beginning screening is unknown. Some data suggest that screening that begins within 3 years of sexual activity or at age 21, whichever comes first, is effective for detection of high-grade lesions.[15] Many other organizations, including the ACOG and the American Academy of Family Physicians (AAFP), recommend routine annual screening beginning once sexually active or when reaching age 18 years. The upper age limit for cervical cancer screening is unclear, with varying recommendations from major organizations. The USPSTF found evidence that yield of screening was low in previously screened women after age 65 years, as long as those women were at low risk for development of cervical cancer. The ACS recommendations suggest stopping cervical cancer screening at age 70 years.[16] The importance of screening itself is clear, but the timing and interval of screening are less clear. The interval between Pap smears is a clinical decision based on risk factors. A study of 31,000 low-risk women aged 30 to 64 years found that screening every 3 years rather than annual screening would produce an average risk for cervical cancer of 3 in 100,000 women, which is the same risk as male breast cancer.[16]

For cervical cancer screening, the Pap smear is an imperfect test. There is a substantial false-negative rate reported for Pap smears, as high as 45% in some studies.[17] False-positive results also occur, and the addition of HPV DNA testing for women aged 30 years or older is an opportunity for reducing costs of screening and for falsely abnormal cytology results.[18] The ACOG currently recommends the use of a combination of cervical cytology and HPV DNA in screening women aged 30 years and older. Women who receive negative results on both tests should be screened no more than every 3 years.[19]

The use of HPV testing for screening has also been studied. HPV testing used as primary screening has theoretic benefits in cost reduction and simplicity for low-income countries where cytology services are scant. In the United States, however, data have shown that HPV testing alone for cervical cancer lacks great specificity given the high prevalence in the general population. In one recent study, the prevalence of HPV was 26.8% in women aged 14 to 59 years, with the age group of 20 to 24 years having a prevalence of 44.8%.[20] The positive predictive value from one study of the HPV test in identifying CIN-2 or CIN-3 lesions and carcinoma was less than 10%.[21] The USPSTF cites insufficient evidence to recommend for or against routine HPV screening.[15]

Diagnosis and Management

The diagnosis of cervical cancer precursors and invasive disease is generally performed during the routine Pap test and pelvic examination, rather than by symptomatic patient presentations. Symptoms of invasive cancer may include abnormal vaginal bleeding, leukorrhea, or pelvic pain, suggesting advanced disease. Abnormal bleeding, especially a history of postcoital bleeding, is a common presenting symptom.

Pap smear results may show cytologic abnormalities of varying degrees, and the terminology for classifying these various lesions was standardized through the 2001 Bethesda System. This system uses the terms low-grade squamous intraepithelial lesion (LSIL) and high-grade squamous intraepithelial lesion (HSIL) to refer to the low- and high-grade precursors to carcinoma. Further diagnosis of these lesions histologically by cervical biopsy, when performed, is classified into CIN 1 for low-grade lesions and CIN 2–3 for high-grade lesions.

Triage of abnormal cervical cytology is defined by the guidelines set forth by the American Society for Colposcopy and Cervical Pathology (ASCCP).[22] In general, women who have atypical squamous cells of undetermined significance (ASCUS) with positive high-risk HPV and those who have LSIL should be triaged to colposcopy.

One of the updates in the new guidelines from 2006 is in the management of these cancer precursors of ASCUS and LSIL in adolescents. This change is due to a higher likelihood of clearance of HPV and resolution of abnormal cytology. The algorithm for this special population is shown in **Fig. 1**.[23]

Adolescents (defined by age 20 years and younger) who have ASCUS with high-risk HPV or LSIL should have repeat cytology at 12 months. At 12 months, a cytology result of HSIL or greater should be referred for colposcopy. If the cytology result is less than the HSIL grade, cytology can again be repeated at 24 months. Guidelines for HSIL cytology results for all women vary from those of ASCUS and LSIL. Management of HSIL results with repeat cytology and HPV testing is inappropriate. Instead, immediate

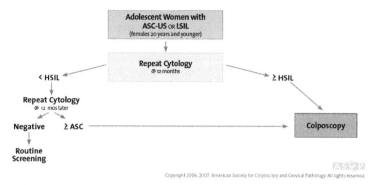

Fig. 1. Guideline for managing adolescent women with either ASCUS or LSIL. (*Reprinted from* The Journal of Lower Genital Tract Disease, Vol. 11, Issue 4, with the permission of the ASCCP © American Society for Colposcopy and Cervical Pathology 2007. No copies of the algorithm may be made without the prior consent of ASCCP. Available at: http://www.asccp.org/.

colposcopy with endocervical sampling or a "see and treat" approach with loop electrosurgical excision procedures (LEEP) is recommended.

In addition to addressing management of abnormal cytology, the 2006 consensus guidelines through the ASCCP also addressed management of women who have cervical intraepithelial neoplasia or adenocarcinoma in situ (AIS) once confirmed through screening algorithms.[24] Treatment of persistent CIN I, and CIN 2–3 at any point, is by way of surgical methods. CIN 1 may be treated with ablative or excisional methods. These include cryotherapy or laser for ablation and LEEP or cold-knife conization for excision. AIS is less common with CIN 2–3, but the incidence is increasing.[25] The usefulness of colposcopic evaluation in AIS is limited, because the visible changes may be minimal, located high in the endocervical canal, or present in multiple noncontiguous "skip" lesions. An excisional procedure, often conization, is thus preferred in women who wish to preserve childbearing status. Hysterectomy is the preferred treatment for those who have completed childbearing.[25]

Staging of cervical cancer is performed by clinical examination of the cervix, and evaluation of the bladder, ureters, and rectum. If the lesion is clearly confined to the cervix on office examination, then only a chest radiograph and evaluation of the ureters by CT urogram are necessary to assign a stage. If this is not possible in the office, examination under anesthesia along with cystoscopy and proctoscopy are necessary.

Early stages of cervical cancer include stage 0 (carcinoma in situ), stage IA (invasion diagnosed only by microscopy), and stage IB (clinically visible lesion confined to the cervix). Stage II tumors extend beyond the uterus, with no parametrial invasion (stage IIA) or with parametrial invasion (stage IIB). The late stages of cervical cancer include stage IIB, stage III (tumor extends to the pelvic wall, or involves the lower one third of the vagina, or causes hydronephrosis or nonfunctioning kidney) and stage IV (tumor has extended beyond the pelvis or has involved [biopsy-proven] the bladder or rectum).[26]

Treatment of Invasive Cervical Cancer

Women who have early-stage cervical cancer may be treated with radical hysterectomy and pelvic lymphadenectomy or with primary radiation and chemotherapy. Treatment of locally advanced disease (stages IIB to IVA) is best performed with primary radiation and concomitant chemotherapy, with randomized trials showing improved prognosis with combined modalities rather than radiation alone. Palliative care should be considered for advanced cervical cancer with distant metastases. The 5-year survival rates are predicted by clinical stage and approach 100% for patients who have stage IA, through 5% to 15% for stage IV. Prognosis is further affected by histologic subtype, age, and medical comorbidities, such as HIV.[27]

OVARIAN CANCER
Epidemiology

In the United States, ovarian cancer is the leading cause of death related to gynecologic malignancy. It is the fifth most common cause of death in women, with an overall prognosis that remains poor. In 2008, there are a predicted 21,650 new ovarian cancer cases and an estimated 15,520 deaths.[28] Most ovarian cancers occur in postmenopausal women, with the largest number of cases occurring in women between 50 and 75 years of age.[29]

Classification of Ovarian Neoplasms

Ovarian tumors are broadly separated into three main categories: epithelial, germ cell, and sex cord. Epithelial stromal tumors are the most common ovarian neoplasms, representing 65% of all ovarian neoplasms. They arise from the epithelial (coelomic) surface of the ovary. Unfortunately, most cases of epithelial cancers are diagnosed in late stages. Germ cell tumors are the second most frequently occurring tumors, composing 20% to 25% of ovarian neoplasms. They may consist of any or all three embryonic layers (ectoderm, mesoderm, or endoderm). In female patients younger than 30 years of age, germ cell tumors are the most frequent ovarian neoplasm. Germ cell tumors are often diagnosed in early stages and are often unilateral in presentation. Because of childbearing potential in this most commonly affected age group, treatment should consider fertility preservation. Finally, sex cord tumors are the third most frequent type of ovarian cancer, composing 6% of all ovarian neoplasms. These tumors may sometimes secrete sex steroid hormones, leading to conditions including amenorrhea, irregular vaginal bleeding, or precocious puberty. Lipoid cell and gonadoblastoma are other rare ovarian neoplasms, occurring at less than 0.1% off all ovarian neoplasms.[30]

Risk Factors and Screening

Women may inquire during routine gynecologic examinations about ovarian cancer screening. Unfortunately, no effective ovarian cancer screening strategy exists for the general population. Serum marker screening (CA-125) and ultrasound screening techniques have been reviewed as potential screening modalities. The USPSTF found that CA-125, pelvic ultrasound, and routine pelvic examinations all fail to reduce mortality from ovarian cancer.[31] Although earlier stage cancers can be detected with multimodality screening, this early detection does not result in a decrease of ovarian cancer mortality. The ACOG has issued statements advising against routine screening, which because of its high false-positive rate leads to an unacceptable number of invasive interventions in women who do not have significant disease.[32] Elevated CA-125 can often occur in benign conditions (**Box 1**).

As with any initial evaluation, a complete history, physical, and pelvic examination should be completed. The history should focus on genetic risks and a detailed family history. An average woman's lifetime risk for ovarian cancer is 1 in 70. Positive family history increases the risk for ovarian cancer. Having one first- or second-degree

> **Box 1**
> **Causes of elevated serum CA-125**
>
> *Benign conditions*
> Benign ovarian cystic and solid tumors
> Leiomyomata uteri
> Endometriosis
> Adenomyosis
> Peritoneal, pleural, or pericardial inflammation
> Intraperitoneal adhesions
> Tuberculous peritonitis
> Pregnancy
> Liver disease
> *Malignant conditions*
> Ovarian cancer
> Metastatic cancer to the ovary
> Metastatic endometrial cancer
> Metastatic cervical cancer
> Breast cancer
> Pancreatic cancer
> Gastrointestinal cancers
> Lung cancer
> Plasma cell dyscrasias
>
> *From* Alektiar K, Fuks Z. Cancer of the ovary. In: Leibel SA, Phillips TL, editors. Textbook of radiation oncology. Philadelphia: Saunders; 2004; with permission.

relative who had ovarian cancer increases the risk by approximately threefold.[33] In screening high-risk populations, the USPSTF finds moderate evidence and recommends that women whose family history is associated with an increased risk for deleterious mutations in the BRCA1 or BRCA2 genes be referred for genetic counseling and evaluation for BRCA testing.[32]

Many other risk factors are based on the "incessant ovulation hypothesis." This hypothesis postulates that ovarian cancer may develop from an aberrant repair process of the surface epithelium during each ovulation cycle.[34] In general terms, more ovulation cycles increase risk, and decreased ovulation lessens risk. Age, parity, menarche, age of menopause, breast-feeding, and birth control or hormonal use history are considered (**Table 2**).

Diagnosis and Management

Most ovarian cancers are diagnosed at advanced stages. Initial symptoms can be nonspecific, and can be seen in many benign gastrointestinal, genitourinary, and gynecologic conditions. Patients and primary care physicians alike should be aware of a pattern of complaints, however, such as abdominal bloating, gastrointestinal complaints, urinary complaints, irregular vaginal bleeding, and increasing abdominal

Table 2
Risk factors for development of ovarian cancer

	Endocrine/Hormonal	Environmental/Dietary	Genetic/Hereditary Syndromes
Increased risk	Uninterrupted ovulation Nulliparity Early menarche Late menopause Exposure to diethylstilbestrol Prior breast cancer	"Industrialized" living Asbestos exposure Obesity Consumption of milk/meat High-fat diet	Hereditary site-specific syndrome Hereditary breast-ovarian syndrome Lynch II syndrome First-degree relative who had breast or ovarian cancer Genetic mutation (eg, *BRCA1, BRCA2*) Gonadal dysgenesis Peutz-Jeghers syndrome
Decreased risk	Multiple pregnancies Early first pregnancy Early menopause Breast-feeding Oral contraceptives	Vegetarian diet High vitamin D levels Higher sunlight exposure Nonsteroidal anti-inflammatory drug use? Mumps? Tubal ligation	
No influence known	Hormone replacement therapy Persistent ovarian cyst Tamoxifen use Medroxyprogesterone acetate	Coffee Tobacco Alcohol Radiation Tranquilizers/hypnotics Infection	

From Staumbaugh M. The ovary. In: Perez CA, Brady LW, Halperin EC, et al, editors. Principles and practice of radiation oncology. 4th edition. Philadelphia: Lippincott Williams & Wilkins; 2004. p. 1934–52; with permission.

girth. Although initial signs can be vague, it is necessary to completely evaluate these common symptoms in clinical context.

The ability to detect adnexal masses by bimanual examination is limited in most women; therefore, we must also understand risk factor stratification and diagnostic guidelines. The primary goal of diagnostic evaluation of adnexal masses is to exclude malignancy. The ACOG and the Society of Gynecologic Oncologists have created guidelines for the management of adnexal masses (**Box 2**).[35] High-frequency, gray-scale transvaginal ultrasonography is the most cost-effective and most accurate imaging technique. Although CT and MRI can detect malignancy, these modalities are more useful for surgical planning, staging, and monitoring of disease once identified. Laboratory considerations include a complete blood count, CA-125, comprehensive metabolic panel, β-HCG, and α-fetoprotein levels.

Ovarian cancer diagnosis requires a thorough surgical exploration. The National Institutes of Health (NIH) Consensus Statement from 1994 suggested referral to a gynecologic oncologist for appropriate staging procedures, because early aggressive cytoreductive surgery and proper staging by physicians who have advanced training in gynecologic cancer offer better survival rates.

Treatment

In women who have completed childbearing and in whom appropriate staging procedures have been completed, a total abdominal hysterectomy with bilateral salpingo-oophorectomy and appendectomy is performed.[36] Unilateral salpingo-oophorectomy and ovarian cystectomy are considered for the following tumors: germ cell tumors, stage I stromal tumors, tumors with low malignancy potential, and stage IA, grade 1 or 2 invasive cancer. Even when patients choose to preserve the uterus and remaining ovary, these patients should undergo complete surgical evaluation and exploration.[37]

Box 2
Society of Gynecologic Oncologists and American College of Obstetricians and Gynecologists referral guidelines for a newly diagnosed pelvic mass

Premenopausal (<50 years old)

CA-125 > 200 U/mL

Ascites

Evidence of abdominal or distant metastasis (by examination or imaging study)

Family history of breast or ovarian cancer (in a first-degree relative)

Postmenopausal (≥50 years old)

CA-125 > 35 U/mL

Ascites

Nodular or fixed pelvic mass

Evidence of abdominal or distant metastasis (by examination or imaging study)

Family history of breast or ovarian cancer (in a first-degree relative)

From Im SS, Gordon AN, Buttin BM, et al. Validation of referral guidelines for women with pelvic masses. Obstet Gynecol 2005;105(1):35–41; with permission.

A discussion of protocol treatment guidelines for each of the ovarian cancers and their particular stages is beyond the scope of this article. Most common, however, is primary cytoreductive surgery and chemotherapy. Aggressive cytoreductive surgery to 2 cm or less of residual tumor significantly enhances survival for patients who have ovarian cancer. Since the mid-1990s, the combination of a platinum agent and a taxane has been accepted as the standard of care in the United States. Radiation therapy is usually reserved for palliative therapy and recurring disease.[38]

FIGO staging remains the most important prognostic variable in determining outcomes in women who have ovarian cancer (**Table 3**). Five-year survival rates are approximately 90% for stage I, 80% for stage II, 15% to 20% for stage III, and less than 5% for stage IV.[37] Additional prognostic considerations include age, histologic grade and subtype, malignant ascites or malignant peritoneal washings, tumor excrescences or ruptured capsule, and volume of residual disease after cytoreductive surgery.[39]

Table 3
International Federation of Gynecologists and Obstetricians stage grouping for primary carcinoma of the ovary (1998)

Stage	Description
I	Growth limited to the ovaries.
IA	Growth limited to one ovary; no ascites. No tumor on the external surface; capsule intact.
IB	Growth limited to both ovaries; no ascites. No tumor on the external surface; capsule intact.
IC	Tumor either stage IA or IB but with tumor on the surface of one or both ovaries, or with capsule ruptured, or with ascites present containing malignant cells, or with positive peritoneal washings.
II	Growth involving one or both ovaries with pelvic extension.
IIA	Extension and/or metastases to the uterus and/or tubes.
IIB	Growth involving one or both ovaries with pelvic extension.
IIC	Tumor either stage IIA or IIB but with tumor on the surface of one or both ovaries, or with capsules ruptured, or with ascites present containing malignant cells, or with positive peritoneal washings.
III	Tumor involving one or both ovaries with peritoneal implants outside the pelvis and/or positive retroperitoneal or inguinal nodes. Superficial liver metastases equals stage III. Tumor is limited to the true pelvis but with histologically verified malignant extension to small bowel or omentum.
IIIA	Tumor grossly limited to the true pelvis with negative nodes but with histologically confirmed microscopic seeding of abdominal peritoneal surfaces.
IIIB	Tumor of one or both ovaries with histologically confirmed implants of abdominal peritoneal surfaces, none exceeding 2 cm in diameter. Nodes negative.
IIIC	Abdominal implants greater than 2 cm in diameter and/or positive retroperitoneal or inguinal nodes.
IV	Growth involving one or both ovaries with distant metastasis. If pleural effusion is present, cytologic test results must be positive to allot a case to stage IV. Parenchymal liver metastasis equals stage IV.

From Pecorelli S, Odicino F, Maisonneuve P, et al. Carcinoma of the ovary. Annual report on the results of treatment of gynaecological cancer, 23rd vol. International Federation of Gynecology and Obstetrics. J Epidemiol Biostat 1998;3:75–102; with permission.

ENDOMETRIAL CANCER
Epidemiology and Etiology

Endometrial cancer is the most common gynecologic cancer in the United States and the fourth most common cancer in women. It is most common in postmenopausal females with a peak incidence occurring between ages 50 and 70. The United States population is aging and obesity rates are climbing; because of these trends the number of endometrial cancer cases is expected to increase. A woman in the United States has an approximately 1 in 30 lifetime risk for developing endometrial cancer. Although most cases of endometrial cancer are diagnosed in early stages, the trend over the past 25 years has shown no statistical improvement in survival rates.[29]

Classification

Histologically, endometrial adenocarcinoma is the most common type of uterine cancer, composing two thirds of the cases, and when typically diagnosed in early stages it has a more favorable outcome. Mucinous carcinomas have a favorable prognosis similar to that of adenocarcinoma. Serous, clear cell, and squamous cell cancers are the most aggressive endometrial cancer cell types, occur more commonly in older women, and are frequently diagnosed in later stages with peritoneal invasion and metastasis.[39]

Clinical Presentation and Risk Factors

Because most cases occur in postmenopausal women, endometrial cancer with common symptoms, including postmenopausal bleeding and chronic vaginal discharge, often prompts a timely work-up with rapid diagnosis. Atypical glandular cells found on Pap screening should also prompt further investigation to rule out the possibility for cervical and endometrial abnormalities. Because the endometrium responds to hormonal stimulation from estrogen, constant proliferation can lead to cellular atypia. Endometrial hyperplasia is divided into two types: simple and complex with or without atypia. Atypical complex hyperplasia is a potential precursor to endometrial cancer. In obesity, adipocytes are capable of converting androstenedione to estrone and high levels of estrogen result.[40] Increasing rates of obesity are believed to contribute to an increase in rates of endometrial cancer. Genetic conditions and tamoxifen are also risk factors to be considered, along with epidemiologic risks (**Table 4**).[41]

Screening

Currently, the ACOG states that screening for endometrial cancer in low-risk patients is neither cost effective nor warranted. High-risk conditions must be identified to understand and determine other screening recommendations. Hereditary nonpolyposis colorectal cancer (HNPCC, also known as Lynch syndrome) increases the risk for endometrial, colon, and ovarian cancers. Prior tamoxifen use (acting as an estrogen antagonist on breast tissue but an estrogen agonist on other tissues) should also be considered as a risk factor.

In regard to screening high-risk patients, the ACS recommends endometrial biopsy starting at menopause and then periodically at the discretion of the physician. On the basis of expert opinion only, a task force organized by the NIH recommends screening patients who have HNPCC. The ACOG leaves screening of patients who have a history of tamoxifen use to the discretion of their physicians.[41]

Diagnosis and Management

A careful history and risk factor evaluation should begin every evaluation for endometrial cancer, along with a detailed physical examination. Pap cytology should be

| Table 4 | |
| Epidemiologic risk factors for endometrial carcinoma | |
Factors	Relative Risk
Chronic estrogenic stimulation	
Estrogen replacement (no progestin)	2–12
Early menarche/late menopause	1.6–4.0
Nulliparity	2–3
Anovulation	No data
Estrogen-producing tumors	No data
Demographic characteristics	
Increasing age	4–8
Caucasian race	2
High socioeconomic status	1.5
European/North American country	2–3
Family history of endometrial cancer	2
Associated medical illness	
Diabetes mellitus	3
Gallbladder disease	3.7
Obesity	2–4
Hypertension	1.5
Prior pelvic radiotherapy	8

From Burke T, Eifel P, Muggia F. Cancers of the uterine body. In: DeVita V, Hellman S, Rosenberg S, editors. Cancer: principles and practice of oncology. 6th edition. Philadelphia: Lippincott Williams and Wilkins; 2001.

updated according to standard age-appropriate guidelines. Primary imaging recommendations include transvaginal ultrasonography, which can accurately show distinguishable patterns of hyperplasia, polyps, and endometrial cancer, and can adequately demonstrate the degree of myometrial invasion. The probability of a postmenopausal woman having endometrial cancer is less than 1.2% if the endometrial lining is less than 4 mm. A meta-analysis of 5892 women demonstrated that endometrial thickness greater than 5 mm identified 96% of cases of endometrial carcinoma.[42] CT scanning is rarely used in early-stage disease but can help confirm advanced-stage III and IV disease. MRI may be more accurate in diagnosing depth of myometrial invasion compared with ultrasound, but with surgical staging the cost effectiveness is questionable.[43]

Tissue evaluation can be performed most easily with an in-office endometrial biopsy (EMB). EMB is fairly accurate in diagnosing endometrial cancer with an 11% false-negative rate, and can spare the patient from the operative risks of anesthesia required for a dilation and curettage (D&C). D&C should ultimately be used for women who are unable to complete an EMB in the office, women who have persisting symptoms and clinical suspicion despite normal EMB, and those who have atypical complex hyperplasia. Other preoperative tests should include a chest radiograph, CA-125 (often elevated in metastatic disease), a complete blood count, a comprehensive metabolic panel, and a urinalysis.

Treatment

Total abdominal hysterectomy and bilateral salpingo-oophorectomy is considered to be the primary treatment of uterine cancer. Sampling of the pelvic and para-aortic lymph nodes is indicated in several circumstances, including clinically enlarged nodes, greater than a 50% myometrial invasion, extrauterine metastasis, involvement of the isthmus/cervix, and for cell types other than adenocarcinoma.[44]

The degree of myometrial invasion, histologic type, and lymphatic and metastatic spread are important prognostic factors. Because these are considered to be major prognostic factors, FIGO changed the staging standards to surgical staging from clinical staging in 1988 (**Table 5**). For those patients who have advanced disease or are poor operative candidates, the FIGO 1971 clinical staging of endometrial cancer is still used (**Table 6**).

Overall 5-year survival rates for endometrial cancer are approximately 75%. Stage I survival is 70% to 90%, stage II survival is 50% to 80%, stage III survival is 30% to 70%, and stage IV survival is 10% to 15%. Histologically, endometrioid adenocarcinomas have a worse prognosis with increasing grade, but overall this group has favorable survival outcomes. Because of the likelihood of systemic spread with serous, clear cell, and squamous cancers, the overall survival rate in this group is less than 35%.[43]

To discuss protocol treatments for each stage and histologic type of endometrial cancer is beyond the scope of this article; however, surgery remains the mainstay of treatment. Adjuvant radiation is also used in endometrial cancer management along with definitive treatment for those patients who have unresectable disease or those who are medically inoperable. Chemotherapy is limited in the treatment of endometrial cancer. Currently a combination of agents, including doxorubicin or Taxol with cisplatin, is showing the most promise toward achieving favorable outcomes.[45]

Table 5
Corpus cancer surgical staging (FIGO 1988)

Stage	Definition
O	Carcinoma in situ (preinvasive)
I	Tumor confined to the uterine corpus
IA	Tumor limited to the endometrium/no myometrial involvement
IB	Invasion to ≤50% of the myometrium
IC	Invasion to >50% of the myometrium
II	Cervical involvement
IIA	Endocervical gland involvement
IIB	Cervical stromal invasion
III	Locoregional spread of tumor
IIIA	Uterine serosa, adnexa, or peritoneal washings/ascites positive for tumor
IIIB	Vaginal Involvement
IIIC	Pelvic or para-aortic lymph nodal involvement
IVA	Invasion of bladder, bowel mucosa, or both
IVB	Distant metastases

Data from Benedet JL, Bender H, Jones H 3rd, et al. FIGO staging classifications and clinical practice guidelines in the management of gynecologic cancers. FIGO Committee on Gynecologic Oncology. Int J Gynaecol Obstet 2000;70(2):209–62.

Table 6 Clinical staging of endometrial cancer (FIGO 1971)	
Stage	Definition
I	Carcinoma confined to the uterine body
IA	Uterine cavity measures 8 cm or less
IB	Uterine cavity is larger than 8 cm
II	Carcinoma involves the uterine body and cervix
III	Carcinoma extends outside the uterus but is confined to the true pelvis
IV	Carcinoma spreads massively to entire pelvic cavity or distant spread
IVA	Tumor involves mucosa of bladder or rectum
IVB	Distant metastasis

Data from Benedet JL, Bender H, Jones H 3rd, et al. FIGO staging classifications and clinical practice guidelines in the management of gynecologic cancers. FIGO Committee on Gynecologic Oncology. Int J Gynaecol Obstet 2000;70(2):209–62.

SUMMARY

The strategies for prevention and detection of gynecologic cancers continue to evolve. Because cancer prevention through screening remains an essential component of primary care, our female patients will increasingly depend on our knowledge of these changes and rely on our education to foster early detection. The exciting addition of the HPV vaccination in prevention of cervical cancer provides hope that similar preventive efforts for ovarian and endometrial cancers will also soon develop.

REFERENCES

1. Atlanta (GA) American Cancer Society: cancer facts and figures 2008. American Cancer Society 2008. Available at: http://www.cancer.org/downloads/STT/2008CAFFfinalsecured.pdf. Accessed June 30, 2008.
2. Tyring SK. Vulvar squamous cell carcinoma: guidelines for early diagnosis and treatment. Am J Obstet Gynecol 2003;189(3 Suppl):S17–23.
3. Madeleine MM, Daling JR, Carter JJ, et al. Cofactors with human papillomavirus in a population-based study of vulvar cancer. J Natl Cancer Inst 1997;89:1516–23.
4. Edwards CL, Tortelero-Luna G, Linares AC, et al. Vulvar intraepithelial neoplasia and vulvar cancer. Obstet Gynecol Clin North Am 1996;23(2):295–324.
5. Stroup AM, Harlan LC, Trimble EL. Demographic, clinical, and treatment trends among women diagnosed with vulvar cancer in the Unites States. Gynecol Oncol 2008;108:577–83.
6. Canavan TP, Cohen D. Vulvar cancer. Am Fam Physician 2002;66:1269–74, 1276.
7. Whitcomb B. Gynecologic malignancies. Surg Clin North Am 2008;88(2):301–17.
8. Landay M, Satmary WA, Memarzadeh S, et al. Premalignant & malignant disorders of the vulva & vagina. In: DeCherney AH, Nathan L, Goodwin TM, Laufer N, editors. Current diagnosis obstetrics and gynecology. 10th Edition. New York: McGraw-Hill; 2007.
9. Ghurani GB, Penalver MA. An update on vulvar cancer. Am J Obstet Gynec 2001;185(2):294–9.
10. Frumovitz M, Bodurka DC. Neoplastic diseases of the vulva: lichen sclerosis, intraepithelial neoplasia, Paget's disease, carcinoma. In: Katz VL, Lentz GM,

Lobo RA, Gershenson DM, editors. Comprehensive gynecology. 5th Edition. Philadelphia: Mosby Elsevier; 2007.

11. Bosch FX, Lorinca A, Munoz N, et al. The causal relationship between human papillomavirus and cervical cancer [review]. J Clin Pathol 2002;55:244–65.

12. Moscicki AB, Shiboski S, Hills NK, et al. Regression of low-grade squamous intraepithelial lesions in young women. Lancet 2004;364:1678–83.

13. Hildersheim A, Hadjimichael O, Schwartz PE, et al. Risk factors for rapid-onset cervical cancer. Am J Obstet Gynecol 1999;180:571–7.

14. Screening for cervical cancer. January 2003. U.S. Preventive Services Task Force. Agency for Healthcare Research and Quality Rockville (MD). Available at: http://www.ahrq.gov/clinic/uspstf/uspscerv.htm.

15. Smith RA, Cokkinides V, von Eschenbach AC, et al. American Cancer Society guideline for the early detection of cervical neoplasia and cancer. CA Cancer J Clin 2002;52(1):8–22.

16. Sawaya GF. Risk of cervical cancer associated with extending the interval between cervical cancer screening. N Engl J Med 2003;349:1501–9.

17. Pairwuti S. False-negative Papanicolaou smears from women with cancerous and precancerous lesions of the uterine cervix. Acta Cytol 1991;35:40–6.

18. Goldie SJ, Kim JJ, Wright TC. Cost-effectiveness of human papillomavirus DNA testing for cervical cancer screening in women aged 30 years or more. Obstet Gynecol 2004;103:619–31.

19. Cervical Cytology Screening. ACOG practice bulletin No 45; August 2003; 102, No. 2.

20. Dunne EF, Unger ER, Sternberg M, et al. Prevalence of HPV infection among females in the United States. JAMA 2007;297:813–9.

21. Zazove P, Reed BD, Gregoire L, et al. Presence of human papillomavirus infection of the uterine cervix as determined by different detection methods in a low-risk community-based population. Arch Fam Med 1993;2:1250–7.

22. Wright TC, Massad LS, Dunton CJ, et al. 2006 guidelines for the management of women with abnormal cervical cancer screening tests. Am J Obstet Gynec 2007; 197(4):346–55.

23. Wright TC, Massad LS, Dunton CJ, et al. 2006 guidelines for the management of women with abnormal cervical cancer screening tests. J Low Genit Tract Dis 2007;11(4):201–22.

24. Wright TC, Massad LS, Dunton CJ, et al. 2006 guidelines for the management of women with cervical intraepithelial neoplasia or adenocarcinoma in situ. Am J Obstet Gynec 2007;197(4):340–5.

25. Wang SS, Sherman ME, Hildesheim A, et al. Cervical adenocarcinoma and squamous cell carcinoma incidence trends among white women and black women in the United States for 1976–2000. Cancer 2004;100:1035–44.

26. ACOG practice bulletin. Diagnosis and treatment of cervical carcinomas. Number 35, May 2002. American College of Obstetricians and Gynecologists. American College of Obstetricians and Gynecologists. Int J Gynaecol Obstet 2002;78:79.

27. Waggoner S. Cervical cancer. Lancet 2003;361(9376):2217–25.

28. Jemal A, Siegel R, Ward E, et al. Cancer Statistics, 2008. Ca Cancer J Clin 2008; 58:71–96.

29. Rubin S, Sabbatini P, Randall M, et al. Ovarian Cancer. In: Pazdur R, Coia L, Hoskins W, et al, editors. Ovarian cancer in cancer management: a multidisciplinary approach. Manhasset (NY): The Oncology Group, CMP Medical; 2007.

30. Coleman RL, Gershenson DM. Neoplastic diseases of the ovary. In: Katz VL, Lentz GM, Lobo RA, Gershenson DM, editors. Katz: comprehensive gynecology. 5th edition. Philadelphia: Mosby; 2007.
31. Screening for ovarian cancer: recommendation statement. May 2004. Agency for Healthcare Research and Quality, Rockville (MD). Available at: http://www.ahrq.gov/clinic/3rduspstf/ovariancan/ovcanrs.htm. Accessed June 30, 2008.
32. American College of Obstetricians and Gynecologists. Committee Opinion No. 280. The role of the generalist obstetrician-gynecologist in the early detection of ovarian cancer. Gynecol Oncol 2002;87(3):237–9.
33. Kerlikowske K, Brown JS, Grady DG. Should women with familial ovarian cancer undergo prophylactic oophorectomy? Obstet Gynecol 1992;80:700–7.
34. Thomas G, Cox J, Ang K. The ovary. In: Perez C, editor. Radiation oncology. St. Louis: Mosby; 2003. p. 757–78.
35. Management of Adenexal Masses. ACOG Practice Bulletin No 83. American College of Obstetricians and Gynecologists. Obstet Gynecol 2007;110:201–14.
36. Staumbaugh M. The ovary. In: Perez C, editor. Principles and practice of radiation oncology. 4th edition. Philadelphia: Linppincott Williams & Wilkins; 2004. p. 1934–52, 63.
37. Im SS, Gordon AN, Buttin BM, et al. Validation of referral guidelines for women with pelvic masses. Obstet Gynecol 2005;105(1):35–41.
38. Karlan B, Markman M, Eifel P. Ovarian cancer, peritoneal carcinoma, fallopian tube cancer in DeVita V, Hellmann S, Robseby S eds. Cancer: principles and practice of oncology 7th Edition. Philadelphia, Lippincott Williams & Wilkins; 2005.
39. Glassburn J, Brady L, Grigsby P. Chapter 62 Endometrium. In: Perez, editor. Principles and practice of radiation oncology. 4th Edition. Philadelphia: Lippincott Williams & Wilkins; 2004.
40. Burke T, Eifel P, Muggia F. Cancers of the uterine body. In DeVita V, Hellman S, Rosenberg S, eds. Cancer principles and practice of oncology 6th Edition. Philadelphia, Lippincott Williams & Wilkins; 2001.
41. Zoorob R, Anderson R, Cefalu C, et al. Cancer screening guidelines. Am Fam Physician 2001;63(6):1101–12.
42. Smith-Bindman R, Kerllikowske K, Feldstein VA, et al. Endovaginal ultrasound to exclude endometrial cancer and other endometrial abnormalities. JAMA 1998; 280:1510–7.
43. Savelli L, Ceccarini M, Ludovisi M, et al. Preoperative local staging of endometrial cancer: transvaginal sonography vs magnetic resonance imaging. Ultrasound Obstet Gynecol 2008;31(5):560–6.
44. Alektiar K, Nori D. Cancer of the endometrium. In: Leibel S, Phillips T, editors. Textbook of radiation oncology. Philadelphia: Saunders; 2004.
45. Humber C, Tierney JF, Symonds RP, et al. Chemotherapy for advanced, recurrent or metastatic endometrial cancer: a systematic review of Cochrane collaboration. Ann Oncol 2007;18:409–20.

Cervical Cancer Screening and Updated Pap Guidelines

Johanna B. Warren, MD[a],*, Heidi Gullett, MD, MPH[b],
Valerie J. King, MD, MPH[a]

KEYWORDS

- Cervical cancer • Screening • Pap testing
- HPV • Dysplasia • Guidelines • Abnormal pap

EPIDEMIOLOGY

Worldwide, cervical cancer accounts for 10% of all cancers, ranking as the third most commonly diagnosed neoplasm.[1] Among developing countries, cervical cancer accounts for 15% of all cancers and ranks second in incidence.[1] High-risk areas worldwide include South America, East and South Africa, and India.[1] In the United States, cervical cancer no longer is the leading cause of cancer deaths for women largely as a result of aggressive cervical dysplasia screening.[2] Cervical cancer still remains, however, an important neoplasm and results in significant mortality for many American women each year.[2] In the United States, more than 10,000 new cases of cervical cancer are diagnosed yearly with more than 3700 deaths per year attributed to the disease.[3] Disparities remain among Hispanic and African American populations within the United States with regard to cervical cancer incidence and mortality.[4] These invasive cancers and deaths are preventable with appropriate screening.

Human papilloma virus (HPV) infections are common with nearly 20 million Americans currently infected and greater than 50% of all sexually active adults infected at some point in their lifetime.[5] Approximately 6.2 million Americans become infected with HPV annually.[5] These infections may resolve spontaneously or may progress to clinically apparent infection, manifesting most notably as cervical dysplasia that can progress to cancer and more common benign genital wart infections.

PATHOPHYSIOLOGY

The normal cervix is comprised of different epithelial cell types, and the pathophysiology of cervical cancer depends on an understanding of the origin and behavior of

[a] Department of Family Medicine, Oregon Health and Science University, 3181 SW Sam Jackson Park Road, Portland, OR 97239-3098, USA
[b] Dayspring Family Health Center, 550 Sunset Trail, Jellico, TN 37762, USA
* Corresponding author.
E-mail address: warrejoh@ohsu.edu (J.B. Warren).

Prim Care Clin Office Pract 36 (2009) 131–149
doi:10.1016/j.pop.2008.10.008
0095-4543/08/$ – see front matter
primarycare.theclinics.com

these cell types and an appreciation of HPV as a causative infectious agent. The mid-cervical canal to upper cervix typically is comprised of mucus-secreting columnar epithelium, originating embryologically from the invaginating müllerian ducts.[6] There is little neoplastic potential for this cell type. Lower in the female genital tract, the vagina and distal ectocervix is comprised of squamous epithelium, often referred to as the original squamous epithelium, as these squamous cells replaced the original müllerian columnar cells when the uterovaginal canal was formed.[6] Again, there is little neoplastic potential for this cell type.

The squamocolumnar junction (SCJ) is the point at which the squamous and columnar cells meet. It typically is found between the central ectocervix and the lower cervical canal, but the location varies throughout a woman's life, from fetal development through menopause. The original SCJ is defined as the location after fetal development at birth. The SCJ is a transformation zone. The normal transformation of one mature cell type to another also is known as metaplasia. When metaplasia is occurring, there is always some neoplastic potential.

In reproductive-aged women, the original SCJ moves out onto the portio of the cervix with hormonal influences. The acidic vaginal pH plus mechanical irritation likely induces the process of squamous metaplasia, resulting in a new SCJ. The area between the original and new squamocolumnar junctions is now referred to as the transformation zone.[7] Immature squamous metaplasic cells in this transformation zone are theoretically the most vulnerable to neoplasia.

Koilocytosis has been described on Papanicolaou (Pap) samples for decades and is recognized as a hallmark of mild dysplasia. In the late 1970s, Meisels and Fortin discovered that HPV was the origin of the koilocytotic atypia.[8] Over the past 4 decades, it has become understood that HPV not only is associated with high-grade cervical lesions but also is considered the causative agent in the development of cervical cancer. The strength of this causal relationship has been described by Bosch and colleagues and is now a well-accepted model for understanding viral-mediated oncogenesis.[9]

HPV infections primarily affect young women. HPV subtypes 6, 11, 16, and 18 are considered the high-risk subtypes and are known to be etiologic agents in the development of neoplastic changes in the transformation zone of the cervix. The technology available to detect these subtypes has changed Pap testing and cervical cancer screening dramatically (discussed later). HPV infection with subtypes 6 and 11 is responsible for 25% of all cervical intraepithelial neoplasia type 1 (CIN 1) and 90% of all anogenital condyloma. Infection with subtypes 16 and 18 is responsible for 25% of all CIN 1 and 70% of all CIN 2 and CIN 3. Subtypes 16, 18, 31, 33, and 45 are found in 63% to 97% of invasive cervical cancers.[10] Other risk factors for development of cervical cancer are listed in **Box 1**.

Although HPV infection is now viewed as an infectious disease, akin to many sexually transmitted diseases, it is difficult to pinpoint when the virus is contracted by any individual woman. In addition, the natural history of each subtype of HPV can vary based on many cofactors, only some of which are modifiable. These factors can make definitive discussions with patients challenging. Exposure to HPV is common, but cervical cancer is uncommon. Moreover, clinically detectable cytologic HPV changes also are uncommon. In 1991, Bauer and colleagues described that 46% of women at a university health center tested positive for high-risk HPV, but only approximately 5% of had cytologic changes caused by this HPV infection.[11] Most HPV infections are transient, with 70% of young women clearing a newly acquired HPV infection within the first 12 months after infection.[12]

The acute low-grade histologic manifestation of a new infection with a high-risk HPV subtype usually is considered CIN 1. These changes usually are transient, with most

Box 1
Risk factors for cervical cancer
Cigarette smoking
Dietary and nutritional factors
Early age at first sexual intercourse
Family history of cervical cancer
History of chlamydia, trichomonas, or herpes simplex virus infection
Inadequate screening
Immunodeficiency, including HIV infection
Multiparity
Persistent HPV infection
Use of oral contraceptives.

women able to clear the infection on their own. CIN 2 and CIN 3, however, are accepted as cervical cancer precursors. Data from the ASCUS-LSIL Triage Study (ALTS) and previous work by Koutsky and colleagues essentially have refuted the idea that CIN 1 progresses to CIN 2, which then progresses to CIN 3 and then to invasive cervical cancer.[10] After immune recognition and clearance of HPV, most low-grade histologic CIN 1 and CIN 2 lesions seem to regress. One study found that the regression rate of CIN 2 in adolescents was up to 84% at 24 months.[13]

In more invasive disease, a higher-grade lesion of CIN 2 or CIN 3 likely develops in an area adjacent to a low-grade HPV infection and then the higher-grade lesion progresses toward cervical cancer.[14–17] Many of the cofactors identified as risk factors, and perhaps several yet to be determined, play a role in the persistence of the high-risk HPV infection in otherwise immunocompetent women. It also is not entirely clear what cascade of events must occur in the presence of such a persistent high-grade infection to promote this aberrant cellular activity toward cancer.

A preventive HPV vaccine has become available in recent years and is marketed under the trade name, Gardasil. It targets the high-risk HPV subtypes 6, 11, 16, and 18 and is designed to induce an immune response before infection with HPV.[18] It is ideal to administer the vaccine before viral exposure, but it also is effective to administer it once a patient tests positive for a high-risk HPV subtype or has an abnormal Pap smear that indicates HPV infection. The rationale behind postinfection vaccine administration is to protect women against infection with one of the other subtypes. The vaccine also provides some cross-protection to additional HPV subtypes that are not among the four covered by the vaccine. The vaccine is FDA approved for administration to women between ages 9 and 26 and has a safe profile with the most common side effect of injection site soreness. Clinical trials currently are underway to investigate therapeutic HPV vaccines that target HPV serotypes 16 and 18 infections by inducing cytotoxic T-lymphocyte responses and killing dysplastic cells.

CERVICAL CANCER SCREENING
Recommendations

Cervical cancer screening with cervical cytology reduces the incidence of and mortality from cervical cancer.[19] Cervical cancer screening is effective because the disease generally has a long preinvasive stage that can be detected before the development of frank carcinoma and metastasis of the disease. The U.S. Preventive Services Task Force (USPSTF) issued its most recent screening recommendations in January 2003 that also were endorsed by the National Cancer Institute. The USPSTF recommendations were based on a high-quality systematic review of the medical literature.[20] The USPSTF strongly recommends cervical cancer screening for women who are sexually active and have a cervix. Their recommendation states that the most benefit from screening is likely to occur by screening women within 3 years of onset of sexual activity or age 21, whichever occurs first. Cervical cancer screening is recommended every 3 years. The USPSTF found little benefit of screening at more frequent intervals for most women. The USPSTF recommends against routine screening of women over age 65 who have had recent adequate screening and who are not otherwise at high risk for cervical cancer. Their analysis indicates that there are likely to be more harms than benefits from routine screening in this age group. These harms include excess biopsies and treatment of lesions that are unlikely to progress and psychologic distress. They also recommend against routine screening for women who have had a total hysterectomy for benign disease and do not, therefore, have a cervix. In their 2003 recommendation, they found insufficient evidence to recommend for or against newer screening modalities, such as liquid-based cytology or HPV DNA testing. In 2003, however, the National Institute for Clinical Excellence in the United Kingdom recommended liquid-based cytology as the primary method for processing samples.[21] Screening recommendations from other United States groups differ slightly from those of the USPSTF. **Table 1** summarizes the key differences between recommendations from the USPSTF, the American College of Obstetricians and Gynecologists (ACOG), and the American Cancer Society (ACS).[22,23]

Collection Devices for Cytologic Screening

A systematic review of 34 randomized trials of cervical smear collection devices by Martin-Hirsch and colleagues was published in 1999.[24] It supports the use of the extended-tip spatula to sample the ectocervix and a cytobrush-type device to sample the endocervix. They conducted a meta-analysis, which demonstrated that the relatively blunt Ayre's spatula is ineffective for collection of endocervical cells compared with extended-tip spatulas. Use of the Ayre's spatula alone also results in less effective detection of dyskaryosis. The combination of a spatula plus a cytobrush device improves collection of adequate cervical samples. This group of investigators also updated their systematic review as a Cochrane review in 2000, including two additional trials.[25] Their conclusions from the earlier review essentially were unchanged, as they found that the combination of a spatula plus a cytobrush is more than 3 times as likely to detect endocervical cells than a spatula alone and approximately twice as likely to detect endocervical cells than the broom-type Cervex-Brush alone.

Increasing Adherence to Appropriate Screening

Advice and recommendations from clinicians are critical determinants of a woman's participation in cervical cancer screening.[3] The 2000 National Health Interview Survey reported that among women who had visited a physician but had not undergone Pap testing, more than 85% reported that their doctor did not recommend the test.[3] In a Cochrane review published in 2002, Forbes and colleagues studied interventions designed to increase uptake of cervical cancer screening among women.[26] Their review included 27 randomized controlled trials and eight quasirandomized trials. They reported that invitations for screening, including sending letters to women, were effective for increasing uptake of screening. Although the review found that

Table 1
Cervical cancer screening guidelines of United States organizations

	USPSTF (2003)	ACOG (2003)	ACS (2002)
Age for initiation of screening	Age 21, or within 3 years of initiation of sexual activity, whichever comes first	Approximately 3 years after onset of sexual intercourse but no later than age 21	Approximately 3 years after onset of sexual intercourse but no later than age 21
Frequency of screening			
• Conventional Pap	At least every 3 years	Annually. May extend interval to every 2–3 years for women age 30 and over who have had three negative cytology tests	Annually. May extend interval to every 2–3 years for women age 30 and over who have had three negative cytology tests
• Liquid-based cytology	Insufficient evidence	Annually. May extend interval to every 2–3 years for women age 30 and over who have had three negative cytology tests	Every 2 years. May extend interval to every 2–3 years for women age 30 and over who have had three negative cytology tests
• With HPV testing	Insufficient evidence	Every 3 years with negative HPV testing and negative cytology	Every 3 years with negative HPV testing and negative cytology
Age for cessation of screening	Age 65 and older with a history of negative cytology and who are not at increased risk for cervical cancer	Inconclusive evidence upon which to establish an upper age limit	Age 70 and older with 3 or more recent, consecutive negative tests and no abnormal tests within the prior 10 years
Screening after total hysterectomy	Discontinue if hysterectomy was for benign reasons.	Discontinue if hysterectomy was for benign reasons and no prior history of high-grade CIN	Discontinue if hysterectomy was for benign reasons and no prior history of high-grade CIN

educational interventions could be helpful, it is not clear whether or not there was a particular format that was most effective.

INTERPRETATION OF PAPANICOLAOU TESTING
Bethesda Guidelines and Specimen Adequacy

Pap testing of the cervix is a sampling of the endocervix and ectocervix. Conventional Pap smears transfer cellular material collected from the cervix onto a glass slide, which then is sprayed with an alcohol fixative for specimen transport. Newer liquid-based Pap testing allows collection of cellular material in a liquid suspension that is transported to a cytology laboratory where it is transferred to a glass slide and prepared for analysis.

The Bethesda System Terminology, designed to standardize the reporting system for Pap testing, was originally published in 2001. These guidelines were updated in 2006 and published again in 2007.[27] An important innovation of the Bethesda guidelines in 2001 was that the Pap report should comment on the quality of the specimen submitted for analysis. Specimen adequacy affects the sensitivity and specificity of that specimen for identification of cytologic abnormalities. Under this system, a specimen is labeled "satisfactory for evaluation" or "unsatisfactory for evaluation." At least 8000 squamous cells on a conventional smear or 5000 squamous cells on a liquid specimen must be present to meet cellularity requirements for classification as satisfactory.[28] Additionally, at least 10 squamous metaplastic or 10 endocervical cells ensures that the specimen represents elements of the transformation zone which is the most vulnerable zone to neoplastic changes.[28] If a specimen is labeled unsatisfactory, a reason is reported. In addition to insufficient cellular material, reasons for unsatisfactory specimens include broken slides and improper specimen labeling. Abnormalities still may be reported if they are visualized, even with unsatisfactory specimens.

The American Society for Colposcopy and Cervical Pathology (ASCCP) has developed an algorithm for managing unsatisfactory Pap tests (**Figs. 1** and **2**).[29] In brief, a Pap test lacking endocervical cells, with borderline cellularity, or with obscuring blood or inflammation should be repeated in 6 months if a patient has a prior abnormal Pap with CIN or a glandular abnormality, a positive HPV test within the past 12 months, no cervical visualization during the Pap test, or if the cytology reading on a prior Pap was obscured for any reason.[29] If an HPV test was performed with the Pap test and returned negative, a repeat Pap may be delayed for an additional 12 months.[29] With an unsatisfactory Pap for other reasons, clinicians should treat any underlying infections and repeat the Pap in 2 to 4 months.[29]

Despite the standardization with the Bethesda system, local variations among laboratories exist. Clinicians should know which resources laboratories have, which Pap collection methods are preferred for processing, and, most importantly, their pathologist.

Description and Interpretation of Cytologic Results

This section describes the terms that are used on standard Pap reports along with their interpretation:

- Negative for intraepithelial lesion or malignancy
- Atypical squamous cells of undetermined significance (ASCUS)
- Atypical squamous cells, cannot exclude high-grade squamous intraepithelial lesion (ASC-H)
- Low-grade squamous intraepithelial lesion (LSIL)
- High-grade squamous intraepithelial lesion (HSIL)
- Atypical glandular cells (AGC)

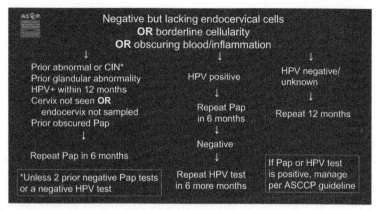

Fig. 1. Pap adequacy algorithm. Managing women with negative Paps lacking endocervical cells or other quality inticators. (*Reprinted from* The Journal of Lower Genital Tract Disease, Vol. 11, Issue 4, with the permission of ASCCP © American Society for Colposcopy and Cervical Pathology 2007. No copies of the algorithms may be made without the prior consent of ASCCP. Available at: http://www.asccp.org/.)

Negative for intraepithelial lesion or malignancy is the terminology that represents a negative, or benign, Pap test result. Many pathologists, however, also report non-neoplastic findings with this designation. These findings typically represent reactive cellular changes associated with inflammation, infection, or atrophy. Common organisms identified include *Trichomonas vaginalis*, *Actinomyces* species, and fungal organisms consistent with *Candida* species; shifts in flora suggestive of bacterial vaginosis often are seen.[28]

Atrophic cells can be visualized on normal Pap specimens and are an expected finding if a specimen is taken from a postmenopausal woman who is not using any hormonal replacement therapy. It is unusual to see a large number of endocervical or squamous metaplastic cells in a postmenopausal woman, as the SCJ regresses into the endocervical canal as a woman progresses through menopause. It often is unnecessary to repeat Pap testing on postmenopausal women who have specimens that are unsatisfactory for this reason.

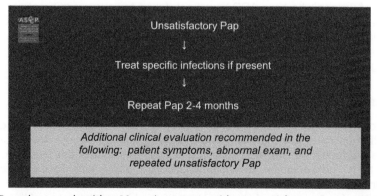

Fig. 2. Pap adequacy algorithm. Managing women with an unsatisfactory Pap test (*Reprinted from* The Journal of Lower Genital Tract Disease, Vol. 11, Issue 4, with the permission of ASCCP © American Society for Colposcopy and Cervical Pathology 2007. No copies of the algorithms may be made without the prior consent of ASCCP. Available at: http://www.asccp.org/.)

Finally, glandular cells (eg, endometrial cells) may be reported. Benign endometrial tissue may extend to where the tip of the broom or brush collection device collects the glandular cells during sample collection. Postmenopausal women using hormone replacement therapy may commonly have this finding. Although usually benign, few women over age 40 who have findings of glandular cells may have an underlying endometrial hyperplastic or neoplastic process. It is thus important to remember to interpret all Pap screening test results in the context of individual patients.

ASCUS represents a sample of cells that is not entirely normal but does not meet criteria for a squamous intraepithelial lesion (SIL).[30] This category spans the range of aggressive reactive changes to those that quantitatively may fall just short of the definition of SIL. Testing for HPV is useful particularly when thinking about this cytologic abnormality, as it can influence the management of these patients. The ALTS trial data showed that up to 63% of women who had ASCUS tested positive for high-risk HPV. Moreover, up to 20% of women who had ASCUS cytology actually had CIN 2 or CIN 3 histology,[31] and up to 0.2% of these women had invasive cancer.[27]

ASC-H should not be confused with ASCUS. The prevalence of high-grade disease with invasive lesions is much higher with ASC-H than with ASCUS, and this cytology result should be considered equivalent to HSIL. There is no role for high-risk HPV testing with this cytology, as infection is assumed. ALTS trial data showed that 41% of women who had ASC-H had CIN 2 or worse pathology.[15]

LSIL is a common finding. The incidence in the United States in 2003 was nearly 3% and likely is increasing.[27] According to a meta-analysis published in 2006, LSIL cytology represents a high-risk HPV infection in just under 80% of cases.[27] It is not uncommon to find infection with multiple HPV subtypes underlying these cellular changes. The ALTS trial showed that the cumulative 2-year risk of CIN 2 or CIN 3 was equivalent for LSIL (27.6%) and ASCUS with high-risk positive HPV infection (26.7%).[15]

HSIL represents moderate to severe dysplasia and carcinoma in situ. This finding is believed a genuine cancer precursor, with a 70% to 75% chance of a CIN 2 or CIN 3 result on biopsy. Nearly all (99%) HSIL cytologic results are associated with high-risk HPV infection.[17] If untreated, at least 30% of women who have HSIL have progression to invasive cancer.[15,27]

AGC are uncommon but should not be confused with ASCUS. These glandular cells may be of endometrial or endocervical origin. Pathologists may report the result as AGC–not otherwise specified, AGC–favor neoplasia, or adenocarcinoma in situ. Up to 40% of women who have AGC have been found to have a significant neoplasia, such as adenocarcinomas of the cervix, endometrium, ovary, and fallopian tubes.[27] Glandular neoplasia often co-exists with squamous disease (CIN). Because of the wide spectrum of neoplastic origins of AGC, testing for HPV subtypes is only one of the diagnostic modalities that must occur with this cytologic result.[32]

MANAGEMENT OF ABNORMAL RESULTS

As discussed previously, screening recommendations vary based on certain population characteristics. Once a Pap screening test is obtained, the result also must be interpreted with respect to patients' individual characteristics of age and pregnancy status. These summarized recommendations for management of cervical cancer screening tests are drawn from the 2006 ASCCP guideline algorithms (**Figs. 3–12**).[33] Discussion of management of abnormal histology is beyond the scope of this article; however, the ASCCP histology guideline algorithms are included for reference in **Figs. 13–18**.[34] As with all clinical recommendations, clinicians should be astute to recurring updated changes.

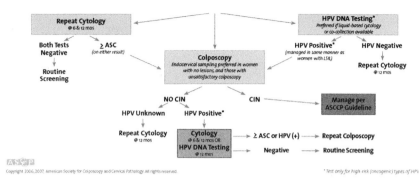

Fig. 3. 2006 ASCCP cytology algorithms. Management of Women with Atypical Squamous Cells of Undetermined Significance (ASC-US). (*Reprinted from* The Journal of Lower Genital Tract Disease, Vol. 11, Issue 4, with the permission of ASCCP © American Society for Colposcopy and Cervical Pathology 2007. No copies of the algorithms may be made without the prior consent of ASCCP. Available at: http://www.asccp.org/.)

The categories of cytologic abnormalities obtained during cervical cancer screening via a Pap test are discussed previously. This documentation is used for cytologic descriptions. If colposcopy and subsequent biopsy are indicated, histologic results are returned using CIN terminology. Management of these abnormalities must be conducted with a different set of histology algorithms (see **Figs. 13–18**).[34]

Normal Papanicolaou Test Results

When a normal Pap test result is obtained with a satisfactory specimen in women up to age 30, the ASCCP recommends repeating the screening examination in 1 year. In women 30 years and older, a mandatory high-risk HPV test may be obtained, and if patients have normal cytology and a negative HPV test, Pap screening may be safely spaced to every 3 years.[33]

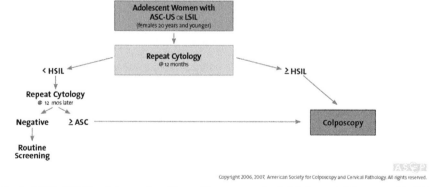

Fig. 4. 2006 ASCCP cytology algorithms. Management of Adolescent Women with Either Atypical Squamous Cells of Undetermined Significance (ASC-US) or Low-grade Squamous Intraepithelial Lesion (LSIL). (*Reprinted from* The Journal of Lower Genital Tract Disease, Vol. 11, Issue 4, with the permission of ASCCP © American Society for Colposcopy and Cervical Pathology 2007. No copies of the algorithms may be made without the prior consent of ASCCP. Available at: http://www.asccp.org/.)

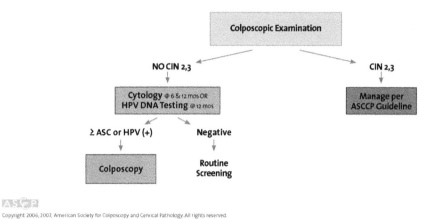

Fig. 5. 2006 ASCCP cytology algorithms. Management of Women with Atypical Squamous Cells: Cannot Exclude High-grade SIL (ASC-H). (*Reprinted from* The Journal of Lower Genital Tract Disease, Vol. 11, Issue 4, with the permission of ASCCP © American Society for Colposcopy and Cervical Pathology 2007. No copies of the algorithms may be made without the prior consent of ASCCP. Available at: http://www.asccp.org/.)

Abnormal Cytology

When a screening Pap result signifies abnormal cytology, additional management is based on patient age and pregnancy status and type of abnormality noted. The 2006 ASCCP guidelines for abnormal cytology management are included for reference in **Figs. 3–12**.[33]

Atypical Squamous Cells of Undetermined Significance

In women under age 21, a Pap should be repeated in 1 year without additional management.[33] In women aged 21 and older, reflexive HPV testing may be used to guide management of this abnormality or repeat cytology may simply be performed at 6 and 12 months.[33] If HPV testing is negative, the Pap may be repeated in 1 year; however, if HPV testing is positive, a clinician should proceed with colposcopy.[33] **Figs. 3–12** review these recommendations in an algorithmic format.

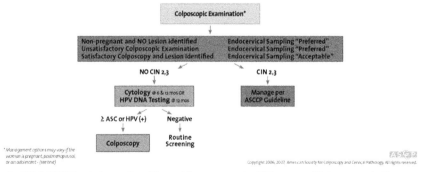

Fig. 6. 2006 ASCCP cytology algorithms. Management of Women with Low-grade Squamous Intraepithelial Lesion (LSIL). (*Reprinted from* The Journal of Lower Genital Tract Disease, Vol. 11, Issue 4, with the permission of ASCCP © American Society for Colposcopy and Cervical Pathology 2007. No copies of the algorithms may be made without the prior consent of ASCCP. Available at: http://www.asccp.org/.)

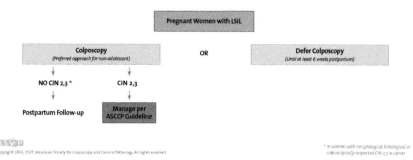

Fig. 7. 2006 ASCCP cytology algorithms. Management of Pregnant Women with Low-grade Squamous Intraepithelial Lesion (LSIL). (*Reprinted from* The Journal of Lower Genital Tract Disease, Vol. 11, Issue 4, with the permission of ASCCP © American Society for Colposcopy and Cervical Pathology 2007. No copies of the algorithms may be made without the prior consent of ASCCP. Available at: http://www.asccp.org/.)

Atypical Squamous Cells, Cannot Exclude High-grade Squamous Intraepithelial Lesion

Regardless of age, colposcopic examination should be performed for ASC-H given its strong link with high-grade dysplasia (discussed previously).[33] Additional management based on colposcopic and histologic findings can be reviewed in the ASCCP histology guidelines (see **Figs. 13–18**).[34]

Low-grade Squamous Intraepithelial Lesion

In women under age 21, the Pap should be repeated in 1 year without further management.[33] In women aged 21 and older, colposcopic examination should be performed.[33] For pregnant patients, colposcopy may be deferred until at least 6 weeks post partum if desired, although colposcopy in nonadolescents during pregnancy is the preferred approach.[33] These recommendations can be visualized in **Figs. 3–12**. Endocervical sampling also is recommended if patients are not pregnant and no lesion is identified or if colposcopy is unsatisfactory.[34] Additional recommendations based on colposcopic and histologic findings are included in the ASCCP histology guidelines (see **Figs. 13–18**).[34]

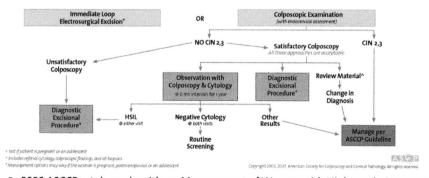

Fig. 8. 2006 ASCCP cytology algorithms. Management of Women with High-grade Squamous Intraepithelial Lesion (HSIL). (*Reprinted from* The Journal of Lower Genital Tract Disease, Vol. 11, Issue 4, with the permission of ASCCP © American Society for Colposcopy and Cervical Pathology 2007. No copies of the algorithms may be made without the prior consent of ASCCP. Available at: http://www.asccp.org/.)

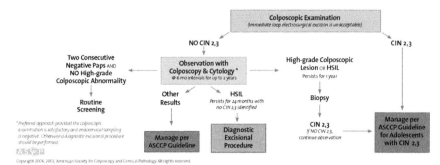

Fig. 9. 2006 ASCCP cytology algorithms. Management of Adolescent Women (20 Years and Younger) with High-grade Squamous Intraepithelial Lesion (HSIL). (*Reprinted from* The Journal of Lower Genital Tract Disease, Vol. 11, Issue 4, with the permission of ASCCP © American Society for Colposcopy and Cervical Pathology 2007. No copies of the algorithms may be made without the prior consent of ASCCP. Available at: http://www.asccp.org/.)

High-grade Squamous Intraepithelial Lesion

Women who have HSIL on Pap smear may be managed by colposcopy or immediate diagnostic excision procedure if they are not adolescents and not pregnant.[33] Adolescents and pregnant patients should be managed by colposcopy initially[33] (see **Figs. 3–12** for complete algorithm). Additional recommendations based on colposcopic and histology findings are included in the ASCCP histology guidelines (see **Figs. 13–18**).[34]

Atypical Glandular Cells

Women who have a Pap diagnosis of AGC should be managed with colposcopy, HPV testing, and endometrial sampling (see **Figs. 3–12**).[35] If only atypical endometrial cells are noted on a Pap, a clinician may proceed with endometrial and endocervical sampling, followed by colposcopy if no endometrial abnormality is detected.[35]

Use of Referral/Consultation

In many instances, primary care clinicians, many of whom also perform diagnostic excisional procedures, manage office-based gynecology. It is necessary, however, for such clinicians to work with consultants in managing complex patients,

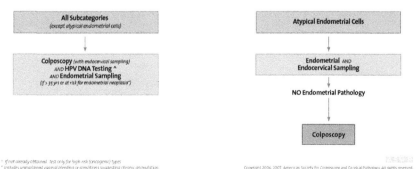

Fig. 10. 2006 ASCCP cytology algorithms. Initial Workup of Women with Atypical Glandular Cells (AGC). (*Reprinted from* The Journal of Lower Genital Tract Disease, Vol. 11, Issue 4, with the permission of ASCCP © American Society for Colposcopy and Cervical Pathology 2007. No copies of the algorithms may be made without the prior consent of ASCCP. Available at: http://www.asccp.org/.)

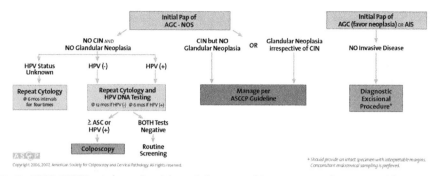

Fig. 11. 2006 ASCCP cytology algorithms. Subsequent Management of Women with Atypical Glandular Cells (AGC). (*Reprinted from* The Journal of Lower Genital Tract Disease, Vol. 11, Issue 4, with the permission of ASCCP © American Society for Colposcopy and Cervical Pathology 2007. No copies of the algorithms may be made without the prior consent of ASCCP. Available at: http://www.asccp.org/.)

especially those who have complicated histories that may not be addressed within the ASCCP guidelines. Furthermore, the ASCCP guidelines note instances where consultation, including review of all Pap and histology slides, is appropriate. For example, requesting review of previous cytology and histology for patients who have a CIN 1 diagnosis preceded by an HSIL or AGC Pap is a reasonable management option (see **Figs. 13–18**).[33]

Use of Cryotherapy and Excisional Procedures

The ASCCP algorithms clearly delineate management guidelines for abnormal histology (see **Figs. 13–18**).[34] Such treatment may consist of cryotherapy, loop electrosurgical excision procedure (LEEP), or cold knife conization. According to the ASCCP, indications for cryotherapy include diagnosis of CIN 2 or CIN 3 with a satisfactory colposcopy and no prior history of high-grade histology.[34] A diagnostic excisional procedure, such as LEEP, is recommended for recurrent CIN 2 or CIN 3 or an initial CIN 2 or CIN 3 diagnosis with an unsatisfactory colposcopy.[34] For adolescents, observation is preferred for CIN 2 with a satisfactory colposcopy.[34] If CIN 3 is suspected, however, or if colposcopy is unsatisfactory, treatment via cryotherapy or excision is

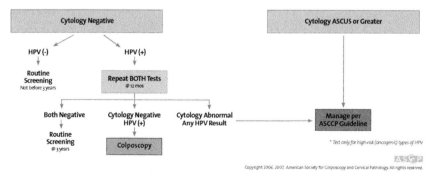

Fig. 12. 2006 ASCCP cytology algorithms. Use of HPV DNA Testing* as an Adjunct to Cytology for Cervical Cancer Screening in Women 30 Years and Older. (*Reprinted from* The Journal of Lower Genital Tract Disease, Vol. 11, Issue 4, with the permission of ASCCP © American Society for Colposcopy and Cervical Pathology 2007. No copies of the algorithms may be made without the prior consent of ASCCP. Available at: http://www.asccp.org/.)

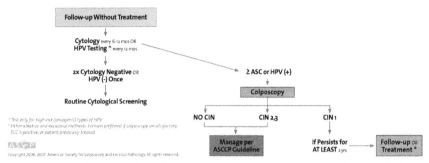

Fig. 13. 2006 ASCCP histology algorithms. Management of Women with a Histological Diagnosis of Cervical Intraepithelial Neoplasia Grade 1 (CIN 1) Preceded by ASC-US, ASC-H or LSIL Cytology. (*Reprinted from* The Journal of Lower Genital Tract Disease, Vol. 11, Issue 4, with the permission of ASCCP © American Society for Colposcopy and Cervical Pathology 2007. No copies of the algorithms may be made without the prior consent of ASCCP. Available at: http://www.asccp.org/.)

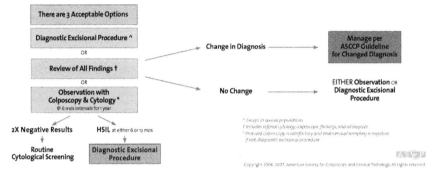

Fig. 14. 2006 ASCCP histology algorithms. Management of Women with a Histological Diagnosis of Cervical Intraepithelial Neoplasia-Grade 1 (CIN 1) Preceded by HSIL or AGC-NOS Cytology. (*Reprinted from* The Journal of Lower Genital Tract Disease, Vol. 11, Issue 4, with the permission of ASCCP © American Society for Colposcopy and Cervical Pathology 2007. No copies of the algorithms may be made without the prior consent of ASCCP. Available at: http://www.asccp.org/.)

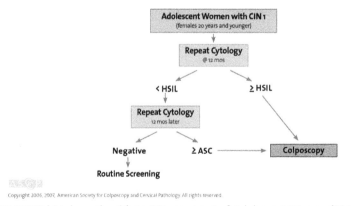

Fig. 15. 2006 ASCCP histology algorithms. Management of Adolescent Women (20 Years and Younger) with a Histological Diagnosis of Cervical Intraepithelial Neoplasia-Grade 1 (CIN 1). (*Reprinted from* The Journal of Lower Genital Tract Disease, Vol. 11, Issue 4, with the permission of ASCCP © American Society for Colposcopy and Cervical Pathology 2007. No copies of the algorithms may be made without the prior consent of ASCCP. Available at: http://www.asccp.org/.)

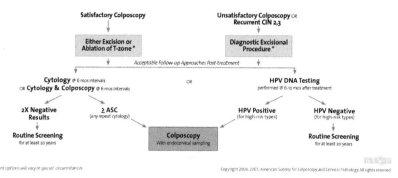

Fig. 16. 2006 ASCCP histology algorithms. Management of Women with a Histological Diagnosis of Cervical Intraepithelial Neoplasia - (CIN 2,3). (*Reprinted from* The Journal of Lower Genital Tract Disease, Vol. 11, Issue 4, with the permission of ASCCP © American Society for Colposcopy and Cervical Pathology 2007. No copies of the algorithms may be made without the prior consent of ASCCP. Available at: http://www.asccp.org/.)

recommended.[34] Finally, if adenocarcinoma in situ is diagnosed via a diagnostic excisional procedure, hysterectomy is the preferred management approach.[34]

Post-treatment Screening Follow-up

After a LEEP or cryotherapy procedure, the ASCCP recommends HPV testing at 6 to 12 months after treatment, cytology at 6-month intervals, or cytology and colposcopy at 6-month intervals.[34] Additional follow-up after these initial screening recommendations can be reviewed in the 2006 Consensus Guidelines algorithm (see **Figs. 13–18**).[34]

CONDYLOMA OR GENITAL WARTS

Condyloma, or genital warts, also are caused predominantly by low-risk types of HPV (reviewed in a 2008 Centers for Disease Control and Prevention report).[5] Genital warts typically appear as small raised lesions in the genital or rectal area of men and women. In most cases, a normal immune system clears this infection within 2 years, although some infections linger with persistence or enlargement of the lesions.[5] Approximately 1% of all sexually active Americans have genital warts at any given time.[5] These lesions may be treated by topical prescription medications (eg, podofilox) or by

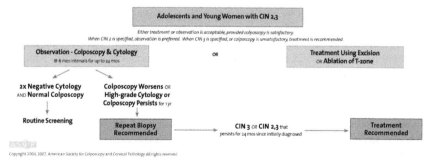

Fig. 17. 2006 ASCCP histology algorithms. Management of Adolescent and Young Women with a Histological Diagnosis of Cervical Intraepithelial Neoplasia - Grade 2,3 (CIN 2,3). (*Reprinted from* The Journal of Lower Genital Tract Disease, Vol. 11, Issue 4, with the permission of ASCCP © American Society for Colposcopy and Cervical Pathology 2007. No copies of the algorithms may be made without the prior consent of ASCCP. Available at: http://www.asccp.org/.)

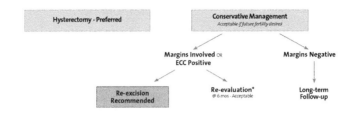

Fig. 18. 2006 ASCCP histology algorithms. Management of Women with Adenocarcinoma in-situ (AIS) Diagnosed from a Diagnostic Excisional Procedure. (*Reprinted from* The Journal of Lower Genital Tract Disease, Vol. 11, Issue 4, with the permission of ASCCP © American Society for Colposcopy and Cervical Pathology 2007. No copies of the algorithms may be made without the prior consent of ASCCP. Available at: http://www.asccp.org/.)

cryotherapy.[5] Observation also is acceptable for monitoring spontaneous clearance. Additionally, the HPV vaccine (discussed previously) covers 90% of the HPV types known to cause condyloma.[36]

VULVAR AND VAGINAL CANCERS

Vulvar and vaginal cancers are rare, accounting for less than 5% and 2% of all gynecologic cancers, respectively, on a yearly basis.[4] In the United States in 2004, there were 1130 cases of new vaginal cancers and 3631 newly diagnosed cases of vulvar cancer.[4] Both of these types of neoplasms are believed secondary to HPV infection; thus, it is critical to inspect the vulva and vagina during routine gynecologic examinations and during colposcopic examinations. In particular, the vulva and vagina should be examined thoroughly when a Pap smear and colposcopic examination are discordant.

PATIENT EDUCATION

Cervical cancer screening and the subsequent management of abnormal Pap test results often are accompanied by significant anxiety for patients. The diagnosis of a sexually transmitted infection, such as HPV, often is overwhelming for women, as may be the subsequent testing they must undergo for further evaluation. Educating patients about cervical cancer screening and the process for management of abnormal results is critical. Such counseling should focus particularly on minimizing risk factors for future HPV infections (discussed previously).[35] Excellent patient handouts are available through the ASCCP, the Centers for Disease Control, and the American Academy of Family Physicians.[37–39]

SUMMARY

Cervical cancer and its dysplasia precursors account for significant morbidity and mortality in women worldwide. HPV infection is common, preventable, and now widely accepted as the causative agent with oncogenic potential in the development of cervical cancer. Screening via Pap testing is critical, and interpretation of test results with knowledge of patiens risk factors is imperative. Many evidence-based guidelines for screening, interpretation, and management have been developed and are widely available for use.

REFERENCES

1. Public Health Agency of Canada. Epidemiology of cervical cancer. Available at the PHAC website: http://www.phac-aspc.gc.ca/publicat/ccsic-dccuac/pdf/chap_2_e.pdf. May 2003; Accessed July 3, 08.
2. Centers for Disease Control and Prevention. Cervical cancer statistics. Available at the CDC web site: http://www.cdc.gov/cancer/cervical/statistics. March 2008 Accessed July 3, 08.
3. Centers for Disease Control and Prevention. Women more likely to undergo cervical cancer screening recommended by a physician. Available at the CDC web site: http://www.cdc.gov/od/oc/media/pressrel/r050510.htm. May 10, 2005 Accessed July 3, 08.
4. Centers for Disease Control and Prevention. Vulvar and vaginal cancers. national gynecologic cancer awareness campaign. Available at the CDC web site: http://www.cdc.gov/cancer/vagvulv. March 2008 Accessed July 3, 08.
5. Centers for Disease Control and Prevention. Genital HPV infection. Available at the CDC web site: http://www.cdc.gov/STD/HPV/STDFact-HPV.htm. April 2008 Accessed July 3, 08.
6. Kurman RJ, editor. Blaustein's pathology of the female genital tract. 4th Edition. New York: Springer-Verlag; 1994. p. 3–12.
7. Ferris DG, Cox JT, O'Connor DM. Modern colposcopy: textbook and atlas. 2nd Edition. Dubuque(IA): Kendall/Hunt Publishing; 2004. p. 15–20.
8. Ferris DG, Cox JT, O'Connor DM. Modern colposcopy: textbook and atlas. 2nd Edition. Dubuque(IA): Kendall/Hunt Publishing; 2004. p. 7–8.
9. Bosch FX, Lorincz A, Munoz N. The causal relation between human papillomavirus and cervical cancer. J Clin Pathol 2002;55:244–65.
10. Koutsky LA, Holmes KK, Critchlow CW. Cohort study of risk of cervical intraepithelial neoplasia grade 2 or 3 associated with cervical papillomavirus infection. N Engl J Med 1992;327:1272–8.
11. Bauer HM, Ting Y, Greer CE. Genital human papillomavirus infection in female university students as determined by PCR-based method. J Am Med Assoc 1991;265:472–7.
12. Ho GYF, Bierman R, Beardsley L. Natural history of cervicovaginal papillomavirus infection in young women. N Engl J Med 1998;338(7):423–8.
13. Castle PE, Cox JT, Jeronimo J. An analysis of high-risk human papillomavirus DNA-negative cervical precancers in the ASCUS-LSIL triage study (ALTS). Obstet Gynecol 2008;111:847–56.
14. ASCUS-LSIL Triage Study (ALTS) Group. Results of a randomized trial on the management of cytology interpretations of atypical squamous dells of undetermined significance. Am J Obstet Gynecol 2003;188:1383–92.
15. ASCUS-LSIL Triage Study (ALTS) Group. A randomized trial on the management of low-grade squamous intraepithelial lesion cytology interpretations. Am J Obstet Gynecol 2003;188:1393–400.
16. Guido R, Schiffman M, Solomon D. Postcolposcopy management strategies for patients referred with low-grade squamous intraepithelial lesions of undetermined significance: a two-year prospective study. Am J Obstet Gynecol 2003; 188:1401–5.
17. Cox JT, Schiffman M, Solomon D. Prospective follow-up suggests similar risk of subsequent cervical intraepithelial neoplasia grade 2 or 3 amoung women with cervical intraepithelial neoplasia grade 1 or negative colposcopy and directed biopsy. Am J Obstet Gynecol 2003;188:1406–11.

18. Harper DM, Franco EL, Wheeler CM. Sustained efficacy up to 4-5 years of a bivalent L1 virus-like particle vaccine against human papillomavirus types 16 and 18: follow-up from a randomized control trial. Lancet 2006;367:1247–55.

19. U.S. Preventive Services Task Force. Screening for cervical cancer—recommendations and rationale. AHRQ Pub. No. 03–515A. Available at the AHRQ web site: http://www.ahrq.gov/clinic/3rduspstf/cervcan/cervcanrr.pdf. 2003 Accessed July 20, 08.

20. Hartman KE, Hall SA, Nanda K, et al. Screening for cervical cancer. Systematic evidence review. No. 25 (Prepared by the Research Triangle Institute-University of North Carolina Evidence-based Practice Center under contract No. 290-97-0011). Rockville (MD): Agency for Healthcare Research and Quality; January 2002. Available at the AHRQ web site: http://www.ahrq.gov/downloads/pub/prevent/pdfser/cervcanser.pdf. Accessed July 20, 08.

21. National Institute for Clinical Excellence. Liquid-based cytology for cervical screening. Technology appraisal guidance October 2003;69. Available at the NICE web site: http://www.nice.org.uk/Guidance/TA69. Accessed July 20, 08.

22. Saslow D, Runowicz CD, Solomon D, et al. American Cancer Society guideline for the early detection of cervical neoplasia and cancer. CA Cancer J Clin 2002;52:342–62.

23. American College of Obstetricians and Gynecologists. Cervical cytology screening. ACOG practice bulletin No. 45. Obstet Gynecol 2003;102:417–27.

24. Martin-Hirsch P, Lilford R, Jarvis G, et al. Efficacy of cervical-smear collection devices: a systematic review and meta-analysis. [published erratum appears in Lancet 2000 Jan 29;355(9201):414]. Lancet 1999;354(9192):1763–70.

25. Martin-Hirsch P, Jarvis G, Kitchener HC, et al. Collection devices for obtaining cervical cytology samples. Cochrane Database Syst Rev 2000;(Issue 3). Art. No.: CD001036. doi: 10.1002/14651858:CD001036.

26. Forbes C, Jepson R, Martin-Hirsch P. Interventions targeted at women to encourage the uptake of cervical screening. Cochrane Database Syst Rev 2002;(Issue 3). Art. No.: CD002834. doi: 10.1002/14651858:CD002834.

27. Wright TC, Massad LS, Dunton CJ. 2006 Consensus guidelines for the management of women with abnormal cervical cancer screening tests. Am J Obstet Gynecol 2007;197:346–55.

28. Solomon D, Davey D, Kurman R. The Bethesda system 2001: terminology for reporting the results of cervical cytology. J Am Med Assoc 2002;287:2115–9.

29. American Society for Colposcopy and Cervical Pathology. Managing women with negative paps lacking endocervical cells or other quality indicators: pap adequacy algorithm. Available at the ASCCP website: http://www.asccp.org/consensus/pap_adequacy/pap_adequacy.pdf. Accessed August 5, 08.

30. Ferris DG, Cox JT, O'Connor DM. Modern colposcopy: textbook and atlas. 2nd Edition. Dubuque (IA): Kendall/Hunt Publishing; 2004. p. 51–62.

31. Solomon D, Schiffman M, Tarone R. Comparison of three management strategies for patients with atypical squamous cells of undetermined significance: baseline results from a randomized trial. J Natl Cancer Inst. 2001;93:293–9.

32. Wright TC, Massad LS, Dunton CJ. 2006 Consensus guidelines for the management of women with cervical intraepithelial neoplasia or adenocarcinoma In Situ. Am J Obstet Gynecol 2007;197:340–5.

33. American Society for Colposcopy and Cervical Pathology. ASCCP cytology guideline algorithms. Available at the ASCCP website: http://www.asccp.org/consensus/cytological.shtml. 2006 Accessed June 15, 08.

34. American Society for Colposcopy and Cervical Pathology. ASCCP histology guideline algorithms. Available at the ASCCP website: http://www.asccp.org/consensus/histological.shtml. 2006 Accessed June 15, 08.

35. Pruitt SL, Parker PA, Follen M, et al. Communicating colposcopy results: what do patients and providers discuss? J Low Genit Tract Dis 2008;12(2):95–102.
36. Centers for Disease Control and Prevention. HPV vaccine. Available at the CDC web site: http://www.cdc.gov/vaccines/vpd-vac/hpv/vac-faqs.htm. April 2008. Accessed August 3, 08.
37. American Society for Colposcopy and Cervical Pathology. Patient education. Available at the ASCCP website: http://www.asccp.org/patient_edu.shtml. July 2008. Accessed August 4, 08.
38. Centers for Disease Control and Prevention. Human papillomavirus infection. Available at the CDC web site: http://www.cdc.gov/STD/HPV/. July 2008. (Accessed August 4, 08).
39. American Academy of Family Physicians. Human papillomavirus (HPV). June 2007. Available at the familydoctor.org website: http://familydoctor.org/online/famdocen/home/common/sexinfections/sti/389.html. Accessed August 4, 2008.

Depression in Childbearing Women: When Depression Complicates Pregnancy

Sheila M. Marcus, MD[a,b,]*, Julie E. Heringhausen, BSN[c]

KEYWORDS

- Depression • Pregnancy • Infant outcomes • Medication
- Psychotherapy

BACKGROUND AND PREVALENCE

Across the United States, prevalence studies show that one in five women experience an episode of major depressive disorder (MDD) during their lifetime.[1] The onset of depressive symptoms is seen most often between ages 20 and 40, the age range when many women become pregnant.[2] Studies have shown that 10% to 16% of pregnant women fulfill the diagnostic criteria for MDD, and even more women experience subsyndromal depressive symptoms, which frequently are overlooked.[3,4] Because of this correlation with life events, it is important for health care providers to be aware of (1) the frequency of depression in this population; (2) signs, symptoms, and appropriate screening methods; and (3) health risks for the mother and growing fetus if depression is undetected or untreated. A study by Marcus and colleagues in 2003 found that of pregnant women screened in an obstetrics setting who reported significant depressive symptoms, 86% were not receiving any form of treatment. Although most women seek some prenatal care over the course of their pregnancy,[5] many women do not seek mental health services because of stigma; thus, antenatal visits to an obstetrician or primary care provider may provide an opportunity for screening and intervention for depression in this high-risk group. Because management of a depressed, pregnant woman also includes care of her growing fetus, treatment may be complicated and

---

[a] Department of Psychiatry, University of Michigan, Rachel Upjohn Building, 4250 Plymouth Road, Ann Arbor, MI 48109, USA
[b] Child and Adolescent Psychiatry, University of Michigan, University of Michigan Health System, Rachel Upjohn Building, 4250 Plymouth Road, Ann Arbor, MI 48109, USA
[c] University of Michigan Medical School, 1301 Catherine Street, 5124 MS I, Ann Arbor, MI 48109, USA
* Corresponding author. Department of Psychiatry, University of Michigan, Rachel Upjohn Building, 4250 Plymouth Road, Ann Arbor, MI 48109, USA.
E-mail address: smmarcus@umich.edu (S.M. Marcus).

Prim Care Clin Office Pract 36 (2009) 151–165
doi:10.1016/j.pop.2008.10.011   **primarycare.theclinics.com**
0095-4543/08/$ – see front matter © 2009 Elsevier Inc. All rights reserved.

primary care providers should consider a multidisciplinary approach, including an obstetrician, psychiatrist, and pediatrician, to provide optimal care.[6]

CLINICAL FEATURES

The *Diagnostic and Statistical Manual of Mental Disorders, Fourth Edition* (*DSM-IV*) defines the diagnosis of depression using the same criteria for men and women, although research shows some variation in female presentation. MDD diagnosis must include existence of depressed or irritable mood or inability to experience pleasure. In addition, four of the following symptoms must be present: feelings of guilt, hopelessness, and worthlessness; sleep disturbance (insomnia or hypersomnia); appetite or weight changes; attention or concentration difficulties; decreased energy or unexplainable fatigue; psychomotor agitation or retardation; and, in severe cases, thoughts of suicide.[7] Women may present in a clinic with more seasonal depression or symptoms of atypical depression (eg, hypersomnia, hyperphagia, carbohydrate craving, weight gain, heavy feeling in arms and legs, worse mood in the evenings, and initial insomnia).[7] Many of these symptoms overlap with the physical and mental changes experienced during pregnancy, making them difficult to distinguish, and, therefore, they often are disregarded.[8]

IDENTIFICATION IN PRIMARY CARE

Practitioners caring for women should be aware of personal and epidemiologic factors that place women most at risk for perinatal depression. An important primary risk factor is a previous personal history (particularly during pregnancy or post partum) or a family history of depression.[9] Another common risk factor is a woman's perception of limited social support and presence of social conflict. Recent literature shows that even when women report adequate social support, if they also report interpersonal conflict, then they are at a high risk for depression.[10] Obstetricians and primary care providers routinely address social support for pregnant women and encourage strengthening their support networks. Interpersonal conflict also may be important to address in the clinical interview.[10] Asking questions about feeling let down and unloved, feeling tense from arguing, and the frequency of unpleasant and distressing social interactions may be adequate to screen for social conflict and identify women who would benefit from clinical interventions addressing these interpersonal conflicts.[10] Other risk factors for depression include (1) history of physical, emotional, or sexual abuse; (2) history of (or current) cigarette smoking, alcohol consumption, or substance use; (3) stressors, such as financial or occupational obligations; (4) stressful health concerns or relationships;[11] (5) living alone; and (6) ambivalence about the pregnancy.[12]

SCREENING

In 2002, the U.S. Preventive Services Task Force published findings noting that a positive answer to either or both of two universal depression screening questions was a quick and effective way to screen for depression: (1) "Over the past two weeks, have you ever felt down, depressed, or hopeless?" or (2) "Have you felt little interest or pleasure in doing things?" Affirmative answers initiate a more in-depth screening tool to gather more information toward the diagnosis.[13] The two measures used most commonly to screen for depression for adults in ambulatory care are the Beck Depression Inventory (2 to 3 minutes to complete)[14] and the revised Center for Epidemiologic Studies Depression Scale (5 to 10 minutes to complete).[15]

The Edinburgh Postnatal Depression Scale (EPDS) is a screening tool used internationally to assess depression during pregnancy and post partum.[16] The EPDS can screen for postpartum depression as early as early as 3 to 5 days after giving birth with a score greater than 9.5.[17] If a woman scores higher than 15 during pregnancy or 13 post partum, then a further assessment is necessary for a diagnosis of depression.[18] Several screening instruments can be used to assess symptom severity and general functioning. One of these is the BASIS-24, a 24-item scale that measures symptoms and general functioning in six major areas: depression/functioning, relationships, self-harm, emotional lability, psychosis, and substance abuse.[11] Screening tools do not address the duration of symptoms, degree of impairment, or comorbid psychiatric disorders;[19] thus, if a patient scores beyond the cutoff range for any of these tools, *DSM-IV* diagnostic criteria should be assessed through further interview.

Regardless of the screening method used, it is important to further question patients who manifest depressive symptoms upon screening. An experienced practitioner may discern whether a patient requires more definitive treatment or if an elevation is score is due to a transient psychosocial stressor. Katon et al have found that using screening tools in conjunction with "depression caremanagers" may improve the quality of care. Such nurse caremanagers provide education, track adherence with medication and psychotherapy, and support the patients in taking an active role in their illness.[20] In those areas where psychiatrists are available, practices may also benefit from using a collaborative care model with a psychiatric consultant who comanages difficult cases with the primary care clinician during the acute phase of their illness. A recent meta-analysis found that there was a twofold increase in medication compliance over six months with the collaborative care approach compared to patients following only with primary care, and enhanced functional outcomes were noted in these patients two to five years later.[21]

CONSEQUENCES OF DEPRESSION IN PREGNANCY

Unidentified and untreated depression can lead to detrimental effects on mother and child. Suicide is the most catastrophic effect of undertreated depression. In addition, depressed women are more likely to participate in unhealthy practices during pregnancy, such as smoking and illicit substance abuse. These women have higher rates of poor nutrition, in part because of lack of appetite, leading to poor weight gain during pregnancy and risking intrauterine growth retardation. Depressed women are less compliant with prenatal care and feel less invested in the care toward their pregnancy. Finally, women who have depression have increased pain and discomfort during their pregnancies, reporting worse nausea, stomach pain, shortness of breath, gastrointestinal symptoms, heart pounding, and dizziness compared with nondepressed women.[22] Untreated maternal depression in pregnancy has been associated with poor pregnancy and birth outcomes, such as maternal preeclampsia, low birth weight, smaller head circumferences, increased risk for premature delivery, increased surgical delivery interventions, lower Apgar scores, and more admissions to neonatal ICUs.[6,23–25]

Research suggests that maternal depression leads to alteration in a mother's neuroendocrine axis and uterine blood flow, which may contribute to premature delivery, low birth weight, and preeclampsia.[26,27] Negative birth outcomes are associated most highly with depression symptoms in the second and third trimesters.[28] Babies of mothers who suffered from depression during their pregnancy have elevated cortisol and catecholamine levels at birth.[6] These infants cry more often and are more difficult to console than babies born to nondepressed mothers.[25] Babies of women at high risk for depression are shown to have more irregular sleep patterns and longer amounts of time in bed before falling asleep.[29] If depression continues into the postpartum period, the risk for long-term effects on a child, such as poor mother-infant attachment, delayed cognitive and linguistic skills, impaired emotional development, and behavioral issues, exist.[30–32] Studies show these babies are fussier, vocalize their needs less, and make fewer positive facial expressions than infants of nondepressed mothers.[33] If a baby is exposed to a depressed maternal environment during the first 4 months, even if the depressed mother receives treatment later, the child's developmental delay and symptoms remain.[30] As these children grow, perhaps because of early exposure or the continued stressful home environment, they are more likely to have emotional instability and conduct disorders, attempt suicide, and require mental health services themselves.[34,35]

TREATMENT OF DEPRESSION DURING PREGNANCY

There are few current medical standards for treatment of women who have depression during pregnancy, in part because ethical constraints preclude randomized controlled trials using pharmacotherapy during gestation. Some women do not seek treatment, but for those who do, many physicians are unsure of how to balance maternal medication needs with risk for exposure to the growing fetus.[36] Because many pregnancies are unplanned and undetected for some time, all women of childbearing age should have their depression managed as if they are or will become pregnant. Primary care providers should engage in preconception planning with all women of childbearing age who have or are at risk for depressive illness. Treatment planning with regard to the use of pharmacotherapy during conception and the first trimester is among the most important decision points for women and their physicians. Women diagnosed with depression who have been asymptomatic for over a year may wish to attempt to reduce or discontinue their antidepressants a few months before conception and throughout the pregnancy;[37] however, one study found that 60% of women taking antidepressants at the time of their baby's conception had depressive symptoms over the course of the pregnancy.[38] Women should be monitored closely for relapse of depressive symptoms. Of women who discontinued their antidepressants during pregnancy, 68% experienced relapse symptoms compared with 26% of women who continued their medication regimen.[39] If a woman's depression history contains multiple relapses or severe symptoms, including suicide attempts and multiple inpatient psychiatric admissions, it is recommended that she remain on antidepressants for her own safety, regardless of pregnancy status.[37]

Although research studies indicate that no major malformations are associated with antidepressant use during pregnancy, it also is not proved that any specific antidepressant is completely safe. All psychotropic medications cross the placenta and enter the amniotic fluid.[40] General guidelines include some straightforward principles: (1) keep the medication regimen simple, (2) use monotherapy, and (3) avoid medication changes during the pregnancy. Use of multiple medications in sequence and medication augmentation strategies all increase the exposure of the fetus.[6] A woman's prior history to pharmacotherapy should be considered when choosing a medication.[6] Although many factors influence pharmacotherapy during pregnancy, drugs with fewer metabolites, drug-drug interactions, more protein binding (preventing placental passage), and lesser teratogenic risk if known should be prioritized when possible.[6]

SPONTANEOUS ABORTION

Research results are mixed when examining rates of antidepressant use and its relationship to spontaneous abortion, and may be confounded by the effect of the illness itself.[41] One study suggests that women taking antidepressants during pregnancy have a statistically significant higher rate of spontaneous abortion (3.9%) regardless of the type of antidepressant.[41] Another study found that spontaneous abortion rates are elevated for exposure to several different antidepressant classes, but only exposure to bupropion is statistically significant.[42]

TERATOGENICITY

The literature on antidepressant use is growing, particularly regarding the use of selective serotonin reuptake inhibitors (SSRIs) during pregnancy and possible risk for teratogenicity. Although the popular press raises a great deal of controversy regarding the safety of the SSRIs, research to date does not confirm major congenital malformations. Kulin and colleagues[43] found no increased risk for major congenital malformations with in utero exposure to SSRIs, in particular fluvoxamine, paroxetine, and sertraline. An earlier study examining fluoxetine exposure in the first trimester found there was an increase in minor anomalies, such as syndactyly.[44] In 2005, GlaxoSmith Kline[45] published a report based on a claims database study of 815 infants that showed babies born to mothers who were taking paroxetine during their first trimester had a 1.5- to 2-fold increased risk for congenital heart defects, in particular atrial and ventricular septal defects. Einarson and colleagues[46] more recently demonstrated that the rate of cardiac defects for babies exposed to paroxetine in the first trimester and nonexposed infants was the same (0.7%, not statistically significant) and within the expected cardiac malformation risk range for all pregnancies. At the time of this writing, the use of paroxetine remains controversial. Most practitioners avoid its use during pregnancy except for those women who have demonstrated a preferential past positive response to this agent. When paroxetine is used, it is recommended to monitor the fetus with fetal echocardiography.[6]

The National Birth Defects Prevention Study in 2007 found no significant relationship between SSRIs and congenital cardiovascular malformations; however, it did find an association between SSRIs (especially paroxetine during the first trimester) and infants who had anencephaly, craniosynostosis, and omphalocele.[47] Conversely, the Slone Epidemiology Center Birth Defects Study published at approximately the same time noted no increased risk for craniosynostosis, omphalocele, or heart defects with overall SSRI use by pregnant women.[48] This study did find some significant relationships between sertraline and omphalocele and between paroxetine and right ventricular outflow tract obstruction defects.[48] Although these findings indicated some increased risk for specific rare birth defects with specific drug exposure, the overall absolute risk for birth defects with the use of SSRIs is small; therefore, these medications are considered relatively safe for use during pregnancy.[47,48]

NEONATAL ADAPTATION

Studies show that up to 30% of infants exposed to SSRIs in utero during the third trimester are likely to have symptoms of poor neonatal adaptation.[49] These symptoms include short term self-limited jitteriness, tachycardia, hypothermia, vomiting, hypoglycemia, irritability, inconsolable crying, abnormal muscle tone, eating difficulties, sleep disturbances, seizures, and respiratory distress,[49] which leads to an overall increased rate of neonatal ICU admissions for these newborns. Studies assessing neonatal outcomes and complications do not correct for commonly co-occurring risk factors, including maternal smoking or use of alcohol or other substances.[11] Ferreira and collegues,[50] correcting for these confounding variables, found no increased incidence of preterm labor or neonatal ICU admission for babies exposed to SSRIs or venlafaxine in utero; however, some infants did exhibit neonatal adaptation syndrome symptoms.

In a 2006 case-controlled study, infants exposed to SSRIs after 20 weeks' gestation had a 1% increased risk for persistent pulmonary hypertension of the newborn;[51] more research is needed to confirm these findings. Although some international literature suggests tapering SSRIs to avoid late gestation exposure, most practitioners in the United States avoid this, as it predisposes women to a substantially heightened risk for late pregnancy and postpartum morbidity secondary to depression.[52] As with any decision regarding pharmacotherapy during pregnancy, a consideration toward tapering should be considered on an individual basis, considering the risks for maternal illness versus the risk for short-term neonatal withdrawal symptoms.[11]

The bulk of the literature to date does not reveal increased risk for congenital malformations associated with pregnant women taking tricyclic antidepressants (TCAs),[53] which historically were the medications of choice for treatment of depression but currently are not used extensively. Doses of TCAs may need to be increased as much as 1.6 times the prepregnancy dose in the second half of pregnancy to establish therapeutic levels as a result of increased plasma volumes and metabolism.[54] Case reports have presented babies with TCA exposure experiencing temporary withdrawal symptoms within the first 12 hours of life, including jitteriness, irritability, urinary retention, bowel obstruction, and occasionally seizures.[53,55] Nulman and colleagues[56] found no associations between maternal use of TCAs or fluoxetine during pregnancy and long-term effects on global IQ, language, or behavioral development in preschool children. Further research is needed to examine long-term outcomes for these children.

Limited information is available regarding exposure to atypical antidepressants, such as bupropion, mirtazapine, trazodone, and venlafaxine in utero.[53,57] Like SSRIs and TCAs, venlafaxine has been implicated in cases of neonatal withdrawal.[58]

NONPHARMACOLOGIC TREATMENTS

Psychotherapy also has been studied in the treatment of depression and is validated empirically for the treatment of mood disorders.[59] For mild depression, providers commonly suggest interpersonal psychotherapy (IPT) or cognitive behavioral therapy (CBT), both having solid evidence-based outcomes data for the treatment of depression.[60] IPT is useful in addressing resolving conflicts and role transitions. In studies, it has shown to reduce depressive symptoms and improve social adjustment.[59] CBT helps these women correct negative thinking and associated behaviors.[60] Couples counseling also may be indicated in women who have significant marital strain. Women seeking treatment for depression also may benefit from nutrition counseling and regular low-impact exercise.[11,61] Many providers advise pregnant women who take herbal supplements for their depression to cease during pregnancy, because limited safety data in pregnancy exist. Finally, studies have shown that it is safe and effective for pregnant women who have severe depression to participate in electroconvulsive therapy if they and their provider see this as the best therapy option.[62]

POSTPARTUM DEPRESSION
Background, Prevalence, and Clinical Features

Postpartum depression develops in approximately 10% to 20% of women who give birth,[63] with higher percentages in adolescents, mothers of premature infants, and women living in urban areas.[64,65] Women who have low income and limited partner support also are at higher risk.[66,67] Postpartum depression often is undetected and commonly underdiagnosed.[68] Many women expect an adjustment period after having a baby and, therefore, may not recognize that the symptoms of depression are out of the ordinary.[68] They may not want to admit they have a problem, they believe they need to prove they are a good mother, or they believe that seeking treatment will result in immediate removal of their child by child protective services. Many women do not seek treatment because of the combination of demanding newborn care and the lack of energy and motivation that comes with the disease process.[59] Furthermore, after the 6-week postpartum visit, a new mother who received her prenatal care from an obstetrician may not have routine health care scheduled, and she may believe she has nowhere to seek help.[68] If postpartum depression is left untreated, the symptoms last an average of 7 months but can extend into the second year after delivery.[59,68] Depression has a wide impact, influencing all members of families, and can lead to marital distress, family conflict, or loss of income and, in extreme cases, it can result in placement of children in care outside the home.[69]

The *DSM-IV*[7] defines postpartum depression with the same symptom criteria as used for depression before or during pregnancy but specifies that it begin within the first 4 weeks after the baby is born. Onset can occur anywhere between 24 hours after giving birth and several months later.[68] Many epidemiologic studies define postpartum depression as depressive symptom onset within 3 months post partum and others as within the first year after delivery.[70] Depression symptoms often are accompanied by comorbid anxiety and commonly women have many concerns about their efficacy as a mother or are preoccupied with the health, feeding, and sleeping behaviors of their infants. As in pregnancy, MDD with postpartum onset must have the requisite clinical symptoms present for at least 2 weeks.[7]

Continuum of Affective Symptoms During Post Partum

Postpartum depression must be differentiated from the "baby blues" and postpartum psychosis. The baby blues are reported to occur in up to 70% of women after delivery.[71] These women feel sad, weepy, irritable, anxious, and confused, with increased sensitivity, fatigue, sleep disturbances, and appetite changes.[7] The symptoms usually peak approximately 4 days post partum and abate by day 10.[68,69] Although these symptoms may last only a few hours to days, women who experience the baby blues are at a higher risk for developing postpartum depression. In women who were diagnosed with postpartum depression 6 weeks after delivery, two thirds had experienced baby blues symptoms.[72] The baby blues, however, almost always resolve within 2 weeks.

Postpartum psychosis occurs less commonly, having an impact on 0.2% of women of childbearing age.[73] Women may experience hallucinations, delusions, unusual behavior, agitation, disorganized thought, and inability to sleep for several nights.[7,69] Often the hallucinations and delusions center on the baby and immediate intervention is vital to protect the lives of mother and child.[7] Typically this disorder presents within 2 weeks post partum or sooner.[7] Most often, postpartum psychosis is the result of affective psychosis, most commonly bipolar affective disorder.[7] Any woman who has had an episode of postpartum psychosis in a prior pregnancy should be screened carefully for bipolar disorder. Women who have had a prior episode of postpartum psychosis are at a high risk for a subsequent episode. Postpartum psychosis is considered a psychiatric emergency because of the potential for catastrophic suicide or infanticide.[69]

RISK FACTORS AND EPIDEMIOLOGY

Risk factors for postpartum depression should be identified before or during pregnancy and discussed at length between patient and provider. Many women who develop postpartum depression have had antenatal symptoms of depression.[74] Once a woman experiences postpartum depression, she is at risk for depression relapses with or without additional pregnancies.[75] Research shows that women who have had previous episodes of postpartum depression have a 25% risk for recurrence.[76] Experts debate whether or not the rapid decline in reproductive hormone levels after delivery contributes to depression development. Bloch and coworkers found that when a decline of estradriol and progesterone was simulated in nonpregnant women, 63% of the women who had a history of postpartum depression experienced some changes in mood, whereas the women who did not have a history of postpartum depression did not experience any emotional changes. Thus, women who have a history of postpartum depression may be more sensitive to the systemic decrease in gonadal steroids post delivery.[77] Other risk factors for postpartum depression include past depressive symptoms not related to pregnancy, a family history of depression, and factors that influence depression at any time point, including poor social support, social conflict, and life stressors.[78]

IDENTIFICATION AND SCREENING OF POSTPARTUM DEPRESSION

Health care providers can have difficulty differentiating postpartum depression symptoms from the normative adjustment of a woman to a new infant. Physicians should take into account the circumstances (eg, extreme fatigue, even though a baby may be sleeping through the night) and intensity of the symptoms.[68] Routine postpartum visits, and well infant pediatric visits present an ideal time for depression screening.[79] Otherwise, physicians can use a screening question, such as, "Have you had depressed mood or decreased interest or pleasure in activities most of the day nearly every day for the past 2 weeks?"[7] Affirmative responses should cue a provider to screen for other neurovegetative symptoms, including appetite and sleep changes, hopelessness, and difficulty paying attention. Significant impairment in social or occupational functioning should prompt a psychiatric referral. Suicidality or the risk for harm to an infant requires an assessment for inpatient hospitalization. Concomitant illicit substance abuse likewise merits a prompt evaluation. If EPDS scores are lower than 10 on clinical assessment but a patient still has some depressive symptoms, a re-evaluation a few weeks later is recommended.[69] Other disease processes can mimic depression or can occur concomitantly. Patients presenting with symptoms of postpartum depression should routinely be tested for anemia and thyroid function, especially because hypothyroidism and hyperthyroidism occur more frequently post partum and can lead to alterations in mood.[69]

TREATMENT OF POSTPARTUM DEPRESSION

Antidepressant medication and psychotherapy are the foundation of treatment for postpartum depression. SSRIs are medications prescribed most commonly but other agents should be considered with a patient's prior positive treatment response. Because of the high risk for recurrence in women who have a previous history of postpartum depression, one study suggests providing prophylactic sertraline to prevent onset of symptoms.[76] Some literature suggests that women who have postpartum depression may be likely to have a more positive response to serotonergic agents, such as SSRIs and venlafaxine, than to TCAs.[80,81] The antidepressant dose may be started at one half the recommended amount and increased slowly; postpartum women seem more sensitive to the side effects of these medications. Increased anxious symptoms at initiation of medications is a common concern.[82] Once a steady, effective dose is reached, then pharmacotherapy should continue for at least 6 months to prevent a relapse of symptoms.[7] If there is no improvement with antidepressants after 6 weeks of therapy, a psychiatric consultation is appropriate.[69]

Many women are hesitant to take antidepressants while breastfeeding a child. All antidepressants are secreted to some degree into the breast milk; however, ethical concerns prevent large randomized controlled trials in lactating mothers to determine efficacy and safety.[37] Both paroxetine and sertraline have been studied in lactating women, and, as with all medications, are secreted into breast milk. Infant serum levels are very low to undetectable with these agents, however.[83,84] Fluoxetine has higher rates of secretion into breast milk. Because fluoxetine and its metabolite, norfluoxetine, have extremely long half-lives, they can accumulate in an infant's blood, reaching detectable levels.[85] Case reports link maternal fluoxetine use to colic, prolonged crying, and vomiting, so it is not considered the first-line SSRI for breastfeeding women.[86] If a mother has a positive history responding to fluoxetine, the benefit outweighs the risk and it should be continued while monitoring the child for side effects.

A substantial majority of lactating infants have no sequelae despite exposure to SSRIs during lactation. Mothers taking any antidepressant should be mindful of their infant's temperament and behavior, especially premature and sick newborns who may be predisposed to dehydration,[69] and should notify their physician if they notice irritability, difficulty feeding, or disturbed sleep patterns.[37] In general, no adverse effects are noted in infants when breastfeeding mothers take TCAs.[87] Breastfeeding while taking doxepin has been reported to cause severe muscle hypotonia, vomiting, drowsiness, and jaundice in babies, and, therefore, is not recommended.[88] Small case reports of atypical antidepressants have found no negative effects on infants with maternal use of mirtazapine or trazodone,[89,90] increased risk for drowsiness and lethargy with nefazodone (only one case),[91] and increased seizure risk with exposure to bupropion if a baby has a history of seizures.[88,92] Larger studies are needed to explore these effects further. Research on long-term effects of SSRI and TCA exposure through breast milk on children shows no alteration in IQ, language development, or behavior.[88]

For postpartum women who have sleep difficulties, diphenhydramine may be helpful.[93] Lorazepam can be used in for women who have profound sleep disruption; it has fewer active metabolites, reduces nighttime anxiety, and enhances sleep. Lorazepam, however, is excreted into breast milk in low concentrations.[94,95] Several studies have observed that in lactating mothers taking lorazepam, there are no adverse effects on infants and no change in the amount of milk consumed. Caution should be taken when prescribing lorazepam during an infant's first few weeks of life because of the relative immaturity of the hepatic metabolism.[94,95]

Interpersonal therapy (IPT) is ideally suited to postpartum mothers, as almost all women have some concerns regarding role transitions that occur during this important life milestone. IPT effectively targets this transition. Likewise, CBT has shown to reduce depressive symptoms[96] by targeting inappropriate expectations that some women may have, such as the need to be a "perfect" mother or a sense of shame by not being overjoyed with their infant during the immediate postpartum period. Both psychotherapies may be provided in 8- to 12-week periods.[59] Pilot studies currently are exploring the efficacy of the treatment provided over the telephone, to allow women to receive treatment without leaving their home.[97] Many women, especially those who have lactation concerns with pharmacotherapy, may be more comfortable beginning with IPT or CBT.[59] Additionally, behavioral strategies, such as adjusting the sleep schedule (having each member of the marital dyad share some of the nighttime responsibilities) and using the support of other family members to assist with nighttime feedings, may enhance a woman's ability sleep at night.[98]

Debate exists over the prospect of hormone therapy for postpartum depression. One study evaluated the effects of transdermal 17β-estradiol versus placebo and found a significant decrease in depression scores in the estradiol group.[99] One half of the women receiving estradiol, however, also were taking antidepressants, so the effect of hormone therapy alone is unclear. Additionally, the hypercoagulable state of postpartum women may limit the clinical usefulness of estrogen treatments. Prophylactic progesterone (norethisterone enanthate) postpartum compared with placebo demonstrated an increased risk for depressive symptoms in the treatment group.[100] More research is needed to explore hormonal treatment possibilities further.

SUMMARY

Primary care providers need to be aware that depression in women during their childbearing years is common. Routine depression screening, particularly at prenatal care visits, coupled with the use of physician collaborators to assist in connecting women with care is paramount. During prenatal interviews, providers should be aware of risk factors for depression, including previous history of depression and interpersonal conflict. Links have been made between depression during pregnancy and poor pregnancy outcomes, such as preeclampsia, insufficient weight gain, decreased compliance with prenatal care, and premature labor. The literature suggests that overall the risks of SSRIs are small during pregnancy relative to the risk for undertreatment of depression. If depression continues post partum, there is an increased risk for poor mother-infant attachment, delayed cognitive and linguistic skills, impaired emotional development, and behavioral issues. Longer term, these children are more likely to have emotional instability, conduct disorders, and require mental health services. To prevent these outcomes, postpartum depression screening with the EPDS or simple screening questions should be a priority for postpartum follow-up visits. Antidepressant treatments, IPT, adjunctive behavioral treatment, and involving family in the supportive care of postpartum women often are helpful strategies. More research is needed to determine the long-term and developmental effects of antidepressant exposure in children occurring during pregnancy and lactation.

REFERENCES

1. Kessler RC, Zhao S, Blazer DG, et al. Prevalence, correlates, and course of minor depression and major depression in the National Comorbidity Survey. J Affect Disord 1997;45(1–2):19–30.
2. Weissman MM, Olfson M. Depression in women: implications for health care research. Science 1995;269(5225):799–801.
3. Gotlib IH, Whiffen VE, Mount JH, et al. Prevalence rates and demographic characteristics associated with depression in pregnancy and the postpartum. J Consult Clin Psychol 1989;57(2):269–74.
4. Brown MA, Solchany JE. Two overlooked mood disorders in women: subsyndromal depression and prenatal depression. Nurs Clin North Am 2004;39(1):83–95.
5. Marcus SM, Flynn HA, Blow FC, et al. Depressive symptoms among pregnant women screened in obstetrics settings. J Womens Health (Larchmt) 2003; 12(4):373–80.
6. ACOG Practice Bulletin. Clinical management guidelines for obstetrician-gynecologists number 92, April 2008 (replaces practice bulletin number 87, November 2007). Use of psychiatric medications during pregnancy and lactation. Obstet Gynecol 2008;111(4):1001–20.

7. DSM-IV, Association AP. In: Diagnostic and statistical manual of mental disorders. No. 4th. Washington, DC: American Psychiatric Association; 1994.
8. Kumar R, Robson KM. A prospective study of emotional disorders in childbearing women. Br J Psychiatry 1984;144:35–47.
9. Altshuler LL, Cohen LS, Moline ML, et al. Treatment of depression in women: a summary of the expert consensus guidelines. J Psychiatr Pract 2001;7(3): 185–208.
10. Westdahl C, Milan S, Magriples U, et al. Social support and social conflict as predictors of prenatal depression. Obstet Gynecol 2007;110(1):134–40.
11. Ross AS, Hall RW, Frost K, et al. Antenatal & neonatal guidelines, education & learning system. J Ark Med Soc 2006;102(12):328–30.
12. Altshuler LL, Hendrick V, Cohen LS, et al. Course of mood and anxiety disorders during pregnancy and the postpartum period. J Clin Psychiatry 1998;59(Suppl 2): 29–33.
13. USPSTF. Screening for depression: recommendations and rationale. Ann Intern Med 2002;136(10):760–4.
14. Feinman JA, Cardillo D, Palmer J, et al. Development of a model for the detection and treatment of depression in primary care. Psychiatr Q 2000;71(1):59–78.
15. Radloff L. The CES-D scale: a self-report depression scale for research in the general population. Applied Psychological Measurement 1977;1:385–401.
16. Cox JL, Holden JM, Sagovsky R, et al. Detection of postnatal depression. Development of the 10-item Edinburgh Postnatal Depression Scale. Br J Psychiatry 1987;150:782–6.
17. Jardri R, Pelta J, Maron M, et al. Predictive validation study of the Edinburgh postnatal depression scale in the first week after delivery and risk analysis for postnatal depression. J Affect Disord 2006;93(1–3):169–76.
18. Matthey S, Henshaw C, Elliott S, et al. Variability in use of cut-off scores and formats on the Edinburgh postnatal depression scale: implications for clinical and research practice. Arch Womens Ment Health 2006;9(6):309–15.
19. Sharp LK, Lipsky MS. Screening for depression across the lifespan: a review of measures for use in primary care settings. Am Fam Physician 2002;66(6): 1001–8.
20. Katon WJ, Seelig M. Population-based care of depression: team care approaches to improving outcomes. J Occup Environ Med 2008;50(4):459–67 (B).
21. Gilbody S, Bower P, Fletcher J, et al. Collaborative care for depression: a cumulative meta-analysis and review of longer-term outcomes. Arch Intern Med 2006; 166(21):2314–21.
22. Zuckerman B, Amaro H, Bauchner H, et al. Depressive symptoms during pregnancy: relationship to poor health behaviors. Am J Obstet Gynecol 1989; 160(5 Pt 1):1107–11.
23. Chung TK, Lau TK, Yip AS, et al. Antepartum depressive symptomatology is associated with adverse obstetric and neonatal outcomes. Psychosom Med 2001; 63(5):830–4.
24. Wadhwa PD, Sandman CA, Porto M, et al. The association between prenatal stress and infant birth weight and gestational age at birth: a prospective investigation. Am J Obstet Gynecol 1993;169(4):858–65.
25. Zuckerman B, Bauchner H, Parker S, et al. Maternal depressive symptoms during pregnancy, and newborn irritability. J Dev Behav Pediatr 1990;11(4):190–4.
26. Wadhwa PD, Dunkel-Schetter C, Chicz-DeMet A, et al. Prenatal psychosocial factors and the neuroendocrine axis in human pregnancy. Psychosom Med 1996;58(5):432–46.

27. Teixeira JM, Fisk NM, Glover V, et al. Association between maternal anxiety in pregnancy and increased uterine artery resistance index: cohort based study. BMJ 1999;318(7177):153–7.
28. Hoffman S, Hatch MC. Depressive symptomatology during pregnancy: evidence for an association with decreased fetal growth in pregnancies of lower social class women. Health Psychol 2000;19(6):535–43.
29. Heringhausen J, Marcus SM, Muzik M, et al. Neonatal sleep patterns and relationship to maternal depression (submitted). American Association of Child and Adolescent Psychiatry's 55th Annual Meeting. Chicago, IL; 2008.
30. Forman DR, O'Hara MW, Stuart S, et al. Effective treatment for postpartum depression is not sufficient to improve the developing mother-child relationship. Dev Psychopathol 2007;19(2):585–602.
31. Coghill S, Caplan H, Alexandra H, et al. Impact of maternal postnatal depression on cognitive development of young children. Br Med J 1986;292:1165–7.
32. Alpern L, Lyons-Ruth K. Preschool children at social risk: chronicity and timing of maternal depressive symptoms and child behavior problems at school and at home. Dev Psychopathol 1993;5:371–87.
33. Field T. Infants of depressed mothers. Infant Behav Dev 1995;18:1–13.
34. Lyons-Ruth K, Wolfe R, Lyubchik A, et al. Depression and the parenting of young children: making the case for early preventive mental health services. Harv Rev Psychiatry 2000;8(3):148–53.
35. Weissman MM, Prusoff BA, Gammon GD, et al. Psychopathology in the children (ages 6–18) of depressed and normal parents. J Am Acad Child Psychiatry 1984;23(1):78–84.
36. Einarson A, Miropolsky V, Varma B, et al. Determinants of physicians' decision-making regarding the prescribing of antidepressant medication during pregnancy. Paper presented at the Fifteenth International Conference of the Organization of Teratology Information Services (OTIS). Scottsdale (AZ), 2002. p. 355–75.
37. Gonsalves L, Schuermeyer I. Treating depression in pregnancy: practical suggestions. Cleve Clin J Med 2006;73(12):1098–104.
38. Hostetter A, Stowe ZN, Strader JR Jr, et al. Dose of selective serotonin uptake inhibitors across pregnancy: clinical implications. Depress Anxiety 2000;11(2): 51–7.
39. Cohen LS, Altshuler LL, Harlow BL, et al. Relapse of major depression during pregnancy in women who maintain or discontinue antidepressant treatment. JAMA 2006;295(5):499–507.
40. Hostetter A, Ritchie JC, Stowe ZN, et al. Amniotic fluid and umbilical cord blood concentrations of antidepressants in three women. Biol Psychiatry 2000;48(10): 1032–4.
41. Hemels ME, Einarson A, Koren G, et al. Antidepressant use during pregnancy and the rates of spontaneous abortions: a meta-analysis. Ann Pharmacother 2005;39(5):803–9.
42. Chun-Fai-Chan B, Koren G, Fayez I, et al. Pregnancy outcome of women exposed to bupropion during pregnancy: a prospective comparative study. Am J Obstet Gynecol 2005;192(3):932–6.
43. Kulin NA, Pastuszak A, Sage SR, et al. Pregnancy outcome following maternal use of the new selective serotonin reuptake inhibitors: a prospective controlled multicenter study. JAMA 1998;279(8):609–10.
44. Chambers CD, Johnson KA, Dick LM, et al. Birth outcomes in pregnant women taking fluoxetine. N Engl J Med 1996;335(14):1010–5.

45. GlaxoSmithKline. Available at: http://www.gsk.com/media/paroxetine/pregnancy_hcp_letter.pdf. Accessed June 19, 2008.

46. Einarson A, Pistelli A, DeSantis M, et al. Evaluation of the risk of congenital cardiovascular defects associated with use of paroxetine during pregnancy. Am J Psychiatry 2008;165(6):749–52.

47. Alwan S, Reefhuis J, Rasmussen SA, et al. Use of selective serotonin-reuptake inhibitors in pregnancy and the risk of birth defects. N Engl J Med 2007;356(26): 2684–92.

48. Louik C, Lin AE, Werler MM, et al. First-trimester use of selective serotonin-reuptake inhibitors and the risk of birth defects. N Engl J Med 2007;356(26): 2675–83.

49. Koren G, Matsui D, Einarson A, et al. Is maternal use of selective serotonin reuptake inhibitors in the third trimester of pregnancy harmful to neonates? CMAJ 2005;172(11):1457–9.

50. Ferreira E, Carceller AM, Agogue C, et al. Effects of selective serotonin reuptake inhibitors and venlafaxine during pregnancy in term and preterm neonates. Pediatrics 2007;119(1):52–9.

51. Chambers CD, Hernandez-Diaz S, Van Marter LJ, et al. Selective serotonin-reuptake inhibitors and risk of persistent pulmonary hypertension of the newborn. N Engl J Med 2006;354(6):579–87.

52. Einarson A, Selby P, Koren G, et al. Abrupt discontinuation of psychotropic drugs during pregnancy: fear of teratogenic risk and impact of counselling. J Psychiatry Neurosci 2001;26(1):44–8.

53. Altshuler LL, Cohen L, Szuba MP, et al. Pharmacologic management of psychiatric illness during pregnancy: dilemmas and guidelines. Am J Psychiatry 1996; 153(5):592–606.

54. Sharma V. A cautionary note on the use of antidepressants in postpartum depression. Bipolar Disord 2006;8(4):411–4.

55. Schimmell MS, Katz EZ, Shaag Y, et al. Toxic neonatal effects following maternal clomipramine therapy. J Toxicol Clin Toxicol 1991;29(4):479–84.

56. Nulman I, Rovet J, Stewart DE, et al. Neurodevelopment of children exposed in utero to antidepressant drugs. N Engl J Med 1997;336(4):258–62.

57. Einarson TR, Einarson A. Newer antidepressants in pregnancy and rates of major malformations: a meta-analysis of prospective comparative studies. Pharmacoepidemiol Drug Saf 2005;14(12):823–7.

58. Way CM. Safety of newer antidepressants in pregnancy. Pharmacotherapy 2007;27(4):546–52.

59. O'Hara MW, Stuart S, Gorman LL, et al. Efficacy of interpersonal psychotherapy for postpartum depression. Arch Gen Psychiatry 2000;57(11):1039–45.

60. Bhatia SC, Bhatia SK. Depression in women: diagnostic and treatment considerations. Am Fam Physician 1999;60(1):225–34, 239–40.

61. Daley AJ, Macarthur C, Winter H, et al. The role of exercise in treating postpartum depression: a review of the literature. J Midwifery Womens Health 2007; 52(1):56–62.

62. Miller LJ. Use of electroconvulsive therapy during pregnancy. Hosp Community Psychiatry 1994;45(5):444–50 (B).

63. Steiner M. Perinatal mood disorders: position paper. Psychopharmacol Bull 1998;34(3):301–6.

64. Hobfoll SE, Ritter C, Lavin J, et al. Depression prevalence and incidence among inner-city pregnant and postpartum women. J Consult Clin Psychol 1995;63(3): 445–53.

65. Logsdon MC, Usui W. Psychosocial predictors of postpartum depression in diverse groups of women. West J Nurs Res 2001;23(6):563–74.
66. Secco ML, Profit S, Kennedy E, et al. Factors affecting postpartum depressive symptoms of adolescent mothers. J Obstet Gynecol Neonatal Nurs 2007; 36(1):47–54.
67. Shanok AF, Miller L. Depression and treatment with inner city pregnant and parenting teens. Arch Womens Ment Health 2007;10(5):199–210.
68. Epperson CN. Postpartum major depression: detection and treatment. Am Fam Physician 1999;59(8):2247–54, 2259–60.
69. Wisner KL, Parry BL, Piontek CM, et al. Clinical practice. Postpartum depression. N Engl J Med 2002;347(3):194–9 (18).
70. Kendell RE, Chalmers JC, Platz C, et al. Epidemiology of puerperal psychoses. Br J Psychiatry 1987;150:662–73.
71. O'Hara MW, Swain AM. Rates and risk of postpartum depression—a meta-analysis. Int Rev Psychiatry 1996;8:37–54.
72. Hannah P, Adams D, Lee A, et al. Links between early post-partum mood and post-natal depression. Br J Psychiatry 1992;160:777–80.
73. Harlow BL, Vitonis AF, Sparen P, et al. Incidence of hospitalization for postpartum psychotic and bipolar episodes in women with and without prior prepregnancy or prenatal psychiatric hospitalizations. Arch Gen Psychiatry 2007; 64(1):42–8.
74. Milgrom J, Gemmill AW, Bilszta JL, et al. Antenatal risk factors for postnatal depression: a large prospective study. J Affect Disord 2008;108(1–2):147–57.
75. Cooper PJ, Murray L. Course and recurrence of postnatal depression. Evidence for the specificity of the diagnostic concept. Br J Psychiatry 1995;166(2): 191–5.
76. Wisner KL, Perel JM, Peindl KS, et al. Prevention of recurrent postpartum depression: a randomized clinical trial. J Clin Psychiatry 2001;62(2):82–6.
77. Bloch M, Schmidt PJ, Danaceau M, et al. Effects of gonadal steroids in women with a history of postpartum depression. Am J Psychiatry 2000;157(6):924–30.
78. Wisner KL, Stowe ZN. Psychobiology of postpartum mood disorders. Semin Reprod Endocrinol 1997;15(1):77–89.
79. Gjerdingen DK, Yawn BP. Postpartum depression screening: importance, methods, barriers, and recommendations for practice. J Am Board Fam Med 2007;20(3):280–8.
80. Cohen LS, Viguera AC, Bouffard SM, et al. Venlafaxine in the treatment of postpartum depression. J Clin Psychiatry 2001;62(8):592–6.
81. Wisner KL, Peindl KS, Gigliotti TV, et al. Tricyclics vs. SSRIs for postpartum depression. Arch Womens Ment Health 1999;1:189–91.
82. Wisner KL, Perel JM, Peindl KS, et al. Effects of the postpartum period on nortriptyline pharmacokinetics. Psychopharmacol Bull 1997;33(2):243–8.
83. Stowe ZN, Owens MJ, Landry JC, et al. Sertraline and desmethylsertraline in human breast milk and nursing infants. American Journal of Psychiatry 1997; 154(9):1255–60.
84. Spigset O, Carleborg L, Norstrom A, et al. Paroxetine level in breast milk. J Clin Psychiatry 1996;57(1):39.
85. Kristensen JH, Ilett KF, Hackett LP, et al. Distribution and excretion of fluoxetine and norfluoxetine in human milk. Br J Clin Pharmacol 1999;48(4):521–7 (B).
86. Lester BM, Cucca J, Andreozzi L, et al. Possible association between fluoxetine hydrochloride and colic in an infant. J Am Acad Child Adolesc Psychiatry 1993; 32(6):1253–5 (B).

87. Yoshida K, Smith B, Craggs M, et al. Investigation of pharmacokinetics and of possible adverse effects in infants exposed to tricyclic antidepressants in breast-milk. J Affect Disord 1997;43(3):225–37.

88. Hale TW. Drug therapy and breastfeeding: antidepressants, antipsychotics, antimanics, and sedatives. Neo Revs 2004;5(10):e451–6.

89. Kristensen JH, Ilett KF, Rampono J, et al. Transfer of the antidepressant mirtazapine into breast milk. Br J Clin Pharmacol 2007;63(3):322–7.

90. Verbeeck RK, Ross SG, McKenna EA, et al. Excretion of trazodone in breast milk. Br J Clin Pharmacol 1986;22(3):367–70.

91. Yapp P, Ilett KF, Kristensen JH, et al. Drowsiness and poor feeding in a breast-fed infant: association with nefazodone and its metabolites. Ann Pharmacother 2000;34(11):1269–72.

92. Chaudron LH, Schoenecker CJ. Bupropion and breastfeeding: a case of a possible infant seizure. J Clin Psychiatry 2004;65(6):881–2.

93. Ringdahl EN, Pereira SL, Delzell JE Jr, et al. Treatment of primary insomnia. J Am Board Fam Pract 2004;17(3):212–9.

94. Summerfield RJ, Nielsen MS. Excretion of lorazepam into breast milk. Br J Anaesth 1985;57(10):1042–3.

95. Johnstone MJ. The effect of lorazepam on neonatal feeding behaviour at term. Pharmatherapeutica 1982;3(4):259–62.

96. Milgrom J, Negri LM, Gemmill AW, et al. A randomized controlled trial of psychological interventions for postnatal depression. Br J Clin Psychol 2005;44(Pt 4):529–42 (A).

97. Flynn HA, Henshaw E, O'Mahen H, et al. In: Team UoMDoPP Personalizing CBT for perinatal depression: results of a qualitative study on improving intervention engagement and effectiveness. Ann Arbor. 2008.

98. Gay CL, Lee KA, Lee SY, et al. Sleep patterns and fatigue in new mothers and fathers. Biol Res Nurs 2004;5(4):311–8.

99. Gregoire AJ, Kumar R, Everitt B, et al. Transdermal oestrogen for treatment of severe postnatal depression. Lancet 1996;347(9006):930–3.

100. Lawrie TA, Hofmeyr GJ, De Jager M, et al. A double-blind randomised placebo controlled trial of postnatal norethisterone enanthate: the effect on postnatal depression and serum hormones. Br J Obstet Gynaecol 1998;105(10):1082–90.

Intimate Partner Violence

Adam J. Zolotor, MD, MPH[a,b,*], Amy C. Denham, MD, MPH[a],
Amy Weil, MD[c,d]

KEYWORDS

- Intimate partner violence • Domestic violence
- Child abuse and neglect

Intimate partner violence (IPV) is a common, serious, and preventable public health problem. IPV includes psychologic, physical, or sexual harm by a current or former partner or spouse. It occurs between married and unmarried couples and between heterosexual and same-sex couples. The Centers for Disease Control and Prevention (CDC) defines IPV as inclusive of the following forms of violence

> Psychologic/emotional violence—involves trauma to a victim caused by acts, threats of acts, or coercive tactics. Psychologic/emotional abuse can include, but is not limited to, humiliating a victim, controlling what a victim can and cannot do, withholding information from a victim, deliberately doing something to make a victim feel diminished or embarrassed, isolating a victim from friends and family, and denying a victim access to money or other basic resources.
>
> Physical violence—the intentional use of physical force with the potential for causing disability, injury, harm, or death. Physical violence includes, but is not limited to, scratching, pushing, shoving, throwing, grabbing, biting, strangulation, shaking, slapping, punching, burning, use of a weapon, and use of restraints or one's body, size, or strength against another person.

This work was support by the Sunshine Lady Foundation Child Maltreatment Doctoral Fellowship

[a] Department of Family Medicine, University of North Carolina School of Medicine, CB #7595, Chapel Hill, NC 27599-7595, USA

[b] Injury Prevention Research Center, CB# 7505, University of North Carolina, Chapel Hill, NC, USA

[c] Department of Medicine, Division of General Medicine and Epidemiology, University of North Carolina School of Medicine, 5039 Old Clinic Building, CB # 7110, Chapel Hill, NC 27599-7110, USA

[d] Beacon Child and Family Program, CB# 7600, University of North Carolina School of Medicine, Chapel Hill, NC, USA

* Corresponding author. Department of Family Medicine, University of North Carolina School of Medicine, CB #7595, Chapel Hill, NC 27599-7595.

E-mail address: ajzolo@med.unc.edu (A.J. Zolotor).

Prim Care Clin Office Pract 36 (2009) 167–179
doi:10.1016/j.pop.2008.10.010

primarycare.theclinics.com

Sexual violence—divided into three categories: (1) use of physical force to compel a person to engage in a sexual act against his or her will whether or not the act is completed; (2) attempted or completed sex act involving a person who is unable to understand the nature or condition of the act, to decline participation, or to communicate unwillingness to engage in the sexual act (eg, because of illness, disability, or the influence of alcohol or other drugs or because of intimidation or pressure); and(3) abusive sexual contact.[1]

EPIDEMIOLOGY

IPV is pervasive. Population-based estimates demonstrate that 32 million Americans have been affected by IPV.[2] The prevalence and incidence of IPV can be measured on a continuum from rare events, such as death, to more common events, such as self-reported pushing, slapping, and intimidation. It also is useful to consider how this pervasive phenomenon affects clinical practice.

The ecologic model of IPV considers IPV a result of a complex set of circumstances from risk factors that occur at the level of the victim, the perpetrator, their relationship, the family, the community, and society. Risk factors at the level of individual victims include female gender, young age, history of IPV, history of sexual assault, history of child abuse victimization, heavy alcohol or drug use, unemployment, depression, and racial or ethnic minority status.[2–4] Relationship level risk factors include income or educational disparity and male control of relationship (eg, psychologic or economic).[5] Community level risk factors include poverty, poor social cohesion, and weak sanctions, including minimal legal penalties or rare successful prosecutions.[6] Societal level risk factors include traditional gender norms and general acceptance of violence for conflict resolution.

Anonymous telephone surveys afford the best estimate of incident and prevalent IPV. The most comprehensive national assessment of IPV from a national telephone survey is from the Behavioral Risk Factor Surveillance System 2005 IPV module. This survey of more than 70,000 United States adults demonstrated that one in four women and one in seven men report a lifetime threatened or completed physical or sexual IPV. In the same survey, 1.4% of women and 0.7% of men reported such victimization within the past year. When IPV is defined more broadly to include a variety of physical and psychologic acts of violence, estimates for any IPV are as high as one in five men and women.[7] Telephone surveys, however, may underestimate the true extent of IPV because of recall bias and social desirability bias, and the estimates for IPV may vary because of survey instruments, operational definitions, and arbitrary cut points.

The National Crime Victimization Survey estimates that 467,000 people are victims of criminal IPV each year. The Survey includes only IPV reported to law enforcement authorities and, therefore, most likely grossly underestimates IPV. More than 80% of IPV incidents reported to law enforcement involve female victims.[8] Death by IPV is a rare but tragic event. Using data from the National Violent Death Reporting System in 16 states, the CDC estimated that 1200 IPV homicides occurred in 2005. The rate of IPV homicide is 0.8 per 100,000 persons. The rate is higher among African Americans (1.5/100,000 persons) and American Indians (2/100,000 persons) than Caucasians (0.6/100,000 persons). The majority of IPV victims are women, estimated at 65%.[9] Victims are at a higher risk for mortality if a perpetrator has access to a gun, has previously threatened the victim with a weapon, or uses illicit drugs. If perpetrator and victim have recently separated or if a victim has asked the perpetrator to leave the mutual dwelling, then the victim also is at higher risk for mortality.[10] Clinicians should be alert to these high-risk situations in counseling individuals who are affected by IPV.

Clinicians may see patients who have a history of current or former IPV in medical offices in high numbers. A recent large study of women enrolled in health maintenance organizations found that 44% had a history of IPV.[11] One study of women in pediatric clinics found that 14% of mothers screened positive for at least one of three questions related to severe IPV. Using a longer standard instrument, however, 76% of mothers reported a history of being a victim of psychologic aggression, 32% reported physical assault, 9% reported resultant injury, and 29% reported sexual coercion within the past year.[12] These data suggest that primary care physicians should consider female patients and mothers presenting in an ambulatory care practice setting as having very high risk for current or past IPV.

HEALTH EFFECTS OF INTIMATE PARTNER VIOLENCE

IPV has a significant effect on victims' health, influencing many aspects of physical and mental health. Individuals affected by IPV consistently are more likely than individuals not affected by IPV to report poor health,[13–15] a measure that correlates with long-term morbidity and mortality. Physical and mental health effects of IPV persist for many years beyond the period of abuse,[5,14] and a longer duration of abuse is associated with worse health outcomes.[16] Physical, sexual, and psychologic/emotional IPV all have adverse health effects.[14–16] The physical and mental health consequences of IPV occur in male and female victims, but women are more likely to report negative physical and mental health effects.[15]

Physical Health

Injuries

Injury is a direct health effect of IPV. Approximately 2 million injuries in women and 600,000 in men are attributable to IPV each year.[17] Approximately 42% of women and 20% of men who experience IPV report that they suffered an injury during their most recent victimization, although less than one third of these injuries are brought to the attention of health care providers. Women are more likely than men to be injured when victimized by an intimate partner, and they tend to have a greater severity of injury. Minor injuries, such as scratches and bruises, are most common, but more serious injuries, such as lacerations, broken bones, sprains, strains, and head injuries, also occur in a significant proportion of victims of IPV.[2]

There is no pathognomonic pattern of injury that suggests IPV; however, certain patterns of injury are suggestive and should raise clinicians' suspicion of intentional injury. Central injuries, such as injuries to the head, neck, breast, or abdomen, are more likely the result of IPV.[18] Trauma to the face, orbital fractures, and dental injuries are especially common.[18,19] Musculoskeletal injuries to the extremities, including fractures, sprains, or dislocations, account for more than one quarter of injuries attributable to IPV.[19] Clinicians should maintain an index of suspicion for IPV when patients present with these types of injuries.

In addition to the acute effects of injury, survivors of IPV also suffer long-term sequelae of inflicted injury. For example, women who have had repeated head trauma may have long-term symptoms of traumatic brain injury. Victims who have sustained injuries from strangulation may have problems with swallowing or speech.[20]

Other physical health effects

Individuals exposed to IPV experience increased risk for several acute and chronic health conditions not directly attributable to trauma, such as sexually transmitted infections,[20,21] cervical dysplasia,[20] unplanned pregnancy,[21] arthritis,[17] migraine,[22] asthma,[17,22] stroke, high cholesterol, heart disease,[17] irritable bowel syndrome and functional gastrointestinal disorders,[13,23] fibromyalgia, chronic fatigue syndrome, and temporomandibular joint syndrome.[17] Victims of IPV also are more likely to have chronic pain syndromes[20,24] and are more likely to have multiple somatic complaints, including stomach pain, back pain, menstrual problems, headaches, chest pain, dizziness, fainting spells, palpitations, shortness of breath, constipation, generalized fatigue, and insomnia.[22]

For many of these health conditions, the mechanism through which IPV increases risk is unknown but probably is multifactorial. Contributing factors may include the direct effect of physical trauma, the long-term accumulated stress of physical and psychologic trauma, and increased prevalence of behavioral risk. Regardless of etiology, it is useful for clinicians to know the constellation of conditions and symptoms that frequently present in victims of IPV. When a patient presents with frequent somatic complaints or other conditions consistent with IPV, a clinician should consider inquiring about IPV not only because intervention may be beneficial to a patient but also because knowledge of IPV could influence the treatment plan and help the clinician understand barriers to treatment adherence.

Mental Health

In addition to the physical health effects (described previously), victims of IPV frequently suffer chronic mental illness.[15] Although mental health consequences are seen whether or not abuse is physical, sexual, or psychologic, some data suggest that mental health outcomes are the worst for individuals who experience sexual IPV.[14]

Individuals who experience IPV are at increased risk for depression,[24] an effect seen with physical, sexual, and emotional IPV[14,16] and in men and women.[15] They also are at increased risk for suicidal thoughts and attempts.[13] Alcohol abuse and illicit drug use also are more common among individuals who experience IPV.[15–17,20]

Posttraumatic stress disorder (PTSD) is prevalent, occurring in 31% to 84% of women exposed to IPV.[25] Symptoms of PTSD, including emotional detachment, sleep disturbances, flashbacks, and mentally replaying episodes of assault, may persist long after the violence is no longer present in a woman's life. Higher rates of PTSD are seen with sexual and physical IPV than with physical IPV alone,[21] and a greater severity and frequency of violence correlates with greater risk for PTSD.[24] The high prevalence of PTSD among survivors of IPV may be a key factor in explaining the relationship between violence and physical health symptoms.[26]

Intimate Partner Violence and Pregnancy

Maternal morbidity and mortality

It is not uncommon for IPV to continue during pregnancy, putting women at risk for several pregnancy-related complications. Women who experience IPV during pregnancy are at increased risk for spontaneous abortion,[20] preterm labor, hypertensive disorders of pregnancy, vaginal bleeding, placental abruption, severe nausea and vomiting, dehydration, diabetes, urinary tract infection and premature rupture of membranes.[27] Pregnancies of couples affected by IPV also are more likely to have been unplanned.[20] IPV also is associated with a short interpregnancy interval in adolescents.[20] Late entry into prenatal care is common among women who are victims of IPV, and the possibility of IPV should be considered in women who receive late or no prenatal care.[20] IPV-related homicide is the leading cause of maternal mortality, accounting for 13% to 24% of all deaths in pregnancy.[20]

Infant morbidity and mortality

Infants affected by IPV during pregnancy also are at risk. Although studies have shown conflicting results, it seems that there is an association between IPV and low birth weight.[27–30] Abuse during pregnancy also seems to increase the risk for prematurity and perinatal death.[31,32]

Disability

A marker of the long-term toll of IPV is the high rate of disability among IPV survivors, approximately twice that of individuals not exposed to IPV.[33] Women who have a history of exposure to IPV report higher rates of disability because of chronic pain, nervous system injuries or disorders, mental illness or depression, chronic disease, and blindness.[33] Victims of IPV report higher use of disability equipment, such as canes or wheelchairs, and are more likely to report activity limitations due to health problems.[17]

Health Risk Behaviors

IPV is associated with several behaviors that confer health risk, which may contribute to the increased physical, mental, and pregnancy-related health risk seen in victims of IPV. More severe violence correlates more strongly with negative health behaviors by victims. IPV victims are more likely to abuse substances, including tobacco, alcohol, and other drugs.[15–17,20] They are more likely to engage in risky sexual behaviors, including unprotected sex, early sexual initiation, multiple sex partners, and trading sex for food, money, or other items.[17,20] Women who are abused are more likely to engage in disordered eating patterns, including overeating and vomiting or use of laxatives for weight control.[20]

Women who have a history of IPV may be perceived to overuse the health care system, with high rates of primary care and emergency department use; however, they commonly report unmet health care needs and troubled patient-physician communication.[20] What providers perceive as a lack of motivation to adhere to health recommendations could be related to the dynamics of violence. Many survivors report that partners interfere with their receipt of health care services,[34] one component in an overall pattern of control of victims' lives by their partners. Recognizing IPV should help providers to understand the barriers and challenges that patients face, allowing them to form a more constructive therapeutic relationship.

SCREENING FOR INTIMATE PARTNER VIOLENCE

As providers become more aware of IPV as a common problem with myriad health consequences, many have begun to screen routinely for IPV. Screening among providers varies as there is no gold standard test for IPV. A recent review of more than 35 existing screening tools underscores the range and confusion in screening for IPV in clinical settings. Many of the tools are too long for practical use in a busy clinic and are more appropriate for research. Shorter tools often lack adequate sensitivity or require follow-up discussion to improve diagnostic usefulness.[35] One study demonstrated that the use of a computer to complete survey-based screening tools is a practical option in emergency department settings.[36]

In parallel, many physicians are reluctant to integrate screening into practice. They are uncomfortable asking about "private" matters, do not feel well equipped to discuss or assist with IPV, or are worried about time, privacy, legal issues, and personal safety. Although many national groups have recommended screening for IPV, rates of screening in primary care settings are estimated at 9% to 11% depending on clinic visit type.[37] A recent study noted more discomfort among male physicians and those in private practice and less discomfort in clinicians practicing for 5 to 10 years, obstetrician/gynecologists, and those working in a hospital setting.[38]

Controversy

In 2004, the U.S. Preventive Services Task Force (USPSTF) assigned screening for IPV a recommendation of level I (insufficient evidence), citing methodologic problems with many studies and lack of proved efficacy of interventions to assist patients. The USPSTF defined successful intervention for IPV in adults as shelter use or leaving the abusive relationship. They found[39]

- No direct evidence that screening leads to decreased disability or premature death
- No existing studies that determine the accuracy of screening tools for identifying family and IPV among children, women, or older adults in general populations.
- Fair to good evidence that interventions reduce harm to children when child abuse or neglect has been assessed
- No studies that have directly assessed the harms of screening and interventions for the family, so cost benefit analysis cannot be conducted[39]

This rigid evaluation of evidence is difficult to apply to IPV screening for several reasons. Screening for IPV should not be compared with radiographic tests for breast cancer or sigmoidoscopy for colon cancer screening but rather to the type of analysis used for more similar and morbid conditions, such as counseling for depression.[40] Many clinicians agree that good evidence for screening for IPV might be hard to obtain. Some clinicians worry that the "insufficient" recommendation would cause even lower detection rates of IPV than before,[41] whereas advocates urge more research to be done. Although evidence does not exist to definitively prove that knowing about IPV reduces harm, common sense and prior experience suggest that knowing about such a difficult, potentially dangerous situation would be helpful toward understanding and assisting patients with health problems and even prevent needless deaths. Smoking cessation counseling may be a good analogy as described by Janssen and colleagues:

> When primary care physicians routinely ask about smoking as part of patient history taking, they do not do so in the belief that asking the question will stop their patients from smoking. Instead, knowledge of smoking status may guide the physician to undertake more frequent monitoring of cardiovascular and pulmonary health status, including measurement of blood pressure, evaluation of exercise tolerance, etc. Similarly, asking about intimate partner violence and obtaining a positive response identifies an opportunity for prevention of health-related sequelae.[42]

Many clinicians were skeptical about the shelter use and departure endpoints identified by the USPSTF. Substantial numbers of patients remain in adverse relationships over time yet may have improved health, especially after disclosure and care of IPV-related medical problems. The American Medical Association, American Academy of Family Physicians, and American College of Obstetricians and Gynecologists recommend IPV screening, whereas the Joint Commission of Accreditation of Health care Organizations mandates patient safety screening for hospital accreditation.

What patients want regarding screening

A recent meta-analysis evaluated qualitative studies regarding women's preferences for IPV screening.[43] Women wanted caregivers to be nonjudgmental, compassionate, and confidential. They wanted the professional to understand the complex, long-term nature of IPV and to understand its social and psychologic ramifications. Women wanted providers to avoid medicalizing the issue and to raise it in a confident, unrushed manner. They wanted confirmation that violence was unacceptable and undeserved and that abuse was not their fault. They hoped the health care professional would bolster their confidence and allow them to progress at their own pace. They did not want to be pressured to disclose, leave the relationship, or press charges. Women wanted to share decision making with providers.[43] They did not want to be told to leave the situation or make us of a shelter, the specific endpoints the USPSTF emphasized. Women prefer to be queried in a patient-centered interview format where a clinician follows up on a patient's own cues rather than checklists.[44] Ninety percent of the teens would not mind being screened by a health care provider; however, those who were most likely to object to screening were victims of physical violence or victims or perpetrators of sexual violence.[45]

Resolution of the conflict

IPV may contribute directly to the health problem (a current injury), exacerbate or cause somatic and psychologic states (PTSD, depression, and anxiety), or explain patient nonadherence (control by perpetrator). Thus, knowing about a woman's experience can be critical to diagnosing and treating her complaints. Asking about violence also educates patients about IPV, may increase recognition of their situation in the future,[46] and informs patients that providers can offer help for these problems. Even though the majority of patients are not currently in an abusive relationship, many have or will experience abuse at some point.

Because it is important to know about violence when providing care, it is recommended that providers assess for violence in all new patients and when it could play a role in determining the differential diagnosis of a medical condition (**Boxes 1** and **2**). Asking about violence before performing a genital examination or during a yearly examination is reasonable. Some institutions have nurses inquire at each appointment in triage when patients are alone. IPV can manifest as many different complaints or problems. Multiple physical complaints, chronic pain, depression, anxiety, substance abuse, or PTSD should prompt consideration of IPV, especially if the examination is inconsistent or treatment is not working.[47–53]

If They Say Yes, Then What?

A positive answer to an IPV screen can feel like a crisis moment because of anxiety generated in a clinician. Most often, abuse is psychologic and ongoing and may not

---

Box 1
Characteristics of good intimate partner violence screening techniques

Always ask about violence in privacy and assure confidentiality

Provide a preface that contextualizes and normalizes your query for the patient

Ask about the past and the present situation

Ask about psychologic and control factors and physical and sexual violence

Ask like you want to know the answer

Ask again if you have clinical suspicion, as patients often will not answer positively to your inquiry the first time or may downplay physical or sexual violence

---

Box 2
Samples of intimate partner violence screening questions

"Because violence is such a common and difficult problem, I ask all my patients if they have ever been harmed emotionally, physically, or sexually in the past or present."

"Many times people complaining of _____ have worse symptoms/more trouble recovering from _____ if they have been exposed to traumatic events. Have you ever been hurt emotionally, physically, or sexually in the past or recently?"

"Do you feel threatened or controlled by a partner, ex-partner, or anyone else in your life?"

"Has your partner or anyone else ever hurt you physically, for example by pushing, shoving, hitting, slapping, or kicking you or by forcing you to have sex?"

---

necessitate crisis-type intervention, and, like other chronic problems, it can be worked on over time. Cementing the therapeutic doctor-patient relationship is crucial and facilitates assessing whether or not a patient is in imminent danger. Patients who may be in severe, acute danger may benefit from seeking additional help if available. Help may come in the form of a hospital-based program, law enforcement (to press formal charges or to begin the process of obtaining a restraining order), community-based IPV organizations that can provide ongoing advocates, or a shelter if patients are worried for their immediate safety. The Violence Against Women Act offers many protections to victims of abuse, independent of their immigration status, and knowing about this law often can assuage patient fears regarding legal action.[54] Frequent office visits can be helpful to continue to care for medical problems, offer support, and assess for safety (**Box 3**).

Safety Assessment

Do patients believe they are in imminent danger? If they answer, "yes," consider contacting the IPV program, law enforcement, or a shelter if available in the community. If possible, empower patients to make these calls. Unfortunately, although patients often know when they are in danger, they are not always correct when they say they are not in danger.[55] One large case-controlled study found that more than one half of the victims of attempted or completed IPV homicides did not suspect they were at risk for harm.[56] To clarify patient safety, clinicians should assess for increasing frequency or severity of violence, prior use or threat of use of a weapon (eg, a knife or gun), assailant use of alcohol or illegal drugs, threat of homicide or suicide, or recent separation. Such patients may be in mortal danger and may benefit from seeking additional help if available.

EFFECTS ON CHILDREN

IPV and child maltreatment (CM) have many overlapping features, risk factors, and consequences. In many cases, they are final common outcomes from family

---

Box 3
Responding to a positive screen for intimate partner violence

Respond with empathy

Establish/continue a collaborative, noncontrolling therapeutic relationship that does not replicate the pattern of abuse

Assist with health

Assess for safety

---

dysfunction, stress, and societal tolerance of violence. Primary care providers are, in some ways, uniquely poised to consider the dynamics of family violence on an entire family unit. In some cases, the best interest of children and parent victims may not be served in the same way.

Co-Occurrence of Intimate Partner Violence and Child Maltreatment

IPV that occurs between partners, one of whom is a parent, often occur in households with CM. CM broadly encompasses child physical abuse, psychologic abuse, neglect, and sexual abuse. Studies that screened for IPV in a population of families affected by CM or for CM in families affected by IPV have clearly demonstrated that IPV and CM often occur in the same homes. Approximately 26% to 73% of families reported to child protective services for CM also are affected by IPV.[57–59] Conversely, families in which a woman is victimized by IPV have rates of CM between 30% and 60%,[57] with some studies reporting rates as high as 100%.[60] Past research estimating rates of co-occurrence of IPV and CM, however, may suffer significantly from selection bias and the lack of an appropriate comparison group. Recently, by using more appropriate comparison populations, several studies have demonstrated relationships between IPV and physical abuse, sexual abuse, and neglect.[61–65]

Harmful Effects of Intimate Partner Violence to Children

IPV can harm children physically and mentally. Children can be considered "collateral damage" in an assault between intimate partners. Nearly one half of homes with CM fatalities have reported IPV.[57,60,62] A single study of child injuries presenting to a pediatric emergency department in a large city demonstrates the range of these collateral injuries. One half of the child victims were under age 2, whereas 59% were being held by a caregiver when injured. Most of the injuries to the child were to the head (25%), face (19%), and eyes (12%). The child's father was most often responsible for the injury (50%), with the child's mother (13%) or mother's boyfriend (10%) found responsible in a smaller percentage of cases.[66] Two studies have demonstrated high emergency department use rates in children whose mothers have a history of IPV.[67,68]

Several longitudinal studies have demonstrated important associations between child and subsequent adult mental health. Child reports of witnessed IPV are associated with increased odds of suicidal ideation[69] and 2.6 times increased odds of suicide attempt.[70] Two reports from a high-risk cohort study have shown that witnessing IPV during childhood leads to more mental health symptoms and more clinical depression, anxiety, and anger.[71,72]

Legal Ramifications

IPV is increasingly important to child welfare agencies because of the direct effects of harm to children (physical and mental) and the risk it poses for CM. At least 40 states, 3 territories, and the District of Columbia include children as a class of protected persons in definitions of IPV. In many states, an act of IPV in the presence of a child confers a harsher penalty. Some states require the reporting of IPV to child welfare agencies under some circumstances.[73]

Practicing primary care providers should understand that IPV is common, it can be harmful to a child's mental and physical health, and it has pervasive psychologic consequences that may be lifelong. It also is related closely to the risk for all forms of CM. Clinicians should understand the IPV reporting laws in their state as issued by child welfare agencies. They also should consider IPV in the differential diagnosis for children's behavioral problems as a cause or contributing factor and understand methods for eliciting a history of IPV from caregiverd. Ultimately, primary care providers may leverage their relationship with a whole family to advocate for adult and child victims of IPV.

SUMMARY

IPV is a common problem, affecting large numbers of women, men, and children who present to primary care practices. It takes on many forms, including psychologic/emotional, physical, and sexual abuse, and its effects on the health of victims and their children are varied. Although many primary care physicians may be uncomfortable inquiring about IPV, a knowledge of patients' IPV victimization may help physicians develop a better understanding of patients' presenting symptoms and health risks, form more effective therapeutic relationships, and work toward reducing the myriad health risks associated with IPV.

REFERENCES

1. Centers for Disease Control and Prevention: National Center for Injury Prevention and Control. Intimate partner violence prevention scientific information: definitions. Available at: http://www.cdc.gov/ncipc/dvp/IPV/ipv-definitions.htm. Accessed July 3, 2008.
2. Tjaden P, Thoennes N. Full report of the prevalence, incidence, and consequences of violence against women: findings from the national violence against women survey. Washington, DC: US Department of Justice; 2000.
3. McCloskey LA, Lichter E, Ganz ML, et al. Intimate partner violence and patient screening across medical specialties. Acad Emerg Med 2005;12(8):712–22.
4. Lehrer JA, Buka S, Gortmaker S, et al. Depressive symptomatology as a predictor of exposure to intimate partner violence among US female adolescents and young adults. Arch Pediatr Adolesc Med 2006;160(3):270–6.
5. Bowen E, Heron J, Waylen A, et al. Domestic violence risk during and after pregnancy: findings from a British longitudinal study. BJOG 2005;112(8):1083–9.
6. Zolotor AJ, Runyan DK. Social capital, family violence, and neglect. Pediatrics 2006;117(6):e1124–31.
7. Straus MA, Gelles RJ. Physical violence in American families: risk factors and adaptations to violence in 8,145 families. New Brunswick (NJ): Transaction; 1990.
8. US Department of Justice. Crime victimization in the United States, 2005 Statistical tables 2007. Washington, DC: US Department of Justice; 2007.
9. Karch DL, Lubell KM, Friday J, et al. Surveillance for violent deaths—National Violent Death Reporting System, 16 states, 2005. MMWR Surveill Summ 2008; 57(3):1–45.
10. Campbell JC, Webster D, Koziol-McLain J, et al. Risk factors for femicide in abusive relationships: results from a multisite case control study. Am J Public Health 2003;93(7):1089–97.
11. Thompson RS, Bonomi AE, Anderson M, et al. Intimate partner violence: prevalence, types, and chronicity in adult women. Am J Prev Med 2006;30(6):447–57.
12. Dubowitz H, Prescott L, Feigelman S, et al. Screening for intimate partner violence in a pediatric primary care clinic. Pediatrics 2008;121(1):e85–91.
13. Ellsberg M, Jansen HA, Heise L, et al. Intimate partner violence and women's physical and mental health in the WHO multi-country study on women's health and domestic violence: an observational study. Lancet 2008;371(9619):1165–72.
14. Bonomi AE, Anderson ML, Rivara FP, et al. Health outcomes in women with physical and sexual intimate partner violence exposure. J Womens Health (Larchmt) 2007;16(7):987–97.

15. Coker AL, Davis KE, Arias I, et al. Physical and mental health effects of intimate partner violence for men and women. Am J Prev Med 2002;23(4):260–8.

16. Bonomi AE, Thompson RS, Anderson M, et al. Intimate partner violence and women's physical, mental, and social functioning. Am J Prev Med 2006;30(6):458–66.

17. Centers for Disease Control and Prevention. Adverse health conditions and health risk behaviors associated with intimate partner violence—United States, 2005. MMWR Morb Mortal Wkly Rep 2008;57(5):113–7.

18. Allen T, Novak SA, Bench LL. Patterns of injuries: accident or abuse. Violence Against Women 2007;13(8):802–16.

19. Bhandari M, Dosanjh S, Tornetta P III, et al. Musculoskeletal manifestations of physical abuse after intimate partner violence. J Trauma 2006;61(6):1473–9.

20. Plichta SB. Intimate partner violence and physical health consequences: policy and practice implications. J Interpers Violence 2004;19(11):1296–323.

21. McFarlane J, Malecha A, Watson K, et al. Intimate partner sexual assault against women: frequency, health consequences, and treatment outcomes. Obstet Gynecol 2005;105(1):99–108.

22. Eberhard-Gran M, Schei B, Eskild A. Somatic symptoms and diseases are more common in women exposed to violence. J Gen Intern Med 2007; 22(12):1668–73.

23. Leserman J, Drossman DA. Relationship of abuse history to functional gastrointestinal disorders and symptoms: some possible mediating mechanisms. Trauma Violence Abuse 2007;8(3):331–43.

24. Dutton MA, Green BL, Kaltman SI, et al. Intimate partner violence, PTSD, and adverse health outcomes. J Interpers Violence 2006;21(7):955–68.

25. Woods SJ. Intimate partner violence and post-traumatic stress disorder symptoms in women: what we know and need to know. J Interpers Violence 2005; 20(4):394–402.

26. Taft CT, Vogt DS, Mechanic MB, et al. Posttraumatic stress disorder and physical health symptoms among women seeking help for relationship aggression. J Fam Psychol 2007;21(3):354–62.

27. Silverman JG, Decker MR, Reed E, et al. Intimate partner violence victimization prior to and during pregnancy among women residing in 26 U.S. states: associations with maternal and neonatal health. Am J Obstet Gynecol 2006;195(1):140–8.

28. Murphy CC, Schei B, Myhr TL, et al. Abuse: a risk factor for low birth weight? A systematic review and meta-analysis. CMAJ 2001;164(11):1567–72.

29. Rosen D, Seng JS, Tolman RM, et al. Intimate partner violence, depression, and posttraumatic stress disorder as additional predictors of low birth weight infants among low-income mothers. J Interpers Violence 2007;22(10):1305–14.

30. McFarlane J. Intimate partner violence and physical health consequences: commentary on Plichta. J Interpers Violence 2004;19(11):1335–41.

31. Sharps PW, Laughon K, Giangrande SK. Intimate partner violence and the childbearing year: maternal and infant health consequences. Trauma Violence Abuse 2007;8(2):105–16.

32. Coker AL, Sanderson M, Dong B. Partner violence during pregnancy and risk of adverse pregnancy outcomes. Paediatr Perinat Epidemiol 2004;18(4):260–9.

33. Coker AL, Smith PH, Fadden MK. Intimate partner violence and disabilities among women attending family practice clinics. J Womens Health (Larchmt) 2005;14(9):829–38.

34. McCloskey LA, Williams CM, Lichter E, et al. Abused women disclose partner interference with health care: an unrecognized form of battering. J Gen Intern Med 2007;22(8):1067–72.

35. Basile KC, Hertz MF, Back SE. Intimate partner violence and sexual violence victimization assessment instruments for use in health care settings: version1. Atlanta (GA): Centers for Disease Control and Prevention, National Center for Injury Control and Prevention; 2007.

36. Rhodes KV, Lauderdale DS, He T, et al. Between me and the computer: increased detection of intimate partner violence using a computer questionnaire. Ann Emerg Med 2002;40(5):476–84.

37. Rodriguez MA, Bauer HM, McLoughlin E, et al. Screening and intervention for intimate partner abuse: practices and attitudes of primary care physicians. JAMA 1999;282(5):468–74.

38. Jaffee KD, Epling JW, Grant W, et al. Physician-identified barriers to intimate partner violence screening. J Womens Health (Larchmt) 2005;14(8):713–20.

39. US Preventive Services Task Force. Screening for family and intimate partner violence: recommendation statement. Ann Intern Med 2004;140(5):382–6.

40. Lachs MS. Screening for family violence: what's an evidence-based doctor to do? Ann Intern Med 2004;140(5):399–400.

41. Marks JS, Cassidy EF. Does a failure to count mean that it fails to count? Addressing intimate partner violence. Am J Prev Med 2006;30(6):530–1.

42. Janssen P, Dascal-Weichhendler H, McGregor M. Assessment for intimate partner violence: where do we stand? J Am Board Fam Med 2006;19(4):413–5.

43. Feder GS, Hutson M, Ramsay J, et al. Women exposed to intimate partner violence: expectations and experiences when they encounter health care professionals: a meta-analysis of qualitative studies. Arch Intern Med 2006;166(1):22–37.

44. McCord-Duncan EC, Floyd M, Kemp EC, et al. Detecting potential intimate partner violence: which approach do women want? Fam Med 2006;38(6):416–22.

45. Zeitler MS, Paine AD, Breitbart V, et al. Attitudes about intimate partner violence screening among an ethnically diverse sample of young women. J Adolesc Health 2006;39(1):119 e111–18.

46. Nicolaidis C. Partner interference with health care: do we want one more piece of a complex puzzle? J Gen Intern Med 2007;22(8):1216–7.

47. Golding JM. Intimate partner violence as a risk factor for mental disorders: a meta-analysis. J Fam Violence 1999;14(2):99–132.

48. Coker AL, Smith PH, McKeown RE, et al. Frequency and correlates of intimate partner violence by type: physical, sexual, and psychological battering. Am J Public Health 2000;90(4):553–9.

49. McCauley J, Kern DE, Kolodner K, et al. The "battering syndrome": prevalence and clinical characteristics of domestic violence in primary care internal medicine practices. Ann Intern Med 1995;123(10):737–46.

50. Roberts GL, Lawrence JM, Williams GM, et al. The impact of domestic violence on women's mental health. Aust N Z J Public Health 1998;22(7):796–801.

51. Petersen R, Gazmararian J, Andersen Clark K. Partner violence: implications for health and community settings. Womens Health Issues 2001;11(2):116–25.

52. Thompson MP, Kaslow NJ, Kingree JB, et al. Partner abuse and posttraumatic stress disorder as risk factors for suicide attempts in a sample of low-income, inner-city women. J Trauma Stress 1999;12(1):59–72.

53. Brokaw J, Fullerton-Gleason L, Olson L, et al. Health status and intimate partner violence: a cross-sectional study. Ann Emerg Med 2002;39(1):31–8.

54. US House of Representatives. Violence Against Women Act. Available at: www.now.org/issues/violence/vawa/vawa1998.html. Accessed July 3, 2008.

55. Weisz A. Assessing the risk of severe domestic violence: the importance of survivor's predictions. J Interpers Violence 2000;15:75–90.

56. Campbell JC, Koziol-McLain J, Webster D, et al. Research results from a national study of intimate partner femicide: the danger assessment instrument. Washington, DC: National Institute of Justice; 2002.

57. Edleson JL. The overlap between child maltreatment and woman battering. Violence Against Women 1999;5:134–54.

58. English DJ, Edleson JL, Herrick ME. Domestic violence in one state's child protective caseload: a study of differential case dispositions and outcomes. Child Youth Serv Rev 2005;27:1183–201.

59. Hazen AL, Connelly CD, Kelleher K, et al. Intimate partner violence among female caregivers of children reported for child maltreatment. Child Abuse Negl 2004; 28(3):301–19.

60. Appel AE, Holden GW. The co-occurrence of spouse and physical child abuse: a review and appraisal. J Fam Psychol 1998;12:578–99.

61. Lee LC, Kotch JB, Cox CE. Child maltreatment in families experiencing domestic violence. Violence Vict 2004;19(5):573–91.

62. Zolotor AJ, Theodore AD, Coyne-Beasley T, et al. Intimate partner violence and child maltreatment: overlapping risk. Brief Treat Crisis Interv 2007;7(4):305–21.

63. Tajima EA. The relative importance of wife abuse as a risk factor for violence against children. Child Abuse Negl 2000;24(11):1383–98.

64. Rumm PD, Cummings P, Krauss MR, et al. Identified spouse abuse as a risk factor for child abuse. Child Abuse Negl 2000;24(11):1375–81.

65. McGuigan WM, Pratt CC. The predictive impact of domestic violence on three types of child maltreatment. Child Abuse Negl 2001;25(7):869–83.

66. Christian CW, Scribano P, Seidl T, et al. Pediatric injury resulting from family violence. Pediatrics 1997;99(2):E8.

67. Duffy SJ, McGrath ME, Becker BM, et al. Mothers with histories of domestic violence in a pediatric emergency department. Pediatrics 1999;103(5 Pt 1):1007–13.

68. Casanueva C, Foushee V, Barth R. Intimate partner violence as a risk for children's use of the emergency room and injuries. Child Youth Serv Rev 2005; 27(11):1223–42.

69. Thompson R, Briggs E, English DJ, et al. Suicidal ideation among 8-year-olds who are maltreated and at risk: findings from the LONGSCAN studies. Child Maltreat 2005;10(1):26–36.

70. Dube SR, Anda RF, Felitti VJ, et al. Childhood abuse, household dysfunction, and the risk of attempted suicide throughout the life span: findings from the Adverse Childhood Experiences Study. JAMA 2001;286(24):3089–96.

71. Dubowitz H, Black MM, Kerr MA, et al. Type and timing of mothers' victimization: effects on mothers and children. Pediatrics 2001;107(4):728–35.

72. Johnson RM, Kotch JB, Catellier DJ, et al. Adverse behavioral and emotional outcomes from child abuse and witnessed violence. Child Maltreat 2002;7(3):179–86.

73. National Clearinghouse on Child Abuse and Neglect Information. Children and domestic violence. Washington, DC: US Department of Health and Human Services; 2004.

Diagnosis and Management of Osteoporosis

Robert W. Lash, MD[a],*, Jane M. Nicholson, MD[b], Lourdes Velez, MD[c],
R. Van Harrison, PhD[d], Jane McCort, MD[e]

KEYWORDS

- Osteoporosis • Bisphosphonates
- Dual-energy x-ray absorptiometry • Osteopenia

Osteoporosis and osteoporotic fractures are significant public health issues that will only grow in importance as the United States population ages. Ten million Americans have osteoporosis and an additional 34 million have low bone mass. Fortunately, there are effective strategies for the prevention, diagnosis, and treatment of osteoporosis.

MAJOR RISK FACTORS

Gender, age, and race all are important risk factors for osteoporotic fractures. Of the 10 million people who have osteoporosis, 8 million are women. In the United States, approximately 56% of postmenopausal women have decreased bone mineral density (BMD) (measured at the hip), and 16% have osteoporosis. In women over 80, the prevalence of osteoporosis is 44%, 10 times higher than women in their 50s.[1] The lifetime probability of a hip fracture for a white woman is 14%; the risk for a white man or a black person of either gender is approximately one third to one half of that figure, estimated at 5% to 7%.[2]

This article is based in part on the following clinical guideline and its update in progress at the time this article was written: McCourt JT, Harrison RV, Smith YR, et al. Osteoporosis—prevention and treatment. Ann Arbor (MI): University of Michigan Health System; 2005.

[a] Division of Metabolism, Endocrinology and Diabetes, Department of Internal Medicine, University of Michigan Medical School, 3920 Taubman Center – Box 0354, Ann Arbor, MI 48109-0354, USA

[b] Department of Obstetrics and Gynecology, University of Michigan Medical School, Ann Arbor, MI, USA

[c] Department of Family Medicine, University of Michigan Medical School, Ann Arbor, MI, USA

[d] Department of Medical Education, University of Michigan Medical School, Ann Arbor, MI, USA

[e] Division of General Medicine, University of Michigan Medical School, Ann Arbor, MI, USA

* Corresponding author.

E-mail address: rwlash@umich.edu (R.W. Lash).

Prim Care Clin Office Pract 36 (2009) 181–198
doi:10.1016/j.pop.2008.10.009
0095-4543/08/$ – see front matter © 2009 Elsevier Inc. All rights reserved.

In addition to age, gender, and race, certain medications (in particular gluco-corticoids) and various medical conditions (eg, renal failure, hypogonadism, and alco-holism) are important secondary causes of osteoporosis. Among women who have osteoporosis, between 30% and 60% have a secondary cause.[2] Solid organ trans-plant is another major risk factor for osteoporotic fractures. Younger women (ages 25 to 44) who have kidney transplants have an 18-fold increase in fractures, with the risk increasing to 34-fold among older transplant recipients.[3]

MORBIDITY, MORTALITY, AND COST

In its 2004 report, the Surgeon General's office estimated that there are 1.5 million os-teoporotic fractures yearly, resulting in 300,000 hospitalizations for just hip fractures and 180,000 resultant nursing home placements.[4] An osteoporotic hip fracture results in 10% to 20% excess mortality over 1 year; 20% of patients who have hip fractures require long-term nursing care.[5,6] Osteoporotic fractures also may result in chronic pain, disability, deformity, or depression. Direct medical costs for the treatment of os-teoporotic fractures are at least $15 billion annually (in 2002 dollars).

DEFINITIONS

Osteoporosis is a systemic skeletal disorder characterized by low bone mass and mi-croarchitectural deterioration of bone tissue predisposing to an increased risk for frac-ture. Although there currently are no practical methods to assess overall bone strength, BMD correlates closely with skeletal load-bearing capacity and fracture risk. The World Health Organization (WHO), therefore, developed definitions based on BMD measurements (**Table 1**). The T score is the number of the SDs from the mean BMD in young adult women. Osteoporosis is defined as T score at any site of less than −2.5 or lower whereas osteopenia is defined as a T score between −1 and −2.5. BMD in the osteoporotic range is a good predictor of increased fracture risk. In contrast, a finding of osteopenia is less helpful as it covers a broad range of BMDs. In addition to T scores, many BMD reports include Z scores, which measure the number of SDs from the mean for women of the same age and cannot be used to make the diagnosis of osteoporosis.

Although there are no standardized diagnostic criteria for osteoporosis in men, most authorities use the WHO criteria of a T score less than −2.5 relative to normal young women. Although men have much higher baseline BMD than women, they seem to have a similar fracture risk for a given BMD.

ETIOLOGY AND NATURAL HISTORY

Bone remodeling is an ongoing, cyclic process of bone formation and resorption. Os-teoclasts first adhere to bone and remove it, followed by osteoblasts that secrete

Table 1 World Health Organization definitions	
Classification	DEXA T score[a]
Normal	≥ -1.0
Osteopenia	> -2.5 and < -1.0
Osteoporosis	≤ -2.5

[a] SD from young normal.

osteoid, resulting in bone formation. Bone loss can occur if there is an imbalance between these two processes. Antiresorptive medications, such as the bisphosphonates, interfere with osteoclast action and are the mainstay of osteoporosis therapy. Anabolic (bone building) therapy currently is limited to recombinant parathyroid hormone (PTH).

Bone has trabecular and cortical components. Trabecular bone predominates in vertebrae and the proximal femur, with cortical bone present in long bone shafts. Trabecular remodeling occurs at a rate of approximately 25% per year whereas the cortical rate is approximately 3% per year. Thus, changes in BMD occur more quickly and have greater clinical implications in trabecular bone. This, in part, explains the prevalence of vertebral and femoral fractures in patients who have osteoporosis.

Bone density in later life depends on the peak bone mass achieved in youth and on the subsequent rate of bone loss. Skeletal mass is maximal in the third decade of life and depends primarily on diet (especially calcium and vitamin D), physical activity, and genetic predisposition.[7,8] During the first few years after menopause, women may have a rapid loss of bone, as much as 5% per year in trabecular bone and 2% to 3% per year in cortical bone. This early postmenopausal loss primarily is the result of increased osteoclast activity and places women at a greater risk than men for osteoporotic fracture. Later, a decline in osteoblast activity predominates and the rate of loss slows to 1% to 2% or less per year.

ASSESSING RISK

BMD, by itself, is an excellent predictor of fracture risk, at least as good as serum cholesterol as a predictor of heart disease and blood pressure as a predictor of stroke.[5] Clinical risk factors also play an important role, however, in the assessment of patients at risk for osteoporotic fractures. Several models have been proposed to stratify osteoporotic risk. One well-regarded model, the FRAX model, is based on WHO data on fracture risk and is available online.[9] **Table 2** and **Box 1** list risk factors and medications associated with osteoporosis and osteoporotic fractures. Patients at highest risk include those who have prior osteoporotic fractures, long-term glucocorticoid use, and solid organ failure or transplant. In addition to these risk factors, the role of falls as a cause of osteoporotic fractures also should be considered when assessing overall fracture risk. **Box 2** lists a variety of factors contributing to increased fall risk. Assessment of these risk factors for low bone density, fractures, and falls are helpful in identifying patients who might benefit from further evaluation, including quantitative measurement of BMD.

RISK FACTORS FOR OSTEOPOROSIS AND OSTEOPOROTIC FRACTURES
White Women

In community-dwelling white women aged 65 and older, osteoporotic fracture is correlated significantly with increasing age, previous fracture of any type after age 50, maternal history of hip fracture, long-acting benzodiazepine or anticonvulsant drug use, previous hyperthyroidism, excessive caffeine intake, standing 4 or fewer hours per day, difficulty rising from a chair, poor vision, and resting tachycardia.

Black Women

Risk factors for hip fracture in black women aged 45 and older include lowest quintile in body mass index (BMI), use of aids in walking, and history of stroke.

Table 2
Clinical risk categories for osteoporosis and osteoporotic fractures (for use with Box 1)

Extremely high risk	High risk
Prior osteoporotic fracture[a] (fracture without significant trauma) Glucocorticosteroid use[b] (prednisone ≥7.5 mg/d or equivalent for ≥6 months) Solid organ transplant[c] (pre or post, especially within first 2-3 y)	Glucocorticosteroid use[b] (prednisone ≥ 5 mg/day or equivalent, for ≥ 3 months) Woman older than 65 or men older than 70 Postemenopausal women or older men with at least one of the following • Personal history of low impact fracture • Family history of fracture hip, wrist, or spine (first-degree relative age ≥ 50 y) • Currently smoking • BMI < 20 • Recent weight loss >10% • Multiple risk factors for falling, (see **Box 2**)

<table>
<tr><td colspan="2" align="center">Moderate risk</td></tr>
<tr>
<td>Hormonal conditions
• Hypogonadism
• Late menarche (age > 15 y)
• Early menopause (age < 45 y)
• Premenopauseal amenorrhea, (eg, anorexia nervosa, exercise, or hyperprolactinemia but not polycystic ovary syndrome or pregnancy)
• Cushing's syndrome
• Hyperparathyroidism (primary or secondary)
• Thyrotoxicosis
Gastrointestinal and nutritional factors
• Gastrectomy
• Low gastric acid (eg, atrophic gastritis, proton pump inhibitors, H$_2$-blockers)
• Impaired absorption
  Celiac disease
  Bariatric surgery
  Inflammatory bowel disease (Crohn's disease more than ulcerative colitis)
  Pancreatic insufficiency
• Heavy alcohol use</td>
<td>Medications (see **Box 1**)
Family history of osteoporosis
Other significant associations
• Severe liver disease
• Chronic kidney disease
• Type 1 diabetes mellitus
• Multiple myeloma
• Rheumatoid arthritis
• Hemochromatosis
• Long-term immobilization
• Prior smoking
Other possible associations
• Addison's disease
• Amyloidosis
• Thalassemia (major > minor)
• Multiple sclerosis
• Nephrolithiasis
• Sarcoidosis
• Depression</td>
</tr>
</table>

[a] Prior fracture is more predictive of future fracture than is BMD.
[b] Glucocorticoids produce the greatest bone loss in the initial 6–12 months of use, average 4%–5%.
[c] Bone loss can be as much as 10% in the first year after transplant.

Falls

Among the elderly, one third of community-dwelling and one half of nursing home residents fall each year. Among such falls, 2% result in hip fracture and up to 5% result in other fractures. Low femoral BMD and low BMI are major risk factors for fall-related injury. Major injuries are more likely in a fall from an upright position or a fall laterally with direct impact to the hip.

Glucocorticoids

The etiology of glucocorticoid-induced osteoporosis and associated fractures is not fully understood but is multifactorial and different from postmenopausal osteoporosis.

Box 1
Medications with risk for bone loss or fracture

Definite risk

Immunosuppressants

- Glucocorticoids (systemic >> inhaled,[a] intranasal, topical, and others)
- Cyclosporin A (Gengraf or Neoral)
- Tacrolimus (Prograf)
- Mycophenolate (CellCept)

Hormonal and antihormonal agents

- Depot medroxyprogesterone acetate (Depo-Provera)[b]
- Tamoxifen, before menopause
- Aromatase inhibitors (anastrozole [Arimidex] or letrozole [Femara])
- GnRH therapy (leuprolide [Lupron] or goserelin [Zoladex])
- Pioglitazone (Actos) and rosiglitazone (Avandia)

Miscellaneous

- Anticonvulsants (phenytoin or phenobarbital > carbamazepine or valproic acid)[b]
- Heparins (unfractionated > low molecular weight)

Possible risk

Lithium

Selective serotonin reuptake inhibitors

Antipsychotics (may cause hyperprolactinemia)

Excessive supplemental fluoride

Proton pump inhibitors

Topiramate (may cause metabolic acidosis)

>, greater than; >>, much greater than.
[a] Inhaled beclomethasone (>1600 µg daily) is associated with risk for bone loss and fracture (inhaler dose range approximately 40–100 µg per spray).
[b] BMD loss related to depot medroxyprogesterone acetate seems to be reversible or nearly reversible. There are minimal data on reversibility of associated fracture risk.

Bone resorption is increased, possibly as a result of stimulation of osteoclast differentiation. Meanwhile, bone formation is reduced resulting from inhibition of osteoblasts. Calcium balance becomes negative, owing to a decrease in gastrointestinal absorption and an increase in urinary loss. Also, glucocorticoids inhibit production of sex steroid hormones, which adversely affects bone remodeling. Glucocorticoid-induced myopathy and inactivity caused by underlying illness may contribute to a decline in BMD by reduction in skeletal loading and to an increase in fracture risk related to greater fall risk.

Bone loss is most rapid during the first 6 to 12 months of commencement of glucocorticoid therapy. In early menopause, trabecular bone is affected more than cortical bone. In chronic glucocorticoid use, fracture risk is higher for a given BMD than in postmenopausal osteoporosis, suggesting that there are glucocorticoid-induced qualitative bone defects. Bone loss associated with glucocorticoid therapy occurs

| Box 2 |
Risk factors for falling
Decreased leg or arm muscle strength
Diminished vision
Environmental hazards for falls
Frailty, unable to rise from chair unassisted
History of falls
Impaired cognition
Impaired gait, balance, or transfer skills
Impaired range of motion
Increasing age
Low physical function
Postural hypotension
Use of any psychotropic medication

in a dose-dependent manner, increasing with greater duration of use or magnitude of dose. The threshold for significant risk seems to be oral prednisone (7.5 mg or more [or equivalent]) for 6 months or longer. Lower doses over extended periods, however, including prolonged use of higher-dose inhaled steroids also may lead to bone loss. Other risk factors for glucocorticoid-induced osteoporosis and associated fractures include decreased BMD before glucocorticoid therapy, the underlying disease resulting in glucocorticoid use, postmenopausal state, older age, and previous fracture.

Organ Failure and Transplantation

Patients who have organ failure, in particular liver and kidney, are at a significant risk for osteoporosis and fracture. The risk is increased further after transplantation, where bone loss in the first year is reported to be as high as 10%. This phenomenon most likely is the result of greater steroid use, although other medications, such as cyclosporin A and tacrolimus, may be factors.

DIAGNOSTIC TESTING

Dual-energy x-ray absorptiometry (DEXA) currently is the test of choice for measuring BMD. The technique compares penetration of two different x-ray sources through soft tissue and bone, then subtracts soft tissue, leaving an estimate of skeletal BMD. A study typically takes less than 10 minutes, and radiation exposure is approximately at 3–4 mrem/site. By comparison, background radiation is approximately 300 mrem per year. Although various skeletal sites can be assessed by DEXA, BMD of the non-dominant hip is the best predictor of hip fracture and is an excellent predictor of vertebral or wrist fracture. There is accelerated loss of vertebral bone early in menopause and early in glucocorticoid use; thus, spine BMD measurements may be helpful particularly in these settings. BMD measurement by DEXA may be spuriously elevated by several factors. Vertebral compression fractures typically result in a smaller vertebral body with no change in the total amount of calcium but resulting in a false increase in BMD. Vertebral osteophytes, degenerative joint disease, and aortic calcifications can also falsely raise vertebral BMD measurements whereas hip measurements tend to have fewer artifacts.

Medicare and many other major insurers typically cover DEXA scans for patients at higher risk, including all women aged 65 or older and patients who have primary hyperparathyroidism, vertebral abnormalities, or chronic glucocorticoid use. Medicare at this time does not cover BMD testing for premenopausal women or for postmenopausal women under 65 receiving estrogen. Follow-up studies are covered, usually at 2-year intervals, although more frequently when indicated (eg, chronic glucocorticoid use). Medicare covers a follow-up BMD test every 2 years (>23 months since last BMD test) to monitor response in those patients undergoing Food and Drug Administration (FDA)-approved treatment of osteoporosis. The decision to obtain a screening DEXA study should be made on the basis of a patient's overall risk of osteoporosis or osteoporotic fractures. **Table 3** lists recommendations for screening and follow-up DEXA studies based on the presence of the clinical risk factors outlined in **Table 2**.

Follow-Up Dual-Energy X-ray Absorptiometry Studies

When deciding if and when to repeat a DEXA scan, the following factors should be considered:

- The patient's clinical risk factors for progression of bone loss and for fracture
- Results from prior DEXA scans
- Whether or not a repeat study will change management or potentially improve compliance with therapy

Table 3 lists recommendations for repeat DEXA studies based on individual patient risk factors, previous DEXA result, and current treatment. More frequent follow-up is indicated early in glucocorticoid use and after transplantation if patients are not on antiosteoporotic therapy. In these settings, a DEXA study at intervals of 6 to 12 months is appropriate. At the other end of the clinical spectrum, an argument can be made to forego follow-up DEXA studies in patients on bisphosphonates who have mild osteoporosis and no evidence of fractures.

When possible, serial measurements should be performed on the same equipment or on a machine by the same manufacturer. The precision error of DEXA on the same machine, that is, the reproducibility of a reading on repeat measurement, is approximately 1%. The 95% CI on any measured change, therefore, is approximately 2.8%. Thus, for a woman who has a 2.0% decrease in BMD, the 95% CI is −4.8 to +0.8%. BMD loss with aging is approximately 1% per year. The mean annual increase in lumbar BMD during the early years of treatment with bisphosphonates typically is approximately 3% (range 0 to 10%). A change of 10% in BMD corresponds to a change of 1.0 in the T score.

Because of these issues regarding the precision and reproducibility of DEXA scans, a minimum 2-year interval between scans provides more meaningful information on bone loss than yearly determinations of BMD. This interval is supported by an analysis of women who lost BMD during the first year of treatment with alendronate or raloxifene; these women were likely to gain BMD with continued treatment.[10] For example, women who took alendronate and lost more than 4% in hip BMD during the first year had an 83% chance of an increase in hip BMD during the second year. A similar phenomenon was seen even in those who received placebo.

Other Diagnostic and Monitoring Modalities

Quantitative calcaneal ultrasound devices are portable and inexpensive. Because of these advantages, they often are used in informal osteoporosis screening programs,

Table 3
Screening and management based on clinical risk for osteoporosis and osteoporotic fractures

Clinical Risk (From Table 2)	Order First DEXA?[a]	Reassess Risk	Repeat DEXA?[a]	Management Based on DEXA[b]		
				T-score < −2	T-score −2 to −1	T-score > −1
Extremely high	Yes	1 y	Consider in 1 y	Treat	Treat	Consider preventive therapy[c]
High	Yes	1 y	If prior T > −1, wait at least 3–5 y	Treat	Consider preventive therapy[c]	Lifestyle[d]
Moderate	Consider	1–2 y	If prior T ≤ −1, wait at least 2 y	Treat	Lifestyle[d]	Lifestyle[d]
All others	No	1–2 y				

[a] Order DEXA only if results will affect patient management: not already receiving full therapy; possible candidate for teraparatide; fractures occurring despite treatment; considering discontinuation of therapy; and so forth.

[b] Lowest T score from femoral neck, total hip, or any combination of lumbar vertebra.

[c] If patient has had fracture without significant trauma, consider other causes of bone abnormality (eg, malignancy).

[d] Lifestyle: ensure adequate intake of calcium and vitamin D and weight-bearing exercise.

such as health fairs. A meta-analysis, however, suggests limited value of ultrasound screening. For example, a positive study in an otherwise healthy 65-year-old woman raises the likelihood of DEXA-confirmed osteoporosis from a population-based pre-test estimate of 22% to only 34%. Conversely, a negative study reduces the likelihood of osteoporosis from 22% to 10%.[11] T scores provided by ultrasound are not equiv-alent to DEXA T scores and, therefore, should not be used for diagnostic purposes. Rather, patients who have abnormally low ultrasound T scores should be evaluated by DEXA for more definitive diagnosis.

Biochemical markers of bone resorption are used in research settings and to assess the effectiveness of antiresorptive therapy. In the latter situation, a decrease in these markers to premenopausal levels usually occurs after 2 to 3 months of therapy. There also are data suggesting that elevated levels of bone resorption makers in older women are an independent risk factor for fractures.[12] Bone markers are not a reliable predictor of BMD, however, and are not a substitute for DEXA in women at risk. Gen-erally, their use in the diagnosis of osteoporosis is not recommended.

PREVENTION OF OSTEOPOROSIS
General Prevention

All patients should be encouraged to eat a balanced diet that includes adequate cal-cium and vitamin D (using supplements when necessary), engage in regular physical activity, avoid heavy alcohol consumption, and refrain from smoking. Specific recom-mendations for calcium and vitamin D intake are discussed later.

Glucocorticoid-Induced Osteoporosis Prevention

Various guidelines for osteoporosis prevention differ in specifics but agree on the fol-lowing principles: patients should be on the lowest effective daily dose of glucocorti-coid for the shortest period of time and, when possible, patients should use inhaled or topical steroids rather than oral preparations, although high-dose inhaled steroids also are shown to cause bone loss.

All patients taking glucocorticoids should be considered candidates for preventive therapy, regardless of dose or duration. Patients who have no history of bone loss and who are on lower doses for shorter durations (eg, prednisone less than 5 mg daily for fewer than 3 months) should be given calcium and vitamin D supplementation. Pa-tients who have pre-existing bone loss should be considered for bisphosphonate ther-apy. Patients on higher doses of glucocorticoids (prednisone more than 7.5 mg daily for longer than 6 months) also should receive bisphosphonates, as they have been shown to prevent glucocorticoid-related bone loss at the lumbar spine and femoral neck and to reduce the risk for vertebral fractures.[13]

EVALUATION OF SECONDARY CAUSES

Although most cases of osteoporosis are postmenopausal or idiopathic, there are sev-eral secondary causes (see **Table 2**). Many of these are treatable (eg, hypogonadism, hyperparathyroidism, and malabsorption) or important to diagnose (eg, renal failure and multiple myeloma). Therefore, a focused evaluation for secondary causes usually is indicated (**Box 3**).

Vitamin D deficiency (defined as <30 ng/mL) increasingly is recognized as contrib-uting to bone loss. More than 50% of postmenopausal women treated for osteoporo-sis are vitamin D deficient.[14] Vitamin D deficiency is not limited, however, to patients who have osteoporosis. Nearly 50% of young women probably are vitamin D deficient particularly at the end of winter.[15] A study of Boston health professionals

---

Box 3
Evaluation for secondary causes of osteoporosis and osteopenia

All patients

Consider measuring serum calcium, alkaline phosphatase, renal function, liver function, and thyrotropin

Premenopausal amenorrhea not the result of pregnancy or polycystic ovary syndrome

Estradiol and follicle-stimulating hormone

Based on clinical situation

Urinary calcium

25-hydroxyvitamin D

Intact PTH with calcium (evaluation for primary or secondary hyperparathyroidism)

24-h urine-free cortisol or 1-mg dexamethasone suppression

Evaluate for occult malignancy, such as multiple myeloma, bony metastases, and so forth

Men

Consider measuring serum testosterone

---

demonstrated that 32% were vitamin D deficient.[16] Based on these findings, assessment of vitamin D levels, empiric vitamin D supplementation (discussed later), or both should be considered in patients who have osteoporosis.

Secondary hyperparathyroidism (normal or low calcium with elevated PTH) should be considered in patients who have renal insufficiency or when inadequate intake or absorption of calcium or vitamin D is suspected. Calcium hyperexcretion may lead to negative calcium balance and often can be treated with thiazide diuretics. Subclinical hypercortisolism is not traditionally believed a risk factor for bone loss, but a recent prospective study suggests it may be more common than previously suspected.[17,18] Thiazolidinediones also are implicated in increased fracture risk.[19–21]

WHOM TO TREAT

When deciding which patients who have decreased BMD should be treated, providers should consider patients' future risk for bone loss and fracture and BMD. For example, patients who have T scores between −1.0 and −2.0 and who have additional risk factors, such as glucocorticoid use or significant liver disease, should be considered for treatment. **Table 3** provides guidelines for patient management depending on BMD and clinical risk factors. Patients who already have had an osteoporotic fracture may be treated on that basis alone, although a DEXA scan may be useful for other reasons, such as excluding a pathologic fracture resulting from metastatic disease.

NONPHARMACOLOGIC THERAPY
Exercise

Observational data and clinical trials indicate that weight-bearing activities, such as aerobics, walking, and resistance training, all are effective at increasing spine BMD.[22,23] The studies are of limited quality (primarily because of difficulty of blinding patients), however, and exercise does not seem to reduce the risk for osteoporotic fractures.

Fall Prevention

Prevention of falls requires attention to the many risk factors (see **Box 2**), including medications, gait, vision, and environmental hazards (eg, poor lighting, area rugs, and lack of handrails in bathrooms). In addition to addressing possible medical causes of falls, providers should consider the potential value of an occupational therapy assessment to reduce fall risk.[24]

Hip Protectors

Hip protectors are anatomically designed plastic shields or pads worn in side pockets of special underwear. In spite of multiple randomized trials, the benefit of hip protectors remains unclear.[25–27] Hip protectors often are difficult to put on and uncomfortable to wear; therefore, compliance may play a role in reducing their potential effectiveness.

PHARMACOLOGIC THERAPY

In assessing the effectiveness of different pharmacologic therapies for osteoporosis, clinical (fractures) and radiologic (changes in BMD) endpoints have been used. Although clinical endpoints are preferable, they are not always practical. For example, the studies that demonstrated the effectiveness of bisphosphonates and estrogen over placebo in reducing hip fractures required more than 10,000 patients. Thus, many studies rely on changes in BMD as a surrogate marker. Although low BMD is an excellent predictor of fracture risk in postmenopausal women, increases in BMD show an inconsistent relationship to fracture.

Each of the available classes of antiresorptive agents (bisphosphonates, selective estrogen receptor modulators, estrogens, and calcitonin) and the only available anabolic agent (recombinant PTH) reduce vertebral fracture rates in postmenopausal women, independent of effects on BMD. Most of these medications also show reduced fracture risk at combined nonvertebral sites. Although this term includes hip fractures, it also includes other sites, such as ribs and wrist. Currently, the only medications with clinical data supporting reduction of hip fractures are alendronate, risedronate, zoledronic acid, and estrogen.[13]

Calcium

Adequate calcium intake is required to achieve maximal peak BMD in early and middle years and to maintain bone density in later life. Calcium supplementation alone, however, has not consistently shown reduction in fracture risk in postmenopausal or glucocorticoid-induced osteoporosis. Commonly used supplements include calcium carbonate and calcium citrate. Calcium carbonate is absorbed best in an acidic environment and, therefore, should be taken with food. It also may be less effective in persons using stomach acid-reducing medications, such as H_2-receptor blockers or proton pump inhibitors, although the clinical significance of this observation is unclear. Calcium citrate generally is more expensive than calcium carbonate but does not require an acidic gastric pH for its absorption. The risk for nephrolithiasis does not increase in patients taking physiologic doses of calcium.[13,28]

Vitamin D

Vitamin D refers to a group of fat-soluble steroid hormones and prohormones that influence calcium by their effects on intestine, kidneys, and bones. Cholecalciferol (D3) is produced by skin exposed to UV light and is the form of vitamin D present in fish. D3 and ergocalciferol (D2) can be synthesized and are used in vitamin supplements and to fortify foods such as milk. D2 and D3 are converted to the active form of vitamin D, calcitriol, or 1,25-dihydroxyvitamin D, by hydroxylation first in the liver and then the kidney.

The recommended daily allowance for vitamin D is 400 to 800 IU, although most authorities recommend the higher dose for patients who have osteoporosis. This amount is produced by sun exposure to hands, arms, and face for 10 to 30 minutes a day, 2 to 3 times a week. Most multivitamins contain vitamin D, typically 400 IU. Many calcium supplements contain vitamin D, and most milk is vitamin D fortified. Vitamin D is fat soluble, thus toxicity can result from excess, probably at doses greater than 2000 IU per day.

The elderly, who may be outdoors less than those who are younger, and who have age-related reduction in the ability of skin to produce vitamin D, are at particular risk for vitamin D deficiency. Also at risk are those persons who reside at higher latitudes, where the amount of UV light exposure during the winter is inadequate for vitamin D synthesis.[15] Patients who have malabsorption, renal insufficiency, liver failure, or other causes of secondary hyperparathyroidism or osteomalacia may require pharmacologic forms of vitamin D and, therefore, may benefit from referral to an endocrinologist.

In spite of many studies and meta-analyses, the effects of calcium and vitamin D on fracture risk remain unclear.[13,15,29] Most studies that have shown vitamin D (along with calcium) effective in preventing fractures have used higher doses of vitamin D (800 IU daily as opposed to 400 IU), and have included patients who had lower baseline levels of vitamin D. The Women's Health Initiative (WHI) examined the effects of calcium and vitamin D supplementation on a lower risk population and found no fracture reduction in the intention-to-treat group. The women who were more compliant with their study medications, however, had a 29% reduction in hip fracture.[30] In spite of the lack of definitive data, calcium and vitamin D supplementation remain standard of care in the treatment of osteoporosis.

Bisphosphonates

Bisphosphonates are analogs of pyrophosphate, bind to hydroxyapatite crystals in bone, and inhibit bone resorption by their effects on osteoclasts. Among all treatments for osteoporosis, bisphosphonates have the largest data set for reduction of fracture risk, including postmenopausal women, men, and in the setting of glucocorticoid use. Bisphosphonates are available in oral (alendronate, risedronate, and ibandronate) and intravenous (zoledronic acid) forms. Although each of these medications has been shown to reduce fractures in placebo-controlled trials, comparative studies looking at fracture risk have not been done. A recent systematic review of therapy for osteoporosis concludes that each of the bisphosphonates reduces vertebral fractures, and alendronate, risedronate, and zoledronic acid reduce hip fractures.[13] Risedronate and alendronate also reduce vertebral fractures in patients on chronic glucocorticoid therapy. Peer-reviewed data for zoledronic acid in this setting are not yet available.

The optimal duration of bisphosphonate therapy for osteoporosis is not known. A study using 10-year data on alendronate therapy demonstrates its ongoing safety and effectiveness, although the study included only 164 alendronate-treated women.[31] The long half-life of the bisphosphonates suggests that their effects may persist after discontinuing therapy. To address this issue, the FLEX trial randomized women who had been on alendronate for 5 years to receive 5 additional years of alendronate or placebo.[32] Women in the placebo group lost some BMD but remained above their pre-alendronate baseline. There was no difference found in overall fractures or in vertebral fractures detected radiographically. The placebo group did have, however, a small increase in clinically detected vertebral fractures. This difference was largest in women who had lower baseline BMDs or prior vertebral fractures, suggesting that women who had milder osteoporosis might be able to discontinue bisphosphonates after 5 years of therapy, with appropriate monitoring of BMD.

The bisphosphonates are associated with adverse effects. Oral bisphosphonates trials have reported esophageal complications ranging from heartburn and acid reflux to esophageal ulceration and perforation. Although these more serious complications are rare, patients who have esophageal disorders may not be good candidates for oral bisphosphonates. Proper administration of oral bisphosphonates should be reviewed with patients. Zoledronic acid is associated with a small increase in atrial fibrillation.[33] The significance of this finding is difficult to interpret, as the overall rate of atrial fibrillation was equal in the treatment and placebo groups. The incidence of atrial fibrillation, however, believed "serious" was higher in the treatment group.[34] More recently, a large trial comparing the incidence of atrial fibrillation in patients on oral bisphosphonates with case controls showed no difference.[35]

Osteonecrosis of the jaw (ONJ) has emerged as a more serious complication of high dose bisphosphonate therapy. ONJ is defined as an area of exposed bone on the maxilla, mandible, or palate that does not heal within 8 weeks. Although a rare occurrence in the past, many cases have been reported since 2003, primarily in patients who received high doses of intravenous bisphosphonates in the setting of cancer treatment.[36] Data from patients taking oral bisphosphonates for osteoporosis have been more reassuring. Fewer than 50 cases have been reported among patients taking oral bisphosphonates, and no cases have been reported in clinical trials covering 60,000 patient years of therapy.[37] Based on these and other studies, the estimated risk for patients taking oral bisphosphonates of developing ONJ is estimated to be less than 1:100,000. The risk is less clear for zoledronic acid therapy for osteoporosis, although the risk again seems small. In the HORIZON trial, only two cases of ONJ were reported among more than 7500 women: one each in the placebo and treatment groups. Current recommendations suggest patients receive any necessary invasive dental work before beginning bisphosphonate therapy, in particular intravenous therapy. The safety of bisphosphonates for women in childbearing years and in pregnancy is not known.

Raloxifene

Raloxifene is a nonsteroidal selective estrogen receptor modulator. It binds to estrogen receptors and inhibits bone resorption without significantly stimulating the endometrium. The Multiple Outcomes of Raloxifene Evaluation trial, which included 7705 patients, demonstrated a vertebral fracture relative risk of 0.7 after 3 years of use by postmenopausal women with osteoporosis.[38] There was a nonsignificant trend for reduction in nonvertebral or hip fracture risk. Raloxifene use also was associated with a reduction in estrogen receptor-positive breast cancer incidence, but no increase in vaginal bleeding or breast pain was seen. The risk for venous thrombosis is approximately the same as with estrogen replacement. No data are reported for the use of raloxifene in glucocorticoid-induced osteoporosis. Raloxifene is not recommended for use in premenopausal women.

Estrogen

Estrogen acts directly on estrogen receptors in bone causing reduced bone turnover and bone loss. Estrogen typically is given as a single agent to women who do not have a uterus and with progestins to women who have not had hysterectomies. For many years, estrogen replacement therapy routinely was given to postmenopausal women. The publication of the WHI, in 2002, however, demonstrated that postmenopausal estrogen therapy had beneficial and deleterious effects.[39] One beneficial effect was a 34% reduction in hip fractures among the 8506 women receiving estrogen and progestin. This was a particularly interesting finding in that the women in the WHI, although postmenopausal, were not selected for participation based on decreased bone density. Further analysis demonstrated a 35% reduction in vertebral fractures, a 29% reduction in wrist fractures, and a 24% reduction in total fractures.[40] Given the size and design of the WHI, the overall bone health of its participants, and the reduction in fracture risk, a strong case can be made that estrogen has the best evidence supporting its role in fracture reduction in postmenopausal women.

Oral contraceptive pills may be used for osteoporosis prevention in premenopausal women who have hypoestrogenemic amenorrhea, especially those receiving glucocorticoids. Attention also must be given to dietary issues, however, including the possibility of an eating disorder. The relationship between bone health and polycystic ovarian syndrome is debated, but premenopausal women who have polycystic ovary syndrome generally are not hypoestrogenemic, thus probably not at increased risk for osteoporosis.

Preparations and formulations, identified as bioidentical hormones, do not have evidence to support a benefit in fracture reduction, or even safety, when compared with FDA-approved sources of estrogen. Considering that more than 16,000 patients were needed to show clinical differences between estrogen and placebo in the WHI, it is unlikely that studies comparing estrogen with any bioidentical formulation will be performed in the near future. Women who wish to use bioidentical hormones should be aware that they are using unproved therapy from the perspectives of safety and effectiveness.

Calcitonin

Calcitonin is a polypeptide hormone that inhibits osteoclast-mediated bone resorption. The Prevention of Recurrence of Osteoporotic Fractures (PROOF) study was of sufficient size (n = 1255) to demonstrate a reduction in vertebral fracture risk.[41] The dropout rate was surprisingly high, however. Calcitonin does not seem to reduce nonvertebral or hip fractures or fractures in patients on glucocorticoid therapy.[13] Calcitonin, in small studies, has been found to significantly reduce the pain of acute vertebral fractures.[42]

Parathyroid Hormone

Teriparatide, a recombinant protein containing the first 34 amino acids of human PTH, is the only available anabolic agent for the treatment of osteoporosis. Although PTH, when secreted continuously (as in primary hyperparathyroidism), stimulates osteoclast activity, intermittent administration has a stimulating effect on osteoblast activity, resulting in increased BMD.

Teriparatide, in a randomized trial with 1637 postmenopausal women, reduced vertebral fractures by 65% and nonvertebral fractures by 53%.[43] There was no reduction in hip fracture, but the total number of fractures was only nine. Teriparatide is given as a daily injection for 24 months, after which the beneficial effects on BMD tends to diminish. For this reason, a course of teriparatide frequently is followed by bisphosphonate therapy, as a way of consolidating gains. Combining PTH and alendronate may reduce the anabolic effects of the former.[44] Teriparatide has been associated with an increased incidence of osteosarcoma in rats given high doses over an extended period of time. Given this concern, it should not be used in patients who have a history of bony malignancy or in those at risk. Tariparatide use typically is reserved for patients who have severe osteoporosis and pre-existing fractures and may be considered in patients who have clinically failed bisphosphonate therapy or are unable to tolerate bisphosphonates.

Combination Therapy

Although combination therapy has theoretic appeal, studies have yet to demonstrate a clinical benefit in combining antiosteoporotic medications.[45] As discussed previously, combination therapy with PTH and alendronate seems to blunt the anabolic effects of PTH. Studies also have investigated the effects of combining bisphosphonate therapy with estrogen[46] and raloxifene.[47] Although combination therapy, in some studies, results in an incremental increase in BMD, consistent decreases in fractures have not been demonstrated. There is a theoretic risk of oversuppression of bone remodeling (frozen bone) with combination therapy, resulting in increased bone brittleness and fragility. This does not seem to have emerged as a clinical concern in long-term studies of bisphosphonate use.[31] No guidelines exist for the use of combination therapy; however, it may be worth considering for patients who have significant, ongoing bone loss in spite of compliance with calcium, vitamin D, and a single antiresorptive agent.

Denosumab

Denosumab is a human monoclonal antibody that binds to receptor activator for nuclear factor κB ligand (RANKL) on the surface of osteoblast precursors, preventing them from activating osteoclasts. Administration of denosumab twice yearly to postmenopausal women who have low BMD resulted in increases in BMD at spine and hip, similar to those seen with alendronate.[48] Fracture trials are now in progress. Denosumab is not yet approved for clinical use.

OSTEOPOROSIS IN MEN

Osteoporosis in men is under-recognized and undertreated.[49,50] One third of all hip fractures occur in men, and the 1-year mortality rate is twice that of women.[51] An American College of Physicians Systematic Review identifies the following as risk factors for osteoporotic fractures: age greater than 70, BMI less than 20 to 25 kg/m^2, weight loss in excess of 10%, physical inactivity, previous osteoporotic fracture, prolonged glucocorticoid use, and androgen-deprivation therapy. Cigarette smoking is risk factor for low BMD and probably fracture, whereas alcohol use is a risk factor for fracture, with less definitive effects on BMD.[50]

Men who have one or more of these risk factors probably should be screened for with osteoporosis by DEXA scan. Because hypogonadism and vitamin D deficiency are common in older men, measurement of both hormones is recommended. Treatment should include calcium and vitamin D supplementation with weight-bearing exercise as tolerated. Bisphosphonates have been shown to reduce vertebral fractures as measured by radiologic studies and are considered first-line therapy in men who have osteoporosis.[52] Tariparatide also has been shown to reduce vertebral fractures.[53] Testosterone has been shown to increase lumbar spine BMD but a reduction in fractures has not been shown.[53] Given the potential complications of testosterone therapy in older men, it should be reserved for patients who have clinically significant manifestations of hypogonadism.

SUMMARY

Osteoporosis is a common disorder resulting in significant morbidity and mortality. Clinical risk factors, including chronic glucocorticoid use and solid organ failure or transplant, can be used to identify those patients most likely to have osteoporosis, with confirmation of diagnosis made by DEXA scan. Patients who have decreased bone mass, including osteopenia, are candidates for calcium and vitamin D supplementation. Patients who have more severe bone loss should be screened for secondary causes and started on medical therapy. First-line therapy for most patients who have osteoporosis is a bisphosphonate, which has been shown to reduce fracture risk at the spine and hip. Estrogen has been shown to be effective at reducing hip fractures in women. Recombinant PTH generally is reserved for patients who have failed, or are not candidates for, bisphosphonate therapy. Follow-up DEXA studies should be reserved for patients in whom a change in BMD will make a difference in therapy.

REFERENCES

1. CDC. National Health and Nutrition Examination Survey: Osteoporosis. Available at: http://www.cdc.gov/nchs/data/nhanes/databriefs/osteoporosis.pdf. Accessed September 1, 2008.
2. NIH Consensus Development Panel on Osteoporosis Prevention, Diagnosis, and Therapy. Osteoporosis prevention, diagnosis, and therapy. JAMA 2001;285(6): 785–95.
3. Ramsey-Goldman R, Dunn JE, Dunlop DD, et al. Increased risk of fracture in patients receiving solid organ transplants. J Bone Miner Res 1999;14(3):456–63.
4. Services UDoHaH. Bone health and osteoporosis: a report of the surgeon general. Rockville (MD): Office of the Surgeon General; 2004.
5. Center JR, Nguyen TV, Schneider D, et al. Mortality after all major types of osteoporotic fracture in men and women: an observational study. Lancet 1999; 353(9156):878–82.
6. Salkeld G, Cameron ID, Cumming RG, et al. Quality of life related to fear of falling and hip fracture in older women: a time trade off study. BMJ 2000;320(7231): 341–6.
7. Gilsanz V, Gibbens DT, Carlson M, et al. Peak trabecular vertebral density: a comparison of adolescent and adult females. Calcif Tissue Int 1988;43(4):260–2.
8. Marshall D, Johnell O, Wedel H. Meta-analysis of how well measures of bone mineral density predict occurrence of osteoporotic fractures. BMJ 1996;312(7041): 1254–9.
9. FRAX. Available at: http://www.shef.ac.uk/FRAX. Accessed January 2, 2009.
10. Cummings SR, Palermo L, Browner W, et al. Monitoring osteoporosis therapy with bone densitometry: misleading changes and regression to the mean. Fracture Intervention Trial Research Group. JAMA 2000;283(10):1318–21.
11. Nayak S, Olkin I, Liu H, et al. Meta-analysis: accuracy of quantitative ultrasound for identifying patients with osteoporosis. Ann Intern Med 2006;144(11):832–41.
12. Garnero P, Sornay-Rendu E, Claustrat B, et al. Biochemical markers of bone turnover, endogenous hormones and the risk of fractures in postmenopausal women: the OFELY study. J Bone Miner Res 2000;15(8):1526–36.
13. MacLean C, Newberry S, Maglione M, et al. Systematic review: comparative effectiveness of treatments to prevent fractures in men and women with low bone density or osteoporosis. Ann Intern Med 2008;148(3):197–213.
14. Holick MF, Siris ES, Binkley N, et al. Prevalence of Vitamin D inadequacy among postmenopausal North American women receiving osteoporosis therapy. J Clin Endocrinol Metab 2005;90(6):3215–24.
15. Holick MF. Vitamin D deficiency. N Engl J Med 2007;357(3):266–81.

16. Tangpricha V, Pearce EN, Chen TC, et al. Vitamin D insufficiency among free-living healthy young adults. Am J Med 2002;112(8):659–62.
17. Chiodini I, Mascia ML, Muscarella S, et al. Subclinical hypercortisolism among outpatients referred for osteoporosis. Ann Intern Med 2007;147(8):541–8.
18. Nieman LK. Screening for reversible osteoporosis: is cortisol a culprit? Ann Intern Med 2007;147(8):582–4.
19. Meier C, Kraenzlin ME, Bodmer M, et al. Use of thiazolidinediones and fracture risk. Arch Intern Med 2008;168(8):820–5.
20. Short R. Fracture risk is a class effect of glitazones. BMJ 2007;334(7593):551.
21. Kahn SE, Zinman B, Lachin JM, et al. Rosiglitazone-associated fractures in type 2 diabetes: an Analysis from a Diabetes Outcome Progression Trial (ADOPT). Diabetes Care 2008;31(5):845–51.
22. Bonaiuti D, Shea B, Iovine R, et al. Exercise for preventing and treating osteoporosis in postmenopausal women. Cochrane Database Syst Rev 2002;(3): CD000333.
23. Shea B, Bonaiuti D, Iovine R, et al. Cochrane Review on exercise for preventing and treating osteoporosis in postmenopausal women. Eura Medicophys 2004; 40(3):199–209.
24. Close J, Ellis M, Hooper R, et al. Prevention of falls in the elderly trial (PROFET): a randomised controlled trial. Lancet 1999;353(9147):93–7.
25. Parker MJ, Gillespie WJ, Gillespie LD. Effectiveness of hip protectors for preventing hip fractures in elderly people: systematic review. BMJ 2006;332(7541): 571–4.
26. de Rooij SE. Hip protectors to prevent femoral fracture. BMJ 2006;332(7541): 559–60.
27. Holzer G, Holzer LA. Hip protectors and prevention of hip fractures in older persons. Geriatrics 2007;62(8):15–20.
28. Curhan GC, Willett WC, Rimm EB, et al. A prospective study of dietary calcium and other nutrients and the risk of symptomatic kidney stones. N Engl J Med 1993;328(12):833–8.
29. Finkelstein JS. Calcium plus vitamin D for postmenopausal women—bone appetit? N Engl J Med 2006;354(7):750–2.
30. Jackson RD, LaCroix AZ, Gass M, et al. Calcium plus vitamin D supplementation and the risk of fractures. N Engl J Med 2006;354(7):669–83.
31. Bone HG, Hosking D, Devogelaer JP, et al. Ten years' experience with alendronate for osteoporosis postmenopausal women. N Engl J Med 2004;350(12): 1189–99.
32. Black DM, Schwartz AV, Ensrud KE, et al. Effects of continuing or stopping alendronate after 5 years of treatment: the Fracture Intervention Trial Long-term Extension (FLEX): a randomized trial. JAMA 2006;296(24):2927–38.
33. Black DM, Delmas PD, Eastell R, et al. Once-yearly zoledronic acid for treatment of postmenopausal osteoporosis. N Engl J Med 2007;356(18):1809–22.
34. Majumdar SR. Oral bisphosphonates and atrial fibrillation. BMJ 2008;336(7648): 784–5.
35. Sorensen HT, Christensen S, Mehnert F, et al. Use of bisphosphonates among women and risk of atrial fibrillation and flutter: population based case-control study. BMJ 2008;336(7648):813–6.
36. Woo SB, Hellstein JW, Kalmar JR. Narrative [corrected] review: bisphosphonates and osteonecrosis of the jaws. Ann Intern Med 2006;144(10):753–61.
37. Bilezikian JP. Osteonecrosis of the jaw—do bisphosphonates pose a risk? N Engl J Med 2006;355(22):2278–81.

38. Ettinger B, Black DM, Mitlak BH, et al. Reduction of vertebral fracture risk in post-menopausal women with osteoporosis treated with raloxifene: results from a 3-year randomized clinical trial. Multiple Outcomes of Raloxifene Evaluation (MORE) Investigators. JAMA 1999;282(7):637–45.

39. Rossouw JE, Anderson GL, Prentice RL, et al. Risks and benefits of estrogen plus progestin in healthy postmenopausal women: principal results From the Women's Health Initiative randomized controlled trial. JAMA 2002;288(3):321–33.

40. Cauley JA, Robbins J, Chen Z, et al. Effects of estrogen plus progestin on risk of fracture and bone mineral density: the Women's Health Initiative randomized trial. JAMA 2003;290(13):1729–38.

41. Chesnut CH 3rd, Silverman S, Andriano K, et al. A randomized trial of nasal spray salmon calcitonin in postmenopausal women with established osteoporosis: the prevent recurrence of osteoporotic fractures study. PROOF Study Group. Am J Med 2000;109(4):267–76.

42. Blau LA, Hoehns JD. Analgesic efficacy of calcitonin for vertebral fracture pain. Ann Pharmacother 2003;37(4):564–70.

43. Neer RM, Arnaud CD, Zanchetta JR, et al. Effect of parathyroid hormone (1–34) on fractures and bone mineral density in postmenopausal women with osteoporosis. N Engl J Med 2001;344(19):1434–41.

44. Black DM, Greenspan SL, Ensrud KE, et al. The effects of parathyroid hormone and alendronate alone or in combination in postmenopausal osteoporosis. N Engl J Med 2003;349(13):1207–15.

45. Pinkerton JV, Dalkin AC. Combination therapy for treatment of osteoporosis: a review. Am J Obstet Gynecol 2007;197(6):559–65.

46. Greenspan SL, Resnick NM, Parker RA. Combination therapy with hormone replacement and alendronate for prevention of bone loss in elderly women: a randomized controlled trial. JAMA 2003;289(19):2525–33.

47. Johnell O, Scheele WH, Lu Y, et al. Additive effects of raloxifene and alendronate on bone density and biochemical markers of bone remodeling in postmenopausal women with osteoporosis. J Clin Endocrinol Metab 2002;87(3):985–92.

48. McClung MR, Lewiecki EM, Cohen SB, et al. Denosumab in postmenopausal women with low bone mineral density. N Engl J Med 2006;354(8):821–31.

49. Ebeling PR. Clinical practice. Osteoporosis in men. N Engl J Med 2008;358(14):1474–82.

50. Liu H, Paige NM, Goldzweig CL, et al. Screening for osteoporosis in men: a systematic review for an American College of Physicians guideline. Ann Intern Med 2008;148(9):685–701.

51. Kiebzak GM, Beinart GA, Perser K, et al. Undertreatment of osteoporosis in men with hip fracture. Arch Intern Med 2002;162(19):2217–22.

52. Orwoll E, Ettinger M, Weiss S, et al. Alendronate for the treatment of osteoporosis in men. N Engl J Med 2000;343(9):604–10.

53. Orwoll ES, Scheele WH, Paul S, et al. The effect of teriparatide [human parathyroid hormone (1-34)] therapy on bone density in men with osteoporosis. J Bone Miner Res 2003;18(1):9–17.

Menopause

David G. Weismiller, MD, ScM

KEYWORDS

- Menopause • Perimenopause • Hormone therapy • Climacteric
- Vasomotor symptoms • Postmenopausal bleeding

At the beginning of the twentieth century, the average woman's lifespan in the United States was significantly shorter than it is today, and few women lived past menopause. In contrast, most women now live almost one third of their lives after the menopause. In Western society, women have a life expectancy of approximately 80 years. In 2000, an estimated 31.2 million women in the United States underwent the menopausal transition. By the year 2020, the size of this group is estimated to be 45.9 million.

The menopause is the time during a woman's life when her reproductive capacity stops. The ovaries cease functioning and they produce fewer reproductive hormones. The body undergoes a variety of changes on account of this and due to aging. The menopause commonly is marked by unpleasant symptoms, yet, although some may be disabling, none is life threatening. Although menopause is a normal transition encompassing a developmental stage in the life cycle, its resulting decline in endogenous estrogen levels can affect various parts of the body. Estrogen deficiency has been implicated in an increased risk for vasomotor symptoms, urogenital atrophy, cardiovascular disease, osteoporosis, and cognitive decline. To provide optimal health care throughout menopause, clinicians should explore the beliefs, lifestyles, and other factors of aging of women in their 40s well before the menopause.

DEFINITION

The World Health Organization (WHO) defines natural menopause as the permanent cessation of menstruation resulting from the loss of ovarian follicular activity or follicle depletion. Natural menopause is recognized to have occurred after 12 consecutive months of amenorrhea for which there is no other pathologic or physiologic cause. Menopause occurs with the final menstrual period, which is known with certainty only in retrospect a year or more after the event.

An adequate biologic marker for menopause does not exist. Documentation of amenorrhea for at least 1 year with an associated serum follicle-stimulating hormone (FSH) level of greater than 50 IU/mL and a circulating serum estradiol level of less than 50 pg/mL have been used.[1] Women who have not had a spontaneous menstrual period for 1 year are classified as postmenopausal.[2] Clinically, menopause is defined

Department of Family Medicine, The Brody School of Medicine, East Carolina University, Greenville, NC 27858-4353, USA
E-mail address: weismillerd@ecu.edu

Prim Care Clin Office Pract 36 (2009) 199–226
doi:10.1016/j.pop.2008.10.007
0095-4543/08/$ – see front matter © 2009 Elsevier Inc. All rights reserved.
primarycare.theclinics.com

as the cessation of ovarian function. Perimenopause includes the period immediately before menopause (when the endocrinologic, biologic, and clinical features of approaching menopause commence) and the first year after the final menstrual period. Postmenopause is defined as the period after menopause and begins after 12 months of spontaneous amenorrhea. Climacteric refers to the entire transition from the reproductive to the nonreproductive state. Thus, it includes immediate premenopausal, perimenopausal, and postmenopausal women.

NATURAL HISTORY

The average age at menopause is approximately 51 in industrialized societies, with more than 90% of women experiencing cessation of menses by age 55. The age tends to be lower in women who smoke and in those who have had no children. Lower age at menopause also may be related to poor socioeconomic status. Analysis has shown that women who have menstrual cycles averaging less than 26 days reach the menopause 1.4 years earlier than those who have longer cycles. It also is believed that a woman's age at menopause may be a biologic marker of aging and that a later menopause may be associated with greater longevity (**Box 1**). The number of follicles in the ovary determines the age at which the menopause takes place. Counts of ovarian follicles show that the number is greatest in the fetus at 7 months, with a decline to approximately 700,000 at birth. The decline continues steadily until approximately age 40 and then declines more rapidly until after the menopause, when essentially there are no follicles left. Evidence indicates that women who smoke experience menopause 1 to 2 years earlier than nonsmokers.[3–11] Overall, premature menopause (menopause before age 40) occurs in approximately 1% of women.[12]

Most women begin the transition (perimenopause) at approximately age 47. Perimenopause typically consists of a change in the amount or duration of menstrual flow,

---

Box 1
Factors associated with age of menopause

Factors associated with an earlier age of menopause

Current cigarette smoking

Earlier onset (1.5 years)

Previous abdominal hysterectomy

Body weight: thinner women experience a slightly earlier menopause

Living at high altitudes

Undernourished women and vegetarians

Factors not affecting age of menopause

Age of menarche

Socioeconomics status

Ethnicity

Previous use of oral contraceptives

Factors potentially affecting the age of menopause

Maternal age at menopause

Parity

Marital status

a change in the length of the menstrual cycle, and skipped menstrual cycles. All women do not go through the same transition of regular menses to irregular menses to amenorrhea as they approach menopause. In 2001, a panel of experts from the Stages of Reproductive Aging Workshop met to discuss a staging system to classify reproductive aging.[3] This proposed new classification of the transition from reproductive to postmenopausal includes seven stages based on menstrual cycles and plasma FSH levels. The experts proposing this system noted that it is a work in progress and has not been validated in research settings. The Study of Women's Health in the Nation, a multisite study of the natural history of menopause, helps in understanding the transition among several ethnic and racial groups of women in the United States.[13] Primary care providers must consider other factors in addition to menopause in the differential diagnosis of amenorrhea. For example, Mold and colleagues[14] found that night sweats reported by primary care patients were associated with panic attacks, greater body mass index, chronic infection, sleep disturbances, antihistamines, and antidepressants in addition to menopause (**Box 2**).[2]

PHYSIOLOGY

Menstruation ceases as ovarian follicle stores are depleted and ovarian function is diminished. This leads to an eventual decreased production of estrogen by the ovaries

---

Box 2
Facts about the typical perimenopausal and menopausal experience

Average age of perimenopausal transition—47 years

Average age of menopause—51 years

Perimenopausal changes

- Changes in amount or duration of menstrual flow
- Changes in length of menstrual cycle
- Missed menstrual periods

Estrogen deficiency–related menopausal symptoms

- Vaginal dryness and dyspareunia
- Vasomotor symptoms: hot flashes, day sweats, nocturnal sweats

Symptoms reported by middle-aged women that may or may not be associated with menopause

- Fatigue
- Palpitations
- Forgetfulness
- Stiffness and soreness
- Insomnia and sleep disturbances
- Changes in libido
- Headaches and backaches
- Mood swings, irritability, anxiety, depression
- Urinary tract infections
- Urine leakage

and decreased stimulation of the endometrial lining.[15] The neuroendocrinologic initiation of female maturation begins in adolescence, between the ages of 11 and 20, during which secondary sex characteristics appear and somatic growth ceases. This time period encompasses a physical maturation process that culminates in reproductive maturity.[16] Marked alterations in circulating hormone levels have significant multiorgan effects. Sex hormone receptors have been identified in many tissues throughout the female body, distributed within the reproductive organs, breasts, bones, skin and most connective tissue, cardiovascular system, urinary tract, liver, and central nervous system.[17–19]

During the reproductive era, menstrual cycle changes follow a normal, age-related, progressive pattern related to ovarian follicular competence and quantity, which typically results in variations in cycle length.[20–22] Beginning at approximately age 40, women experience longer and often heavier menstrual periods secondary to a gradual increase in serum FSH levels and anovulatory cycles.[23–25] These age-related changes in the menstrual cycle are preceded and paralleled by declining fecundity. The decline in fertility begins at approximately 35 years of age and decreases precipitously after age 40.[25–28] The transition from the reproductive era to the postreproductive state is not as sudden an event as the term, menopause, suggests.[2] The endocrinologic changes and characteristic signs and symptoms associated with natural menopause extend over a period of years and encompass an interval marked with waning function through cessation of menses.

HORMONAL CHANGES WITH ESTABLISHED MENOPAUSE

Many women do not identify themselves as perimenopausal until an overt change, such as menstrual irregularity, occurs. Two early perimenopausal changes include shortening of the follicular phase of the menstrual cycle, resulting in longer periods, and a rise in the circulating serum levels of FSH. The lengthening of the menstrual cycle interval, which begins 2 to 8 years prior to menopause, also is related to decreased serum levels of inhibin, a nonsteroidal inhibitor of pituitary FSH secretion. The hormonal fluctuations that begin in the perimenopausal phase and continue over several years before menopause do not halt suddenly when a woman reaches menopause. Instead, FSH and luteinizing hormone (LH) levels undergo an accelerated rise in the 2 to 3 years before menopause, with estrogen levels declining only within approximately 6 months before menopause. After menopause, when ovarian follicles are depleted, FSH and LH levels continue to rise. Eventually, there is a 20-fold increase in FSH levels and an approximately threefold increase in LH levels, both of which peak in the first 1 to 3 years after menopause.[29] By comparison, ovarian estrogen production does not continue beyond menopause, when ovarian follicles and their estrogen-producing granulose cells are depleted. Androgen-producing theca cells within the ovary remain, yet their production capability is markedly reduced.[30] In ovulating women, ovarian theca cells are the primary source of production of three main androgens:[1] testosterone,[2] androstenedione,[3] and dehydroepiandrosterone (DHEA).[31] The adrenal glands, liver, fat, and skin also contribute to the production of these androgens.[32]

OFFICE ISSUES

Many women who are entering the menopausal years seek answers about how best to maintain their health and address the conditions that often accompany menopause. Goals of effective menopause counseling include (1) an established patient-physician partnership where the physician acts as facilitator of a healthy lifestyle and the patient acts as the decision maker; (2) risk management and disease prevention; (3) self-care; and (4) access to health information from the physician.

Women who seek treatment for menopause-related symptoms, such as hot flashes, may be more anxious and less able to cope with stress than women who do not seek treatment.[33] Hardy and Kuh[34] have suggested that work and family stressors may influence symptom reporting during the menopause transition. Others have suggested that an increase in psychologic symptoms may be associated with current life events and difficulties, in particular those experienced in family life, which often take place concurrently with the menopausal transition.[34,35] To provide appropriate advice and support to their patients, clinicians should recognize that many symptoms associated with menopause, including hot flashes, may begin in the premenopause years, and, for some women, they may be indicative of other psychosocial or medical issues.

In 2000, the Jacobs Institute of Women's Health, the American College of Obstetricians and Gynecologists (ACOG), and the National Committee for Quality Assurance produced new menopause counseling guidelines.[36] The guidelines include principles of patient counseling, topics to cover, information about methods of managing symptoms and diseases of advancing age, and resources for clinicians and women. A task force of the American Association of Clinical Endocrinologists also has published an extensive menopause management guideline (http://www.aace.com/pub/pdf/guidelines/menopause.pdf).[37]

EVALUATION OF PERIMENOPAUSE

Accurate diagnosis of perimenopause allows patients and physicians to predict the onset of menopause. No single element of the history or clinical examination is powerful enough to confirm the probability of being perimenopausal. Besides menstrual history, the most powerful predictor of menopausal status may be age. Analysis of longitudinal data of women at all ages shows the probability of menstruating spontaneously after 12 months of amenorrhea to be less than 2%.[21] The evaluation can be divided into five basic categories: (1) self-assessment, (2) symptoms, (3) family and medical history, (4) physical signs, and (5) laboratory tests.[38]

SELF-ASSESSMENT

The first step in the evaluation of perimenopause should center on a physician asking a woman if she thinks she is starting menopause. Women may base their perceptions of their menopausal status on an awareness of the subtle changes taking place in their bodies.[39] In a cross-sectional study by Garamszegi and colleagues, self-reported menopausal status correlated more accurately with symptoms than menstrual cycle characteristics.[40] There are several standardized questionnaires available for rating the severity of menopausal symptoms and their effect on a patient's quality of life. Two of these questionnaires are available on line: (1) the Menopause Rating Scale (MRS) (http://www.menopause-rating-scale.info/) and the (2) Utian Quality of Life Scale (http://www.menopause.org/Portals/0/Content/PDF/UQOL.pdf). The MRS contains 11 questions and the Utian Quality of Life Scale contains 23; both questionnaires can be completed by patients and scored by a physician. The MRS is available online in multiple languages.

PHYSICAL SIGNS
Vasomotor Symptoms

Climacteric symptoms typically include vasomotor complaints, including hot flashes and night sweats. Hot flashes are the most common symptom of menopause, occurring in approximately 50% of women during the menopause transition; even those women who experience regular menstruation, and approximately 20% of affected women, request treatment for hot flashes.[13,14,41] Most women who have menopausal symptoms experience spontaneous cessation of vasomotor symptoms within 5 years after onset; however, a substantial proportion of women continue to experience symptoms beyond 5 years, and in these cases the long-term effects of using hormone replacement therapy (HRT) (treatment discussed later) must be considered.[42]

Women describe a hot flash as the sudden onset of a sensation of heat, sweating, and flushing that occurs most often in the face and spreads to the head, neck, and chest lasting 1 to 5 minutes. Chills, clamminess, and anxiety also may accompany hot flashes. The frequency and intensity of symptoms vary widely among women, with some experiencing an occasional sensation of warmth whereas others experience frequent episodes of intense heat and drenching sweat that disrupt daily activities and sleep. Night sweats often are hot flashes that occur at night, usually while a woman is sleeping. If night sweats interfere with sleeping patterns, this may correlate with reports of insomnia, fatigue, and irritability among climacteric women.[39]

There seem to be cultural differences in the reporting or experiencing of hot flashes. Hot flashes are more prevalent in African American and Latin American women than in non-Hispanic white women but less common in Chinese and Japanese women.[43] Other variables associated with increased reporting of hot flashes include maternal history, early age of menarche and menopause onset, history of irregular menses, higher body mass index, alcohol use, exposure to hot or humid weather, and cigarette smoking.[13,44,45] Cigarette smoking seems to increase the likelihood of experiencing hot flashes, but most other potential risk factors, including obesity, exercise, and alcohol intake, are not consistently associated.[46] Hot flashes resolve in most women after a few years, yet in 10% to 15% of women, the hot flashes persist for decades or even become lifelong.[47]

The exact mechanism of altered thermoregulation in postmenopausal women who have hot flashes is not known. One theory suggests that changes in estrogen levels associated with menopause alter central nervous system adrenergic neurotransmission and cause abnormal thermoregulation. This theoretically could account for the success of clonidine, an α-adrenergic agonist that decreases central norepinephrine release, in reducing the frequency of hot flashes.[48]

Alternatively, there is some evidence that decreasing estrogen levels during the menopause transition result in changes in serotonergic neurotransmission that may lead to hot flashes. Lower estrogen levels are associated with lower levels of serum serotonin, resulting in an increased sensitivity of hypothalamic serotonin receptors. Stimulation of these receptors can alter the thermoregulatory set point in animals. Mild stressors, such as heat or anxiety, cause a brief release of serotonin that may stimulate central receptors, lower the thermoregulatory set point, and cause hot flashes. A systematic review by Nelson and colleagues supports this hypothesis.[48] It demonstrates that selective serotonin reuptake inhibitors, which increase central serotonin levels, are effective in the treatment of hot flashes.

By far, HRT is the most effective treatment currently available for hot flashes. Overall, women randomized to hormone therapy have 60% to 85% average reductions in hot flash frequency.[49,50] There seems to be a dose-response effect, but low doses often are effective in controlling symptoms.[51] Given the marked efficacy of estrogen for the treatment of hot flashes, whether or not other therapies are needed can be argued. Postmenopausal estrogen therapy reduces the risk for fractures secondary to osteoporosis (absolute risk reduction, 2.09%; number needed to treat [NNT], 48) and colorectal cancer (absolute risk reduction, 0.3%; NNT, 333). It has been shown, however, to increase the risk for cardiovascular disease events (absolute risk increase, 1.42%; number needed to harm, 70) and breast cancer (absolute risk increase, 0.42%; number needed to harm, 238).[52] HRT also is associated with possible unpleasant side effects, including uterine bleeding, breast tenderness, and headache, but these adverse effects are believed worth the dual benefits of symptom relief and potential disease prevention. This reasoning largely has been responsible for the lack of research on the etiology of hot flashes and alternatives to estrogen for treatment.[53]

Urogenital Atrophy

Vaginal dryness sometimes is experienced as a result of decreasing estrogen production during the climacteric. This can lead to urogenital atrophy and changes in the quantity and composition of vaginal secretions. Estimates of the prevalence of vaginal dryness among late perimenopausal women are approximately 20%.[54,55] In Western countries, urinary incontinence affects between 26% and 55% of middle-aged women;[56,57] the cause may be declining estrogen levels. Lower estrogen levels can lead to atrophy of the urethral mucosa and the trigone, the muscle controlling urination, resulting in less control over bladder function.[58] Some studies have found an association between an increased prevalence of urinary incontinence and menopause whereas others have not.[56,59,60]

Psychologic Events

Many hypotheses, including biologic, social, and psychologic bases, have been suggested to explain why depression occurs more frequently in women. Some biochemical support exists for a hormonal role in the development of mood disorders, as the incidence of depressive disorders diverges between men and women beginning at adolescence.[61] Significant evidence indicates that estrogen and progesterone influence the levels of various neurotransmitters that are associated with mood, including serotonin and norepinephrine.[62] Women experience mood disorders linked to the menstrual cycle or pregnancy, including premenstrual syndrome (PMS) and postpartum depression.[63] Women who have PMS have a higher incidence of major depressive disorder and postpartum depression and, although depression has been associated with use of hormonal medication, including oral contraceptives, there also is evidence to suggest that baseline moods improve with hormonal therapy.[64]

Psychosocial factors play an integral role in the development of depression, with happily married women having a slightly lower incidence of depression compared to single women. Other factors, including sexual abuse, a history of domestic violence, miscarriage and abortion, death of a child or spouse, family history of depression, and mothers of children who have attention deficit disorders, also are correlated with depression.[65] Cultural influences may affect the risk for depression in women,[66] with women in the workplace facing multiple and often conflicting roles as mother, spouse, and breadwinner. Concerns in the workplace, such as sexual harassment and nonequal salary with lack of advancement compared with male counterparts, also place women at increased risk for depression.

Although female gender clearly is associated with a higher risk for affective disorders,[67,68] the effect of menopausal status on this risk is controversial. Several longitudinal studies conducted in Europe and North America observing cohorts of women through menopause report no increase in moderate or severe depressive symptoms with the menopause.[35,69-71] More recent studies also reveal no apparent increased depression or decreased well-being at menopause; however, just prior to menopause a small increase in mild symptoms occurs.[72–74] Factors often associated with decreased mood at menopause include previous depression, previous PMS, hysterectomy, psychosocial stressors, negative attitudes toward menopause, and poor health and lifestyle variables, such as smoking and lack of exercise.

Some studies indicate a mild increase in anxiety symptoms, similar to depression, in some women just prior to menopause; however, several well-designed prospective studies found no increased rate of anxiety with menopause.[35,71] Many checklists for menopause symptoms used in epidemiologic studies include nervous tension and irritability. Although the relevance of these symptoms is unclear, they could be caused by a lack of sleep resulting from menopausal symptoms, illness, or stressful life events. Some investigators have suggested that anxious symptoms could result from changes in hormone levels, similar to those during the 10- to 14-day luteal phase of the menstrual cycle[75] and associated with PMS or dysphoric disorder. Women who present to menopause clinics tend to have increased rates of anxiety and other psychologic symptoms;[76,77] however, these symptoms may not be representative of all women.

Significant social events occur during midlife, including changing relationships, maturing children, marital instability or widowhood, and the illness or loss of parents. The time of menopause is a time of transition from childbearing and child rearing to a time of growth, concentration on the marital relationship, and sometimes freedom to travel. It also is a transition to old age, increased risk for illness, and grandparenting. The North American Menopause Society survey from 1998 determined that most women viewed menopause and midlife as the beginning of positive changes in their lives and overall health. More than 75% of surveyed women reported making health-related lifestyle changes, such as smoking cessation, at menopause. Mood disorders or cognitive disruption that coincide with menopause should not be attributed solely to menopause without first evaluating psychosocial, medical, or other issues that may occur at the time of menopause.

Laboratory Tests

Many clinicians rely on the measurement of serum hormone levels, such as FSH, to confirm the diagnosis of perimenopusal and menopausal status. In most clinical scenarios, FSH measurement does not help a clinician make a diagnosis.[38]

Follicle-stimulating hormone

Measurement of serum FSH levels has been used to identify and categorize perimenopausal and postmenopausal women. High FSH levels indicate that menopausal changes are occurring in the ovary. As the ovary becomes less responsive to stimulation by FSH from the pituitary gland (and ultimately produces less estrogen), the pituitary gland increases production of FSH to stimulate the ovary to produce more estrogen. Some clinicians and researchers, however, doubt the clinical value of FSH measurements in perimenopausal women, as FSH levels fluctuate considerably each month depending on whether or not ovulation has occurred.[3,78,79] The assessment of FSH is expensive and misleading. Until a well-validated tool to confirm menopause is available, clinicians should use their clinical judgment in obtaining this assay. By age 55, the likelihood of menopausal status is greater than 90%. If a clinician feels a strong need to obtain a serum FSH level, then the following are recommended:

- In a patient who is not taking oral contraceptive pills, a serum FSH level greater than 50 mIU/mL indicates that menopause probably has been reached

- Obtain a serum FSH level at any time when a woman is taking active oral contraceptive pills. If the FSH is greater than 45 mIU/mL, then menopause probably has been reached.
- If a patient is taking oral contraceptives, obtain an FSH on day 6 of the placebo pill pack. If the serum FSH level is greater than 30 mIU/mL, then menopause probably has been reached.
- Obtain serum estradiol and FSH levels after 2 weeks without the woman taking oral contraceptive pills. An increase in the serum FSH or no change in basal estradiol levels indicates probable menopause.

Estradiol

Recent longitudinal studies have reported that early perimenopausal (change in cycle frequency) women maintained premenopausal estradiol levels whereas late perimenopausal (no menses in previous 3 to 11 months) and postmenopausal women experienced significant declines in estradiol levels.[80] Estradiol can be measured using serum, urine, and saliva. Similar to FSH, estradiol levels are highly variable during perimenopause. A circulating serum estradiol level of less than 50 pg/mL has been used as a threshold for the diagnosis of menopause.

Inhibins

Inhibin A and inhibin B are secreted by the ovary and usually are measured in plasma. Like estradiol, inhibins exert negative feedback on the pituitary gland, reducing FSH and LH secretion. A loss of inhibin contributes to the rise in FSH that occurs with ovarian senescence. The ovaries produce less inhibin B as fewer follicles proceed to maturation, and the number of follicles declines with age.[81] A longitudinal study of hormone levels throughout the menopause transition reported that inhibin B levels decline as women progress through the perimenopause whereas inhibin A levels remain unchanged. At approximately the time of the final menstrual period, inhibin A levels decrease.[80] Further research needs to be conducted to document the benefit of these hormone level assays in making a diagnosis of perimenopause.

OTHER PERIMENOPAUSAL ISSUES
Reproduction

Healthy, lean women of older reproductive age (older than 40) who are nonsmokers can safely use combination estrogen and progestin contraceptives. Benefits include effective contraception and reductions in irregular bleeding and vasomotor symptoms associated with the perimenopausal transition. Available epidemiologic data also suggest potential long-term benefits, including reductions in the risks for fractures among postmenopausal women and for ovarian, endometrial, and colorectal cancers. For women of older reproductive age who are obese, smoke cigarettes, or have hypertension, diabetes, or migraine headaches, however, the cardiovascular risks associated with combination oral contraceptives are considered to outweigh the benefits. For these women, reasonable treatment options include progestin-only and intrauterine contraceptive methods, barrier contraceptives, and sterilization (in women who have completed childbearing or do not want to have children).[82] Regardless of other contraceptive use, consistent use of condoms should be encouraged for all women at risk for sexually transmitted infections. The WHO and the ACOG have developed similar guidelines for addressing the use of combination estrogen and progestin hormonal contraception in women of older reproductive age (**Table 1**).[83,84]

Table 1
Guidelines regarding the use of combination estrogen and progestin contraceptives in women older than 35, according to risk factors[a]

Risk Factor	Guidelines	
	American College of Obstetricians and Gynecologists	**World Health Organization**
Diabetes	Progestin-only or intrauterine contraception should be used[b]	Risk unacceptable
Hypertension	Progestin-only or intrauterine contraception should be used[b]	Risk unacceptable
Migraine	Progestin-only or intrauterine contraception should be used[b]	Risk unacceptable
Obesity	Progestin-only or intrauterine contraception may be safer than combination estrogen and progestin contraception[c]	Benefit usually outweighs risk[c]
Smoking	Progestin-only or intrauterine contraception should be used[b]	Risk unacceptable
None of the above	Healthy women who are nonsmokers doing well with the use of combination contraceptive may continue this method until 50–55 years of age, after weighing the risks and benefits	For women ≥ 40 years of age, the risk for cardiovascular disease increases with age and also may increase with combined hormonal contraceptive use; in the absence of other adverse clinical condition, combined hormonal contraceptives can be used until menopause

[a] Recommendations are from ACOG[82] and the WHO.[84]
[b] This category includes progestin-only oral contraceptives, depot MPA, contraceptive implants, and progestin-releasing and copper intrauterine devices.
[c] Obesity in women 35 years of age and older is not specifically addressed.

Sexuality

One of the myths prevalent in Western society is that aging women (or men) have a reduced interest in and desire for sexual intimacy. There is a lack of clarity regarding possible changes in female sexuality with menopause. Although sexual problems are common in women presenting to menopause or gynecology clinics, the picture is less clear in the general population.[85] Intimacy is a lifelong human need that does not change with age. Although aging and hormonal changes associated with menopause may result in physical symptoms that decrease opportunities for and enjoyment of sexual intimacy, there is no evidence that the importance of sexuality decreases after menopause.

Hot flashes may result in insomnia and a higher incidence of general complaints that reduce a woman's sense of well-being. Atrophic changes in the vagina, in particular vaginal dryness, decreased lubrication in response to sexual stimulation, and reduced vaginal elasticity, often result in dyspareunia. The aging process itself also may be associated with changes in a woman's physical health or that of her partner, and sociocultural and other family issues could reduce emotional well-being. This complex interplay between physical and psychologic dynamics suggests that although hormones have a role in sexuality during and after the menopausal transition, other contributory factors can influence a woman's sexual practice and libido.[86] Bachman and Leiblum reported that libido in 60- to 70-year-old women is not dependent on female sex hormones; rather, personal relationships and life circumstances are predominant determinants of sexuality.[87] Several studies have found that menopausal symptoms are one of many factors affecting sexual interest among women in midlife and older age.[88,89]

The availability of a sexually interested partner has been identified as the single most significant determinant of sexual activity in older women.[90] Marital status also has a significant impact on a woman's sexual activity in her later life. Newman and Nichols reported that only 7% of the 101 menopausal single, widowed, or divorced women they studied reported any sexual activity; by comparison, 54% of the 149 married subjects living with a partner still were sexually active.[91]

In counseling menopausal women, clinicians should initiate a discussion about sexuality and query patients regarding the presence of any symptoms or life changes that are likely to affect their sexuality or sexual experiences. Many women and couples may be unprepared for the gradual changes that occur in sexual functioning caused by aging and may fear that these changes indicate a loss of sexual capability.[86] Educating women about the physiologic and anatomic changes that occur during menopause and promoting communication of their sexual needs and concerns to their partner, if applicable, provide important emotional support. Such a discussion affords the clinicians an opportunity to address existing sexual changes experienced by a woman or her partner and to recommend specific interventions or referral for additional counseling. Most important, such dialogue opens the door for future follow-up on this sensitive and significant life issue.[86]

TREATMENT
Hormonal Replacement Therapy

Estrogen has been used as a hormonal supplement for nearly 60 years to treat menopausal symptoms, and randomized controlled trials indicate that estrogen reduces the frequency of hot flashes by 77% or by approximately 2.5 to 3 hot flashes daily compared to placebo and decreases symptoms associated with vulvovaginal atrophy.[92] Since the results of the Women's Health Initiative (WHI) were published (**Table 2**), use of estrogen, with or without progestin, has declined significantly.[93] In addition, several well-publicized evidence-based studies have been published, all of which have helped to change the face of HRT.[94–97] Based on the best available evidence, hormones are used as therapy to treat menopausal symptoms or as a means of helping to avoid or minimize the risk for certain diseases. HRT effectively relieves the most common menopausal symptoms,[98] and the absolute risk for cardiovascular disease and cancer is low when these drugs are used for short periods of time.[99] In addition, HRT may be appropriate in the prevention or management of osteoporosis, the most common metabolic disease in the United States, and one that is linked directly to declining serum estrogen levels. In several meta-analyses of observational studies, the risk for dementia has been reduced with long-term use of estrogen, whereas in the WHI trial, the hazard ratio for probable dementia was 2.05 in women beyond age 65 who were taking estrogen and progesterone. To date, use of HRT for the prevention or treatment of dementia has not been recommended.

Prior to publication of the evidence-based studies (discussed previously), fairly succinct guidelines existed for using HRT. With better awareness of risks and benefits, such guidelines no longer are useful nor are they easy to generate. The decision to use HRT depends on a woman's current health status and her personal and family

Table 2
Summary of results from the Women's Health Initiative

Outcome	Estrogen Plus Progestin[a]		Number Needed to Treat/Number Needed to Harm
	Relative Risk (95% CI)	Absolute Risk (%)	
Coronary heart disease	1.29 (1.02–1.63)	↑0.43	232
Stroke	1.41 (1.07–1.85)	↑0.44	227
Pulmonary embolism	2.13 (1.39–3.25)	↑0.44	227
Invasive breast cancer	1.26 (1.00–1.59)	↑0.42	238
Colon cancer	0.63 (0.43–0.92)	↓0.3	333
Hip fracture	0.66 (0.45–0.98)	↓0.25	400

[a] In this trial, 16,608 postmenopausal women who did not have a hysterectomy were randomly assigned to receive 0.625 mg of conjugated estrogen plus 2.5 mg of MPA per day or an identical placebo and were followed for an average of 5.2 years.

Data from Rossouw JE, Anderson GL, Prentice RL, et al. Risks and benefits of estrogen plus progestin in healthy postmenopausal women: principle results from the Women's Health Initiative randomized controlled trial. JAMA 2002;288:321–3.

health history, with specific attention to gynecologic cancers and cardiovascular disease. The results of the WHI study cannot be generalized to a population of women in early menopause because the WHI was designed to evaluate HRT in an older population of aging postmenopausal women.

All types and routes of administration of estrogen have been proved effective in improving symptoms of menopause. The benefit of hormone therapy is dose-related and Food and Drug Administration (FDA) guidance should be followed in using HRT at the lowest dose and for the shortest duration possible, although evidence from randomized, controlled trials supporting this guideline is unavailable.[99] Several estrogen and progestin formulations are available, and there is no strong evidence that one formulation is superior to another. Hormones delivered via a transdermal patch are associated with a lower risk for venous thromboembolism compared to oral formulations (**Table 3**). A reasonable starting dose of estrogen for women who are having hot flashes is 0.025 mg of transdermal estradiol, 0.5 mg of oral estradiol, or 0.3 mg of conjugated equine estrogen.[99] Although it is reasonable to believe that the transdermal route of administration of estrogen avoids first-pass hepatic metabolism and, therefore, may reduce thromboembolic risk, no randomized controlled trials to support this concept have been published.

For women who have an intact uterus, a progestin should be combined with estrogen to reduce the risk for endometrial cancer and to prevent endometrial hyperplasia. If a woman is using only intravaginal estrogen, then a progestin is not necessary. Progestins also are unnecessary in women who have undergone total hysterectomy.[99] When used cyclically, a progestational agent should be administered in an adequate dose for 10 to 14 days each month. Common choices of orally administered progestational agents that have been shown to provide endometrial protection include medroxyprogesterone acetate (MPA) (2.5 mg daily or 5 mg for 10 to14 days per month), micronized progesterone (100 mg daily or 200 mg for 10 to 14 days per month), norethindrone (0.35 mg daily or 5 mg for 10 to 14 days per month), or levonorgestrel (0.075 mg daily). The side effects of progestational compounds are difficult to evaluate and vary with the agent administered.[100] Amenorrhea may be achieved by using a low dose of a progestogen administered continuously (daily) in conjunction with estrogen.

Table 3
Selected estrogen and progestin preparations for the treatment of menopausal vasomotor symptoms[a]

Preparation	Generic Name	Brand Name	Doses (mg/day)
Estrogen			
Oral	Conjugated estrogens	Premarin	0.3, 0.45, 0.635, 1.25
	17β-Estradiol	Estrace	0.5, 1.0, 2.0
Transdermal	17β-Estradiol	Alora	0.025, 0.05, 0.075, 0.1 (patch applied twice weekly)
		Climara	0.025, 0.0375, 0.05, 0.075, 0.1 (patch applied weekly)
Vaginal	Estradiol acetate	Femring vaginal ring[b]	0.05, 0.1 (inserted every 90 days)
Progestogen			
Oral	MPA	Provera	2.5, 5.0, 10.0
	Micronized progesterone	Prometrium	100, 200 (in peanut oil)
Vaginal	Progesterone	Prochieve 4%	45
Combination preparation			
Oral sequential[c]	Conjugated estrogens and MPA	Premphase	0.625 conjugated estrogens plus 5.0 MPA
Oral continuous[d]	Conjugated estrogens and MPA	Prempro	0.625 conjugated estrogens plus 2.5–5.0 MPA; 0.45 conjugated estrogens plus 2.5 MPA; or 0.3 or 0.45 conjugated estrogens plus 1.5 MPA
Transdermal continuous[d]	17β-estradiol-norethindrone acetate	Activella	1.0 estradiol plus 0.5 norethindrone
	17β-estradiol-levonorgestrel	Climara Pro	0.045 estradiol plus 0.015 levonorgestrel (patch applied weekly)
	17β-estradiol-norethindrone acetate	CombiPatch	0.05 estradiol plus 0.14 or 0.25 norethindrone (patch applied twice weekly)

[a] Estrogen should be avoided in women who have a history of or are at high risk for cardiovascular disease, breast cancer, uterine cancer, or venous thromboembolic events and in those who have active liver disease. Hormone therapy can cause uterine bleeding, breast tenderness, and headache. Doses of estrogen that are approximately biologically equivalent: 0.625 mg of Premarin, 1.0 mg Estrace, and 0.05 mg of Alora, Climara, or Femring.
[b] Unlike other vaginal preparations listed in **Table 3**, Femring delivers a higher systemic level of estrogen and should be opposed by a progestin in women who have a uterus.
[c] The first 14 pills contain estrogen and the subsequent pills (days 15–28) contain estrogen with progestin.
[d] Each pill or patch contains estrogen and progestin.

More than 30% of women ultimately need to change their pharmacologic regimen to consider its use a success. **Box 3** outlines the FDA-recommended contraindications to HRT and common side effects. Many side effects of HRT are similar to premenstrual symptoms. As women age, their cardiovascular risks increase, indicating a need for greater caution when HRT is concerned. The use of estrogen (in conjunction with a progestational agent in women who have a uterus) should be discussed thoroughly by each woman with her physician.

Box 3
Contraindications and common side effects of hormone replacement therapy

Absolute contraindications

Current, past, or suspected breast cancer

Known or suspected estrogen-sensitive malignant conditions

Undiagnosed genital bleeding

Untreated endometrial hyperplasia

Previous idiopathic or current venous thromboembolism (eg, deep venous thrombosis and pulmonary embolism)

Active or recent arterial thromboembolic disease (eg, angina and myocardial infarction)

Untreated hypertension

Active liver disease

Known hypersensitivity to the active substances of HRT or to any of the excipients

Hypertriglyceridemia[a]

Porphyria cutanea tarda

Relative contraindications

Migraine headaches

History of fibroids

Atypical ductal hyperplasia of the breast

Active gallbladder disease

Common side effects

Breast soreness

Fluid retention and bloating

Nausea

Leg cramps

Headaches

Oily skin and acne

Mood alterations

Irregular bleeding (improves within 6–12 months for most women)

[a] Because of the potential for HRT to elevate triglycerides, its use is considered by some as an absolute contraindication in women who have triglyceride levels greater than 500 mg/dL.[134] Similarly, HRT should be considered relatively contraindicated in women whose triglyceride levels are greater than 300 mg/dL. A triglyceride level of less than 300 mg/dL is not considered a contraindication.

Systemic hormones may not be necessary for all women. Women who find vaginal symptoms most problematic can gain relief by using intravaginal estrogen (eg, creams or suppositories).[101,102] There is significantly reduced systemic absorption via these methods yet the clinical significance of this reduction is not known.

Nonhormonal Pharmacologic and Complementary Treatment

High-quality studies have provided solid evidence that HRT is the most effective treatment for common menopausal symptoms. Concerns about the adverse effects of estrogen have led to an increased interest in alternative therapies for improving menopausal symptoms. In particular, women who have breast cancer who cannot take estrogen are seeking alternatives for symptom control, and estrogen therapy is contraindicated. Women report using a wide variety of complementary and alternative medicine (CAM) therapies, including stress management, nonprescription remedies, chiropractic and naturopathic care, massage therapy, dietary soy, herbs, and acupuncture, to control menopausal symptoms.[103] A growing body of literature with randomized controlled trials is available comparing the efficacy and adverse effects of therapies other than agents composed primarily of estrogen, progestin or progesterone, or androgen for menopausal hot flashes. For simplicity, these are referred to as nonhormonal therapies, although some therapies, such as plant isoflavones, have weak estrogenic and antiestrogenic activities (**Table 4**).

The use of supplements and botanicals in medicine creates special challenges. Many articles about CAM therapies, especially botanicals, published in United States medical journals have come under scrutiny because of the difficulty in properly comparing different preparations. The evidence for several of the CAM therapies women commonly seek generally is supportive and the risk for harm seems low.[104] Lifestyle changes may provide relief, including lowering body temperature by dressing in layers, using a fan, and consuming cold foods and beverages; getting more exercise; losing weight; quitting smoking; and practicing relaxation techniques (eg, meditation, paced respiration, biofeedback, and massage and reflexology).[105]

Androgen Therapy

Normal postmenopausal women have a 50% reduction in serum androstendione as a result of decreased adrenal hormone production, with a consequent testosterone production from peripheral conversion. Concentrations of the adrenal androgens DHEA and DHEA sulfate also decline with aging, independent of menopause; thus, by 40 to 50 years of age, their serum values are approximately one half those of younger women.[106,107] Symptoms attributed to androgen deficiency, including decreased libido, decreased sexual response, decreased sense of well-being, poor concentration, and fatigue, also may be attributable to estrogen deficiency. Accordingly, symptoms attributed to androgen deficiency may be a result of androgen deficiency itself or a deficiency of estradiol.[108]

Conflicting data are available on the effects of androgen replacement therapy on sexual function in menopausal women.[109–113] Administration of testosterone by various routes at supraphysiologic doses has been shown to improve libido, sexual arousal, frequency of sexual fantasies, sexual function, body composition, muscle strength, and quality of life in comparison with administration of estrogen alone. Physiologic replacement testosterone therapy seems to have an inconclusive effect on sexual function in women.[114] Many observations are compatible with androgen therapy, yielding improved bone-related factors, particularly in doses that exceed the normal range.[109,115–119] Adverse effects may occur with androgen replacement

Table 4
Alternatives to estrogen for management of menopausal symptoms

Treatment	Dose (Orally Daily)	Side Effects	Superior to Placebo
Conventional			
Clonidine	0.1–0.4 mg	Drowsiness, dry mouth, constipation, hypotension, insomnia, postural hypotension, reaction to skin patch; to discontinue slowly reduce dose to avoid rebound hypertension, headaches, and agitation	Yes; no long-term studies
Selective serotonin reuptake inhibitors			
Fluoxetine	20–30 mg	Dry mouth, insomnia, sedation, decreased appetite, constipation	Inconsistent effect; few studies, side effects profile significant, no long-term studies
Paroxetine	12.5–25 mg		Yes; no long-term studies
Venlafaxine	37.5–75 mg		Yes; efficacy increases with higher doses but so do side effects; no long-term studies
Gabapentin	900 mg in divided doses	Somnolence, fatigue, dizziness, and palpitations	Yes; no long-term studies
Alternative			
Black cohosh	2–4 mg of terpene glycoside or 4 mL of tincture	Diarrhea and vomiting, skin rash, dizziness, headaches, weight gain. Case reports on autoimmune hepatitis and asthenia	Yes, but inconclusive results, long-term safety not known; caution with estrogen-dependent tumors
Red clover	40–80 mg	Headache, myalgia, arthralgia, nausea, and diarrhea. Contraindicated in bleeding disorders	Inconsistent effect; few studies, long-term safety unknown
Phytoestrogens	34–100 mg	Mastalgia, weight gain, a case report of hypertensive crisis	Inconclusive
Ginseng	200 mg	Insomnia, mastalgia, skin eruptions, gastrointestinal, interacts with warfarin	Few studies
Evening primrose	500 mg	Gastrointestinal, headache, lowers seizure threshold in epileptics	Only one randomized study
Dong quai	450 mg	Photosensitization, warfarin interaction	Only one randomized study
Vitamin E	50–100 mg	Diarrhea, abdominal pain	Only one randomized study

therapy at supraphysiologic levels, as acne, hirsutism, erythrocytosis, and a significant reduction in high-density lipoprotein cholesterol levels have been described.[108]

The FDA has not yet approved use of androgens in women for control of menopausal symptoms. Therefore, such therapy is considered off-label intervention at this time. Several modes of administration exist for possible off-label androgen therapy in menopausal women: (1) oral (methyltestosterone); (2) injection (testosterone enanthate and testosterone cypionate); and (3) topical testosterone (Androderm, AndoGel, and Testim).

Fracture Prevention in Postmenopausal Women

Postmenopausal women are at an increased risk for fracture compared with premenopausal women and men of all ages on account of hormone-related bone loss. The lifetime risk for fracture in white women is 20% for the spine, 15% for the wrist, and 18% for the hip. Observational studies have found that age-specific incidence rates for postmenopausal fractures of the hip increased exponentially after age 50. The incidence of hip fractures is highest in non-Hispanic white women and then decreases successively in Hispanic, Asian, and African American women. Fractures may result in pain, short- or long-term disability, hemorrhage, thromboembolic disease, shock, and death. Vertebral fractures are associated with pain, physical impairment, muscular atrophy, changes in body shape, loss of physical function, and a decreased quality of life. Approximately 13% of people die in the first year after a hip fracture, representing a doubling of mortality compared with people of similar age and no hip fracture.[120] One-half of all older women who have previously been independent become partly dependent after hip fracture, and one third become totally dependent.

Several treatments have been shown to be effective in preventing fractures in postmenopausal women (**Table 5**). Alendronate (Fosamax), risedronate (Actonel), and parathyroid hormone (Forteo) reduce vertebral and nonvertebral fractures compared with placebo. Etidronate (Didronal), ibandronate (Boniva), pamidronate (Aredia), and raloxifene (Evista) reduce vertebral fractures but have not been shown to reduce nonvertebral fractures. There is a trade-off between benefits and harms with raloxifene. Raloxifene has been shown to have a protective effect against breast cancer but increases venous thromboembolic events and stroke compared with placebo.[121] The active treatment group receiving HRT in the WHI study demonstrated a reduction in hip fracture risk (absolute risk reduction, 0.25%; NNT, 400) and all fractures (absolute risk reduction, 2.09%; NNT, 48);[52] however, long-term treatment with HRT for osteoporosis prevention may not be justified when weighed against the increased risk for cardiovascular events and invasive breast cancer. In addition, an analysis of continued health outcomes 3 years after stopping HRT in the active treatment group of the WHI demonstrated the initial benefit of HRT reducing fracture risk was no longer observed after stopping therapy.[122]

It currently is not known whether or not multifactorial nonpharmacologic interventions, including environmental manipulation or regular exercise, reduce the risk for fractures secondary to osteoporosis. Hip protectors may reduce the risk for hip fractures in nursing home residents but compliance tends to be low.

Postmenopauasal Bleeding

Irregular bleeding is common after HRT is initiated and improves within 6 to 12 months for most women.[99] Therefore, switching regimens or formulations prior to completion of 6 months of therapy usually is not helpful. Abnormal bleeding is not easily defined in this group of women but in general, women should be evaluated for the following reasons: (1) they are taking cyclic HRT and experience unusually prolonged or heavy bleeding that occurs near the end of the progestogen phase of the cycle or breakthrough bleeding that occurs at any other time or (2) they are

Table 5				
Selected treatments to prevent fractures in postmenopausal women				
Drug	Dose (Oral Administration—Unless Otherwise Indicated)	Protects Against Vertebral Fractures (Compared to Placebo)	Protects Against Nonvertebral Fractures (Compared to Placebo)	Comments
Alendronate (Fosamax)	10 mg daily or 70 mg weekly	Yes	Yes	May cause severe esophagitis
Parathyroid hormone	20 μg subcutaneous daily in thigh or abdomen for ≤ 2 years	Yes	Yes	Available as teriparatide (Forteo) in the United States
Risedronate (Actonel)	5 mg daily, 35 mg weekly, or 75 mg on 2 consecutive days each month	Yes	Yes	May cause esophagitis
Calcitonin	100 units subcutaneous/intramuscular or 200 units (1 spray) intranasal daily (alternate nostrils)	Yes?	No	May reduce vertebral fractures over 1–5 years
Calcium plus vitamin D	1200 mg/400–800 IU daily	Yes?	Yes?	Studies have had inconclusive results about fracture protection
Ibandronate (Boniva)	2.5 mg daily or 150 mg per month	Yes	No	
Zoledronic acid (Zometa, Reclast)	Zometa—4 mg intravenous infusion over ≥ 15 min every 3–4 weeks; Reclast—5 mg intravenous once yearly	Yes	Yes	Very expensive (>$200)
Vitamin D analogues (alfacalcidol or calcitriol)	0.25–2 μg daily	Yes?	Yes?	Studies have had inconclusive results about fracture protection; alfacalcidol not available in the United States
Raloxifene (Evista)	60 mg daily	Yes	No	Trade-off between benefits and harms
Calcium alone	—	No	No	—
Vitamin D alone	—	No	No	—
Hip protectors	N/A	Yes	No	Low compliance with use
Hormone therapy	N/A	Yes	Yes	Increases risk for invasive breast cancer and cardiovascular events

taking continuous HRT and experience bleeding that persists longer than 6 to 12 months or that occurs after amenorrhea has been established. Postmenopausal women taking HRT for less than 12 months may be observed for 1 year prior to diagnosing abnormal uterine bleeding.

Postmenopausal women who are not taking HRT or who are taking HRT for more than 12 months require prompt directed evaluation for abnormal uterine bleeding, as there is a concern for endometrial cancer. The risk for developing endometrial cancer increases with age. Several modalities are available for evaluation. The gold standard for diagnosing endometrial cancer is dilation and curettage (D&C) (96% sensitivity for the detection of cancer, with a 2% to 6% false-negative rate).[123,124] Analyses have shown that it is more costly and no more accurate in diagnosing endometrial abnormalities than office endometrial biopsy.[125] Saline infusion sonohysterography infuses saline into the uterine cavity during ultrasound to improve the image. The saline separates the two walls of the endometrium, allowing their thickness to be measured and allowing clinicians to evaluate the uterus for intracavitary lesions, such as fibroids or polyps. Hysteroscopy with biopsy provides more information than D&C alone[126] and rivals the combination of saline-infusion sonohysterography and endometrial sampling in its ability to diagnose polyps, submucous fibroids, and other sources of abnormal uterine bleeding.[127] Postmenopausal women who are poor candidates for general anesthesia and those who decline D&C may be offered transvaginal ultrasonography (96% sensitive for detection of endometrial cancer)[124] or saline-infusion sonohysterography (95% to 97% sensitive for detection of endometrial cancer)[128,129] with endometrial biopsy. Results demonstrate that with a normal endometrial thickness of 4 millimeters or less and a pretest probability of 10%, the probability of cancer after a normal transvaginal ultrasonography is 1%. Endometrial thicknesses of 4 and 5 millimeters have sensitivities for uterine cancer of 96%.[124]

The sensitivity of endometrial biopsy for the detection of endometrial abnormalities is reported to be as high as 96%.[130] The procedure is as effective as a D&C for diagnosing malignancy.[131–133] Its advantages include lower cost, no anesthesia requirement, and ability to be carried out easily in an office setting. Unfortunately, 4% to 10% of postmenopausal women may have cervical stenosis, which prevents the insertion of the pipelle into the uterine cavity, and D&C under anesthesia ultimately may need to be performed. Although the endometrial aspirate can detect cancer accurately, it does not detect any structural abnormalities, such as fibroids and polyps. When a biopsy sample is normal and postmenopausal bleeding continues, further evaluation of the endometrium is recommended.

HEALTH-RISK ASSESSMENT AND SCREENING FOR POSTMENOPAUSAL WOMEN

Health maintenance for postmenopausal women has profound societal and economic implications. Increasing the duration of vitality and independence, maintaining quality of life, and decreasing the length of disability of elderly women also decrease the economic burden on the health care system and society. Proactive screening, ongoing patient assessment, and aggressive intervention aid clinicians and patients in preserving optimal patient health after menopause and delaying morbidity as late in life as possible (**Table 6**). Health care providers should strongly encourage patients to quit smoking to prevent lung cancer and cardiovascular disease. Postmenopausal women should be screened for breast cancer risk factors. Risk can be accessed on the basis of family history, fertility or infertility history, and age at menarche, menopause, and first pregnancy. Preventive measures should include an annual clinical breast

Table 6

Counseling on preventive health care

Disease Process	Service	Schedule
Cervical cancer	Papanicolaou (Pap) smear	All women should begin screening approximately 3 years after initiating vaginal intercourse but no later than 21 years of age. Screening should be done annually using conventional cytology or every 2 years if using liquid-based cytology. Beginning at age 30, women who have had 3 consecutive normal Pap tests may be screened every 2 to 3 years. Another reasonable option for women over 30 is to be screened every 3 years (but not more frequently) with the conventional or liquid-based Pap test plus the HPV DNA test. Women who have risk factors, such as diethylstilbestrol (DES) exposure before birth, HIV infection, or a weakened immune system due to organ transplant, chemotherapy, or chronic steroid use, should continue to be screened annually.
		Women 70 years of age or older who have had 3 or more consecutive normal Pap tests and no abnormal Pap test results in the last 10 years may choose to stop having screening. Women who have a history of cervical cancer, DES exposure before birth, HIV infection, or a weakened immune system should continue to have screening as long as they are in good health.
		Women who have had a total hysterectomy also may choose to stop having cervical cancer screening, unless the surgery was done as a treatment for cervical cancer or precancer. Women who have had a hysterectomy without removal of the cervix should continue to follow the guidelines described previously.
Breast cancer	Breast self-examination; clinical breast examination, mammogram	Women aged 40 and older should have an annual mammogram and an annual clinical breast examination; ideally, the clinical breast examination should be scheduled near the time of and before the mammogram; women aged 20 to 39 should have a clinical breast examination every 3 years. Women should know how their breasts normally feel and report any breast change promptly to their health care providers. Breast >self-examination is an option for women starting in their 20s. Women at high risk (greater than 20% lifetime risk) should get an MRI and a mammogram every year. Women at moderately increased risk (15% to 20% lifetime risk) should talk with their doctors about the benefits and limitations of adding MRI screening to their yearly mammogram. Yearly MRI screening is not recommended for women whose lifetime risk for breast cancer is less than 15%.
Ovarian cancer	Pelvic examination	Performed annually starting at age 21 or 3 years after a woman becomes sexually active, whichever comes earlier.
Endometrial cancer	Counseling at annual health examination	The American Cancer Society recommends that at the time of menopause, all women should be informed about the risks and symptoms of endometrial cancer and strongly encouraged to report any unexpected bleeding or spotting to their doctors. For women who have or at high risk for hereditary nonpolyposis colon cancer, annual screening should be offered for endometrial cancer with endometrial biopsy beginning at age 35.

Colorectal cancer	Flexible sigmoidoscopy, colonoscopy, double-contrast barium enema, CT colonography	Beginning at age 50, women at average risk for developing colorectal cancer should use one of the following screening tests designed to find both early cancer and polyps. Flexible sigmoidoscopy every 5 years,* colonoscopy every 10 years, double contrast barium enema every 5 years,* CT colonography (virtual colonoscopy) every 5 years.* (*Colonoscopy should be done if test results are positive.)
Hypertension	Blood pressure measurement	The optimal interval for blood pressure measurement has not been determined and is left to clinical discretion; current expert opinion is that adults believed to be normotensive should receive blood pressure measurements once every 2 years if their last diastolic and systolic blood pressure readings were below 85 and 140 mm Hg, respectively, and annually if the last diastolic blood pressure was 85–89 mm Hg.
Cholesterol	Complete lipoprotein panel: total cholesterol, high-density lipoprotein, triglycerides, low-density lipoprotein (fasting)	Adults aged 20 years or older, once every 5 years
Immunizations	Influenza	Vaccine is strongly recommended for any person aged $\geq$ 6 months who, because of age or underlying medical condition, is at increased risk for complications on influenza; health care workers and other individuals (including household members) in close contact with persons at high risk should be vaccinated to decrease the risk for transmitting influenza to persons at high risk; influenza vaccine also can be administered to any person aged $\geq$ 6 months to reduce the chance of influenza infection.
	Td	Every 10 years
	Pneumovax	Age 65
Bone density	Dual-energy x-ray absorptiometry	The U.S. Preventive Services Task Force (USPSTF) recommends that women aged 65 and older be screened routinely for osteoporosis. The USPSTF recommends that routine screening begin at age 60 for women at increased risk for osteoporotic fractures. The exact risk factors that should trigger screening in this age group are difficult to specify based on evidence. Lower body weight (weight < 70 kg) is the single best predictor of low bone mineral density. There is less evidence to support the use of other individual risk factors (for example, smoking, weight loss, family history, decreased physical activity, alcohol or caffeine use, or low calcium and vitamin D intake) as a basis for identifying high-risk women younger than 65. At any given age, African American women on average have higher bone mineral density than white women and thus are less likely to benefit from screening.

* Colonoscopy should be done if test results are positive.

Data from American Cancer Society. Cancer facts & figures 2008. Atlanta: American Cancer Society; 2008; Levin B, Lieberman DA, McFarland, et al. Screening and surveillance for the early detection of colorectal cancer and adenomatous polyps, 2008: a joint guideline from the American Cancer Society, the US Multi-Society Task Force on Colorectal Cancer, and the American College of Radiology. Published online March 5, 2008. CA Cancer J Clin 2008;58:130–60 and Saslow D, Boetes C, Burke W, et al. for the American Cancer Society Breast Cancer Advisory Group. American Cancer Society guidelines for breast screening with MRI as an adjunct to mammography. CA Cancer J Clin 2007;57:75–89.

examination and annual mammography in women age 40 and older. For cardiovascular disease, it is important to assess family history and modifiable risk factors, such as blood pressure, cholesterol level, diabetes, current smoking, nutrition, and physical inactivity. Physicians must promote colon cancer screening and assess women for cancers of the ovary and uterus. Osteoporosis screening should be discussed after assessing a woman's risk factors. Dual-energy x-ray absorptiometry scanning, which has high precision and reproducibility and low radiation exposure, remains the recommended approach to evaluate bone density.

SUMMARY

Increased public awareness of the benefits of a healthy transition through the menopausal and postmenopausal stages offers women a new perspective on aging and empowers them to take a greater responsibility for their own health and well-being. Primary care physicians are a chief influence on appropriate information regarding menopause and postmenopausal health behaviors, risk assessment, and medical interventions that preserve female patients' health and that prevent premature death and disability. Clinicians can help postmenopausal women identify therapy goals of short-term relief of menopausal symptoms and long-term relief and prevention of osteoporosis and fractures. No intervention is suitable for every woman and each option has different risk and benefit profiles. Physicians must consider each woman's needs and concerns individually and should be cognizant that because a woman's needs can change, re-evaluation is needed.

REFERENCES

1. Hargrove JT, Eisenberg E. Menopause. Med Clin North Am 1995;79:1337–56.
2. Mitchell E, Woods N, Mariella A. Three stages of the menopausal transition: observations from the Seattle Midlife Women's Health Study. Menopause 2000; 7:334–49.
3. Soules MR, Sherman S, Parrott E, et al. Executive summary: Stages of Reproductive Aging Workshop (STRAW). Fertil Steril 2001;76:874–8.
4. McKinlay SM. The normal menopause transition: an overview. Maturitas 1996;23: 137–45.
5. Willett W, Stampfer MJ, Bain C, et al. Cigarette smoking, relative weight, and menopause. Am J Epidemiol 1983;117:651–8.
6. Kaufman DW, Slone D, Rosenberg L, et al. Cigarette smoking and age at natural menopause. Am J Public Health 1980;72:420–2.
7. Brambilla DJ, McKinlay SM. A prospective study of factors affecting age at menopause. J Clin Epidemiol 1989;42:1031–9.
8. Bromberger JT, Matthews KA, Kuller LH, et al. Prospective study of determinants of age at menopause, Am J Epidemiol 1997;145:124–133.
9. Hiatt RA, Fireman BH. Smoking, menopause, and breast cancer. J Natl Cancer Inst 1986;76:833–8.
10. Adena MA, Gallagher HG. Cigarette smoking and the age at menopause. Ann Hum Biol 1982;9:121–30.
11. Gold EB, Bromberger J, Crawford S, et al. Factors associated with age at natural menopause in a multiethnic sample of midlife women. Am J Epidemiol 2001;153: 865–74.
12. Coulam CB, Anderson SC, Annegers JF. Incidence of premature ovarian failure. Obstet Gynecol 1986;67:604–6.

13. Gold EB, Block G, Crawford S, et al. Lifestyle and demographic factors in relation to vasomotor symptoms: baseline results from the Study of Women's Health Across the Nation (SWAN). Am J Epidemiol 2004;159(12):1189–99.

14. Mold JW, Mathew MK, Belgore S, et al. Prevalence of night sweats in primary care patients: an OKPRN and TAFP – Net collaborative study. J Fam Pract 2002;51:452–6.

15. O'Connor KA, Holman DJ, Wood JW. Menstrual cycle variability and the perimenopause. Am J Human Biol 2001;13:465–78.

16. Strauss SS, Clarke BA. Adolescence. In: Lewis JA, Berstein J, editors. Women's Health: a relational perspective across the life cycle. Sudbury (MA): Jones and Bartlett; 1996. p. 65–106.

17. Gorril MJ, Marshall JR. Pharmacology of estrogen and estrogen induced effects on non-reproductive organs and systems. J reprod Med 1986;31(Suppl):842–7.

18. Ingegno MD, Money SR, Thelmo W, et al. Progesterone receptors in the human heart and great vessels. Lab Invest 1988;59:353–6.

19. Wren BG. The menopause and society. In: Wren BG, Nachtigall LE, editors. Clinical management of the menopause. Sydney, Australia: McGraw-Hill Book Company; 1986. p. 1–6.

20. Munster K, Schmidt L, Helm P. Length and variation in the menstrual cycle—a cross-sectional study from a Danish country. Br J Obstet Gynaecol 1992;99:422–9.

21. Treloar AE, Boynton RE, Behn BG, et al. Variation of the human menstrual cycle through reproductive life. Int J Fertil 1967;12:77–126.

22. Vollmann RF. The menstrual cycle. In: Friedman EA, editor. Major problems in obstetrics and gynecology. Philadelphia: WB Saunders; 1977. p. 73–158.

23. MacNaughton J, Banah M, McCloud P, et al. Age-related changes in life follicle stimulating hormone, oestradiol and immunoreactive inhibin in women of reproductive age. Clin Endocrinol 1992;36:339–45.

24. McKinlay SM, Brambilla DJ, Posner JG. The normal menopause transition. Maturitas 1992;4:103–5.

25. Meldrum DR. Female reproductive aging—ovarian and uterine factors. Fertil Steril 1993;59:1–7.

26. Jansen RP. Fertility in older women. International Planned Parenthood Foundation Med Bull 1984;18:1624–6.

27. Menken J, Trussell J, Larsen U. Age and infertility. Science 1986;233:1389–94.

28. van Noord-Zaadstra BM, Looman CWN, Alsbach H, et al. Delaying childbearing: effect of age on fecundity and outcome of pregnancy. BMJ 1991;302:1361–5.

29. Byyny RL, Speroff L. A clinical guide for the care of older women: primary and preventive care. 2nd Edition. Baltimore (MD): Lippincott, Williams & Wilkins; 1996.

30. Eden JA. Androgenic disorders and the menopause. In: Wren BG, Nachtigall LE, editors. Clinical management of the menopause. Sydney Australia: McGraw-Hill Company; 1996. p. 32–40.

31. Speroff L, Glass RH, Kase NG. Menopause and postmenopausal hormone therapy. In: Clinical gynecologic endocrinology and infertility. 6th Edition. Baltimore (MD): Lippincott, Williams & Wilkins; 1999. p. 643–780.

32. Longcope C, Jaffee W, Griffling G. Production rates of androgens and oestrogens in postmenopausal women. Maturitas 1981;3:215–23.

33. Hunter MS, Liao KL. Determinants of treatment choice for menopausal hot flashes: hormonal versus psychological versus no treatment. J Psychosom Obstet Gynaecol 1995;16:101–8.

34. Hardy R, Kuh D. Change in psychological and vasomotor symptom reporting during the menopause. Soc Sci Med 2002;55:1975–88.

35. Kaufert PA, Gilbert P, Tate R. The Manitoba Project: a re-examination of the link between menopause and depression. Maturitas 1992;14:143–55.
36. Jacobs Institute of Women's Health Expert Panel on Menopause Counseling. Guidelines for counseling women on the management of menopause. Washington (DC): Jacobs Institute of Women's Health; 2000.
37. AACE Menopause Guidelines Revision Task Force. American Association of Clinical endocrinologists medical guidelines for clinical practice for the diagnosis and treatment of menopause. Endocr Pract 2006;12:315–37.
38. Bastian LA, Smith CM, Nanda K. Is this woman perimenopausal? JAMA 2003; 289:895–902.
39. Harlow SD, Crawford SL, Sommer B, et al. Self-defined menopausal status in a multi-ethnic sample of midlife women. Maturitas 2000;36:93–112.
40. Garamszegi C, Dennerstein L, Dudley E, et al. Menopausal status: subjectively and objectively defined. J Psychosom Obstet Gynaecol 1998;19:165–73.
41. Jinping X, Bartoces M, Neale VA, et al. Natural history of menopause symptoms in primary care patients:a MetroNet study. J Am Board Fam Pract 2005;18:374–82.
42. Kronenberg F. Hot flashes: epidemiology and physiology. Ann N Y Acad Sci 1990;593:52–86.
43. Avis NE, Stellato R, Crawford S, et al. Is there a menopausal syndrome? Menopausal status and symptoms across racial/ethnic groups. Soc Sci Med 2001;52:345–56.
44. Wylie_rosett J. Menopause, micronutrients, and hormone therapy. Am J Clin Nutr 2005;81:1223S–31S.
45. Li C, Samsioe G, Borgfeldt J, et al. what are the background factors? A prospective population-based cohort study of Swedish women (The Women's Health in Lund Area study). Am J Obstet Gynecol 2003;189:1646–53.
46. Greendale GA, Gold EB. Lifestyle factors: are they related to vasomotor symptoms and do they modify the effectiveness or side effects of hormone therapy? Am J Med 2005;118(Suppl 2):148–54.
47. Grady D, Sawaya GF. Discontinuation of postmenopausal hormone therapy. Am J Med 2005;118(Suppl 2):163–5.
48. Nelson HD, Vesco KK, Haney E, et al. Nonhormonal therapies for menopausal hot flashes: systematic review and meta-analysis. JAMA 2006;295:2057–71.
49. MacLennan A, Lester S, Moore V. Oral estrogen replacement therapy versus placebo for hot flushes: a scientific review. Climacteric 2001;4:58–74.
50. Nelson HD. Commonly used types of postmenopausal estrogen for treatment of hot flashes: scientific review. JAMA 2004;291:1610–20.
51. Ettinger B. Vasomotor symptom relief versus unwanted effects: role of estrogen dosage. Am J Med 2005;118(Suppl 2):74–8.
52. Rossouw JE, Anderson GL, Prentice RL, et al. Risks and benefits of estrogen plus progestin in healthy postmenopausal women: principle results from the Women's Health Initiative randomized controlled trial. JAMA 2002;288:321–33.
53. Tice JA, Grady D. Alternatives to estrogens for treatment of hot flashes—are they effective and safe? JAMA 2006;295:2076–8.
54. Tang GW. The climacteric of Chinese factory workers. Maturitas 1994;19: 177–82.
55. Freedman RR. Physiology of hot flashes. Am J Human Biol 2001;13:453–64.
56. Rekers H, Drogendijk AC, Valkenburg HA, et al. The menopause, urinary incontinence and other symptoms of the genitor-urinary tract. Maturitas 1992;15:101–11.
57. Kuh D, Cardozo L, Hardy R. Urinary incontinence in middle aged women: childhood enuresis and other lifetime risks factors in a British prospective cohort. J Epidemiol Community Health 1999;53:453–8.

58. Greendale GA, Lee NP, Arriola ER. The menopause. Lancet 1999;343:571–80.

59. Milsom I, Ekelund P, Molander U, et al. The influence of age, parity, oral contraception, hysterectomy and menopause on the prevalence of urinary incontinence in women. J Urol 1993;149:1459–62.

60. Sherburn M, Guthrie JR, Dudley EC, et al. Is incontinence associated with menopause? Obstet Gynecol 2001;98:628–33.

61. Herjanic B, Reich W. Development of a structured psychiatry interview for children: agreement between child and parent on individual symptoms. J Abnorm Child Psychol 1982;10:307–24.

62. Halbreich U. Gonadal hormones and antihormones, serotonin and mood. Psychopharmacol Bull 1990;26:291–5.

63. Pearlstein TB, Frank E, Rivera-Tovar A, et al. Prevalence of axis II and axis III disorder s in women with late luteal phase dysphoric disorder. J Affect Disord 1990;20:129–34.

64. Bancroft J, Sartorius N. The effects of oral contraceptives on the well being and sexuality of women. Oxford Review of Reproductive Biology 1990;12:57–92.

65. McCormick LH. Depression in mothers of children with attention deficit hyperactivity disorder. Fam Med 1995;27:176–9.

66. Yonkers KA, Austin LS. Mood disorders: women and affective disorders. Prim Psychiatry 1996;3:27–8.

67. Leibenluft E. Women with bipolar illness: clinical and research issues. Am J Psychiatry 1996;153:163–73.

68. Parry BL. Reproductive factors affecting the course of affective illness in women. Psychiatr Clin North Am 1989;12:207–20.

69. Hallstrom T, Samuelson S. Mental health in the climacteric. The longitudinal study of women in Gothenburg. Acta Obstet Gynecol Scand Suppl 1985;130:13–8.

70. Holte A, Mikkelsen A. Psychosocial determinants of climacteric complaints. Maturitas 1991;13:205–15.

71. Matthews KA, Wing RR, Kuller LH, et al. Influences of natural menopause on psychological characteristics and symptoms of middle-aged healthy women. J Consult Clin Psychol 1990;58:345–51.

72. Cawood EHH, Bancroft J. Steroid hormones, the menopause, sexuality and well being of women. Psychol Med 1996;26:925–36.

73. Gath D, Osborn M, Bungay G, et al. Psychiatric disorder and gynecological symptoms in middle-aged women: A community survey. BMJ 1987;294: 213–8.

74. Porter M, Penney GC, Russell D, et al. A population based survey of women's experience of the menopause. Br J Obstet Gynaecol 1996;103:1025–8.

75. Torgerson DJ, Thomas RE, Reid DM. Mothers and daughters menopausal ages, is there a link. Eur J Obstet Gynecol Reprod Biol 1997;74:63–6.

76. Garnett T, Studd JWW, Henderson A, et al. Hormone implants and tachyphylaxis. Br J Obstet Gynaecol 1990;97:917–21.

77. Hay AG, Bancroft J, Johnstone EC. Affective symptoms in women attending a menopause clinic. Br J Psychiatry 1994;164:513–6.

78. Hee J, MacNaughton J, Bangah M, et al. Perimenopausal patterns of gonadotrophins, immunoreactive inhibin, oestradiol and progesterone. Maturitas 1993;18:9–20.

79. Sherman BM, Korenman SG. Hormonal characteristics of the human menstrual cycle throughout reproductive life. J Clin Invest 1975;55:699–706.

80. Burger HG, Cahir N, Robertson DM, et al. Serum inhibins A and B fall differentially as FSH rises in perimenopausal women. Clin Ecdocrinol Metab. 1991;73: 667–73.

81. Illingworth PJ, Reddi K, Smith KB, et al. The source of inhibin secretion during the human menstrual cycle. J Clin Endocrinol Metab 1991;73:667–73.

82. ACOG practice bulletin. No. 73: use of hormonal contraception in women with coexisting medical conditions. Obstet Gynecol 2006;107:1453–72.

83. Peterson HB, Curtis KM. Long-acting methods of contraception. N Engl J Med 2005;353:2169–75.

84. Medical eligibility criteria for contraceptive use. 3rd Edition. Geneva: World Health Organization; 2004.

85. Sarrell PM, Whotehead MI. Sex and menopause: defining the issues. Maturitas 1985;7:217–24.

86. Robertson R. Sexuality and the menopause. In: Wren BG, Nachtigall LE, editors. Clinical management of the menopause. Sydney, Australia: McGraw Hill Book Company; 1996. p. 41–8.

87. Bachmann GA, Leiblum SR. Sexuality in sexagenarian women. Maturitas 1991;3: 43–50.

88. Avis NE, Stellato R, Crawford S, et al. Is there an association between menopause status and sexual functioning? Menopause 2000;7:297–309.

89. Koster A, Garde K. Sexual desire and menopausal development: a prospective study of Danish women born in 1936. Maturitas 1993;16:49–60.

90. Pfister S, Dougherty P. Growing older. In: Lewis JA, Bernstein J, editors. Women's health: a relational perspective across the life cycle. Sudbury (MA): Jones and Bartlett; 1996. p. 192–236.

91. Newman G, Nichols CR. Sexual activities and attitudes in older persons. JAMA 1960;173:335–41.

92. MacLennan A, Lester A, Moore V. Oral estrogen replacement therapy versus placebo for hot flushes [Cochrane Review on CD-ROM]. Oxford, England: Cochrane Library; 2002. Update Software.

93. Hing E, Brett KM. Changes in US prescribing patterns of menopausal hormone therapy. 2001–2003. Obstet Gynecol 2006;108:33–40.

94. Hulley S, Grady D, Bush T, et al. Randomized trial of estrogen plus progestin for secondary prevention of coronary heart disease in postmenopausal women. Heart and Estrogen/Progestin Replacement Study (HERS) Research Group. JAMA 1998;280(7):605–13.

95. Million Women Study Collaborators The. The Million Women Study: a confidential national study of women's health. Available at: http://www.millionwomenstudy.org/index2.html. Accessed May 6, 2008.

96. The Nurses' Health Study. Available at: http://www.channing.harvard.edu/nhs/?fb_page_id=6548964549&. Accessed August 1, 2008.

97. Nelson HD, Humphrey LL, LeBlanc E, et al. Postmenopausal hormone replacement therapy for primary prevention of chronic conditions. Summary of the evidence for the U.S. Preventive Services Task Force. Agency for Healthcare Research and Quality. Available at: http://www.ahrq.gov/clinic/3rduspstf/hrt/hrtsum1.htm. Accessed August 1, 2008.

98. North American Menopause Society. Estrogen and progestogen use in peri- and postmenopausal women: March 2007 position statement of The North American Menopause Society. Menopause 2007;14:168–82.

99. Institute for Clinical Systems Improvement. Health care guideline: menopause and hormone therapy (HT): collaborative decision-making and management. Available at: http://www.icsi.org/guidelines_and_more/gl_os_prot/womens_health/menopause_and_hormone_therapy/menopause_and_hormone_therapy_ht_collaborative_decision-making_and_management_.html. Accessed May 29, 2008.

100. Greendale GA, Reboussin BA, Hogan P, et al. Symptom relief and side effects of postmenopausal hormones: results from the Postmenopausal Estrogen/Progestin Interventions Trial. Obstet Gynecol 1998;92:982–8.
101. Kelley C. Estrogen and its effect on vaginal atrophy in post menopausal women. Urol Nurs 2007;27(1):40–5.
102. Raz R, Stamm WE. A controlled trial of intravaginal estriol in postmenopausal women with recurrent urinary tract infections. N Engl J Med 1993;329:753–6.
103. Newton KM, Buist DS, Keenan NL, et al. Use of alternative therapies for menopause symptoms: results of a population-based survey [erratum appears in Obstet Gynecol]. Obstet Gynecol 2002;100:18–25.
104. Cheema D, Coomarasamy A, El-Toukhy T. Non-hormonal therapy of post-menopausal vasomotor symptoms: a structures evidence-based review. Arch Gynecol Obstet 2007;276:463–9.
105. North American Menopause Society. Treatment of menopause-associated vasomotor symptoms: position statement of The North American Menopause society. Menopause 2004;11:11–33.
106. Bachmann GA. The hypoandrogenic woman: pathophysiologic overview. Fertil Steril 2002;77(Suppl 4):S72–5.
107. Adashi EY. The climacteric ovary as a functional gonadotropin-driven androgen-producing gland [erratum in Fertil Steril. 1995; 63:684]. Fertil Steril 1994;62:20–7.
108. Braunstein GD. Androgen insufficiency in women: summary of critical issues. Fertil Steril 2002;77(Suppl 4):S94–9.
109. Bachmann G, Bancroft J, Braunstein(Princeton) G. Female androgen insufficiency: the Princeton consensus statement on definition, classification, and assessment. Fertil Steril 2002;77(Suppl 4):660–5.
110. Sherwin BB, Gelfand MM, Brender W. Androgen enhances sexual motivation in females: a prospective, crossover study of sex steroid administration in the surgical menopause. Psychosom Med 1985;47:339–51.
111. Davis SR, McCloud P, Strauss BJ, et al. Testosterone enhances estradiol effects on postmenopausal bone density and sexuality. Maturitas 1995;21:227–36.
112. Sarrel P, Dobay B, Wiita B. Estrogen and estrogen-androgen replacement in postmenopausal women dissatisfied with estrogen-only therapy: sexual behavior and neuroendocrine responses. J Reprod Med 1998;43:847–56.
113. Dobs AS, Nguyen T, Pace C, et al. Differential effects of oral estrogen versus oral estrogen-androgen replacement therapy on body composition in post menopausal women. J Clin Endocrinol Metab 2002;87:1509–16.
114. Shifren JL, Braunstein GD, Simon JA, et al. Transdermal testosterone treatment in women with imparired sexual function after oophorectomu. N Engl J Med 2000;343:682–8.
115. Watts NB, Notelovitz M, Timmons MC, et al. Comparison of oral estrogens and estrogen plus androgen on bone mineral density, menopause symptoms and lipid-lipoprotein profiles in surgical menopause [erratum in Obstet Gynecol. 1995;85(5 Pt 1):668]. Obstet Gynecol 1995;85:529–37.
116. Raisz LG, Wiita B, Artis A, et al. Comparison of the effects of estrogen alone and estrogen plus androgen on biochemical markers of bone formation and resorption in postmenopausal women. J Clin Endocrinol Metab 1996;81:37–43.
117. Need AG, Durbridge TC, Nordin BE. Anabolic steroids in postmenopausal osteoporosis. Wien Med Wochenschr 1993;143:392–5.
118. Hassager C, Riis BJ, Podenphant J, et al. Nandrolone decanoate treatment of post-menopausal osteoporosis for 2 years and effects of withdrawal. Maturitas 1989;11:305–17.

119. Tariq S, Kamel H, Morley J. Dehydroepiandrosterone and pregnenolone. In: Meilke AW, editor. Endocrine replacement therapy in clinical practice. Totowa (NJ): Humana Press; 2003. p. 307–29.

120. Tinetti ME, Inouye SK, Gill TM, et al. Shard risk for falls, incontinence, and functional dependence. Unifying the approach to geriatric syndromes. JAMA 1995; 273(17):1348–53.

121. Vogel VG, Costantino JP, Wickerman DLO, et al. Effects of tamoxifen vs Raloxifene on the risk of developing invasive breast cancer and other disease outcomes: the NSABP Study of Tamoxifen and Raloxifene (STAR) P-2 trial. JAMA 2006;295(23):2727–41.

122. Heiss G, Wallace R, Anderson GL, et al. for the WHI Investigators. Health risks and benefits 3 years after stopping randomized treatment with estrogen and progestin. JAMA 2008;299(9):1036–45.

123. Ben-Yehuda OM, Kim YB, Leuchter RS. Does hysteroscopy improve upon the sensitivity of dilatation and curettage in the diagnosis of endometrial hyperplasis or carcinoma? Gynecol Oncol 1998;68:4–7.

124. Tabor A, Watt HC, Wald NJ. Endometrial thickness as a test for endometrial cancer in women with postmenopausal vaginal bleeding. Obstet Gynecol 2002;99:663–70.

125. Feldman S, Berkowitz RS, Tosteson ANA. Cost-effectiveness of strategies to evaluate postmenopausal bleeding. Obstet Gynecol 1993;81:968–75.

126. Gimpelson RJ. Panoramic hysteroscopy with directed biopsies vs. dilatation and curettage for accurate diagnosis. J Reprod Med 1984;29:575–8.

127. Krampl E, Bourne T, Hurlen-Solbakken H, et al. Transvaginal ultrasonography, sonohysterography and operative hysteroscopy for the evaluation of abnormal uterine bleeding. Acta Obstet Gynecol Scand 2001;80:616–22.

128. O'Connell LP, Fries MH, Zeringue E, et al. Triage of abnormal postmenopausal bleeding: a comparison of endometrial biopsy and transvaginal sonohysterography versus fractional curettage with hysteroscopy. Am J Obstet Gynecol 1998;178:956–61.

129. Mihm LM, Quick VA, Brumfield JA, et al. The accuracy of endometrial biopsy and saline sosohysterography in the determination of the cause of abnormal uterine bleeding. Am J Obstet Gynecol 2002;186:858–60.

130. Stovall TG, Ling FW, Morgan PL. A perspective, randomized comparison of the Pipelle endometrial sampling device with the Novak curette. Am J Obstet Gynecol 1991;165(5 pt 1):1287–90.

131. Grimes DA. Diagnostic dilation and curettage: a reappraisal. Am J Obstet Gynecol 1982;142:1–6.

132. Ong S, Duffy T, Lenehan P, et al. Endometrial pipelle biopsy compared to conventional dilatation and curettage. Ir J Med Sci 1997;166:47–9.

133. Tahir MM, Bigrigg MA, Brookers ST, et al. A randomized controlled trial comparing transvaginal ultrasound, outpatient hysteroscopy and endometrial biopsy with impatient hysteroscopy and curettage. Br J Obstet Gynaecol 1999;106:1259–64.

134. Goldenberg NM, Wang P, Glueck CJ, et al. An observational study of sever hypertriglyceridemia, hypertriglyceridemic acute pancreatitis, and failure of triglyceride-lowering therapy when estrogens are given to women with and without familial hypertriglyceridemia. Clin Chim Acta 2003;332:11–9.

Index

Note: Page numbers of article titles are in **boldface** type.

Prim Care Clin Office Pract 36 (2009) 227–242
doi:10.1016/S0095-4543(09)00009-8
0095-4543/09/$ – see front matter © 2009 Elsevier Inc. All rights reserved.

primarycare.theclinics.com

C

Moving?

Make sure your subscription moves with you!

To notify us of your new address, find your **Clinics Account Number** (located on your mailing label above your name), and contact customer service at:

E-mail: elspcs@elsevier.com

800-654-2452 (subscribers in the U.S. & Canada)
314-453-7041 (subscribers outside of the U.S. & Canada)

Fax number: 314-523-5170

Elsevier Periodicals Customer Service
11830 Westline Industrial Drive
St. Louis, MO 63146

*To ensure uninterrupted delivery of your subscription, please notify us at least 4 weeks in advance of move.

Printed and bound by CPI Group (UK) Ltd, Croydon, CR0 4YY

03/10/2024

01040462-0006